Consultations in Dermatology II

with

Walter B. Shelley

Professor of Dermatology,
University of Pennsylvania School of Medicine

With photographs by Edward F. Glifort

1974

W. B. SAUNDERS COMPANY • Philadelphia • London • Toronto

W. B. Saunders Company: West Washington Square
Philadelphia, Pa. 19105

12 Dyott Street
London, WC1A 1DB

833 Oxford Street
Toronto, Ontario M8Z 5T9, Canada

Consultations in Dermatology with Walter B. Shelley—II   ISBN 0-7216-8214-6

Print No.:   9   8   7   6   5   4   3   2   1

To
Anne

Dearest, best and brightest

Acknowledgments

Elliott Morse and his colleagues at the Library of the College of Physicians of Philadelphia for provisioning and nourishing us.

Doctors Richard G. Bennett, Loren T. Burns, Arnold W. Klein, David A. Paslin, Robert I. Rudolph, Ronald N. Shore, and all our resident physicians for their superb care and study of these patients.

Marion Adamek for flawless copy from a pen-script often occult and indecipherable.

John L. Dusseau and the staff of W. B. Saunders Company for making *Consultations II* come true.

Contents

Consultations:

Preface

The warmth of your response to our first volume of "Consultations" has encouraged us to hope that you would join us again on rounds.

Please do . . . .

1

This **scaly, crusted, erythematous, well-marginated eruption** *of the chest also involves the back, face and scalp. Initiated by a tropical sunburn, it has persisted for 4 months despite a variety of local treatments.*

Biopsy—flaccid, acantholytic bulla formation high in the epidermis.

Pemphigus Erythematosus

This is pemphigus but in masquerade. Blisters and erosions, the dread hallmarks of ordinary pemphigus, are nowhere to be seen. Yet this smoldering scaling erythematous rash springs from the same autoimmune mechanism responsible for pemphigus vulgaris. Indeed, our patient's epidermis shows loss of intercellular cohesion and the consequent fragmentation and splitting. Moreover, immunofluorescent staining would show antiepithelial immunoglobulins present between the epidermal cells as well as in the blood. All these are the microscopic and serologic findings of pemphigus vulgaris also. Then why the phenomenal difference in the clinical picture?

Simply, in pemphigus erythematosus as seen here, the loss of cell cohesion occurs so high in the epidermis that the normal barrier to water loss is destroyed. There is hence a constant seepage of fluid into the scales which gives them a distinctive, somewhat moist gray appearance. By contrast, in pemphigus vulgaris the epidermal split is low, the overlying epidermis retains its normal impermeability, and the intraepidermal exudate, not free to escape, forms the blister or bulla.

Clinically, pemphigus erythematosus most often masquerades as lupus erythematosus. Senear and Usher, the first investigators to give form and substance to this entity, stressed that the gross appearance as well as the facial predilection was reminiscent of lupus. As the years went on, it became evident, moreover, that both diseases could be triggered by sunburn, that both were autoimmune in nature, and now most recently that both have the same immunofluorescent antibody deposits in the dermis. Thus, actually there may be less masquerade than co-identity in

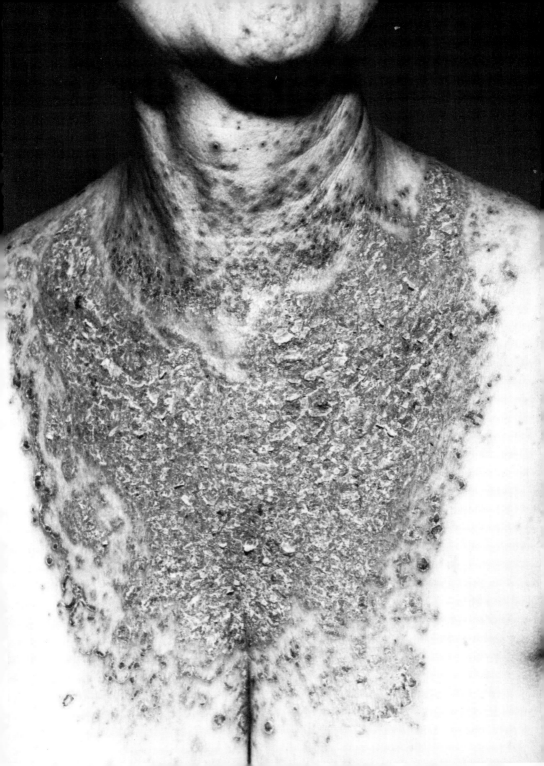

these two diseases. Yet, pemphigus erythematosus is unique, for it does not show the scarring or mucosal involvement so typical of lupus. In any event, the original hybrid name remains accurate.

The sternal and interscapular areas, as well as intertriginous zones, are likewise sites of predilection for this Senear-Usher syndrome, and in these locales, as well as on the face, the masquerade may be that of seborrheic dermatitis. Thus, the French speak so accurately of this form as seborrheic pemphigus. Other diseases showing superficial epidermal clefts and slits such as impetigo, keratosis follicularis and chronic benign familial pemphigus may show a fleeting resemblance, also. On the scalp, pemphigus erythematosus may be so widespread and destructive that in one patient known to us it was diagnosed as a malignancy. His entire scalp was excised before the pemphigus erythematosus was ultimately recognized. And in our patient the masquerade is that of a chronic photosensitivity or sunburn reaction.

From this clinical forum of endless diagnostic debate the laboratory has miraculously lifted us, with its beautiful immunofluorescent demonstration of the specific sign of pemphigus, antiepithelial antibodies. No longer do we have to depend on the Nikolsky sign of our thumb shearing away the upper poorly cohesive epidermis. The answer is in the Tzanck smear showing acantholytic cells, in the biopsy evidence of subcorneal loss of continuity in the epidermal syncytium, and most precisely in the direct and indirect demonstration of intercellular fluorescent antibodies.

Once the diagnosis has been established, careful medical study must reflect an awareness of the fact that autoimmune diseases frequently coexist. Look for lupus erythematosus, myasthenia gravis, thyroiditis or even a thymoma.

Pemphigus erythematosus has a relatively benign course and in limited forms may require little treatment other than high-potency topical steroids. In some, however, the course is more severe and chronic. Months (more likely years) of systemic steroids in appropriate dosage may be required to prevent extension into a widespread or exfoliative process, pemphigus foliaceus, only recently recognized to be the same disease. Clearly the incessant exfoliation was the basis for its descriptive label. It is but rarely that pemphigus erythematosus converts to fatal pemphigus vulgaris, the third species of this epidermolytic family.

Specifically, our patient needs full measure of attention. Repeated local compresses such as a dilute Burow's solution will serve to cleanse and debride the scaling, crusted, inflamed areas. Interim applications of a topical corticosteroid cream should prove soothing and helpful as well. Conversely, occlusive dressings or medicaments are to be eschewed. All areas must be protected from such hazards as significant sun exposure, scrubbing with soap and water, potential sensitizing agents, and contact with those who have a pyoderma, herpes simplex or a fresh vaccination. Although oral antimalarials given prior to exposure reduce the photo-toxic effects of sunlight in this disease, it is doubtful whether they are necessary unless excessive sunlight cannot be avoided. After healing is accomplished, the use of any of a number of sun screens (e.g., para-aminobenzoic acid, benzophenones) against the shorter ultraviolet band or sunburn spectrum (280 to 320 mm.) is valuable. But recall, it is sun-burn, not sun itself, which triggers this disease.

Internally the sovereign and necessary therapy for this patient is either ACTH or corticosteroids. Although the massive doses commonly necessary for the suppression of pemphigus vulgaris are not usually required, long-term full dosage is advisable. After weeks of this therapy the skin should show enough improvement, so that over the months the dose can be tapered gradually. Always the patient must be apprised that, should the dose fall below the requisite maintenance level, new lesions may appear. In that event, a temporary dosage increase may be necessary, followed again by a programmed reduction.

Concomitant systemic antibiotic therapy is desirable in the beginning phase. This may be introduced as erythromycin, or a specific antibiotic may be selected on the basis of culture and sensitivity tests. Once healing begins and the overgrowth of bacteria is reduced, the antibiotic therapy is best discontinued to avoid inducing further ecologic imbalance. Occasionally, candidiasis may supervene and necessitate thymic review as well as appropriate attention with a nystatin or amphotericin B lotion.

The immunologic nature of pemphigus makes rational the use of modern immunosuppressants such as cyclophosphamide, azathioprine or methotrexate, and in some instances dramatic results have been reported following their conjoint use with oral steroids.

No doubt out of the swirl of today's immunologic research, exciting new approaches must surely come with the discovery of precisely why these patients are rejecting their own outer skin.

Shelley, W. B., and Crissey, J. T.: *Classics in Clinical Dermatology with Biographical Sketches.* Charles C Thomas, Springfield, Illinois, 1970, pp. 426–432.
Introduction to Senear and Usher and their classic of 1926 on a pemphigus which mimes both lupus erythematosus and seborrheic dermatitis.

Perry, H. O., and Brunsting, L. A.: Pemphigus Foliaceus. Arch. Derm., *91*:10–23, 1965.
The generalized severe form of pemphigus erythematosus (Senear-Usher).

Senear, F. E., and Kingery, L. B.: Pemphigus Erythematosus. Arch. Derm., *60*:238–252, 1949.
Differential: lupus erythematosus, seborrheic dermatitis, impetigo, dermatitis herpetiformis, dermatitis medicamentosa, erythema multiforme, epidermolysis bullosa, eczema, psoriasis.

Lubowe, I. I., Mandel, E. H., and Zeilicoff, S.: Pemphigus in Familial Incidence: Pemphigus Erythematodes in a Mother and Pemphigus Vegetans in a Daughter. Arch. Derm., *94*:371–371, 1966.
Rare and mysterious.

Petratos, M. A., and Andrade, R.: Pemphigus Erythematosus. Report of a Case in a Child Less Than 6 Years of Age. Amer. J. Dis. Child., *113*:394–397, 1967.
But usually a disease of middle age.

Saikia, N. K., and Macconnell, L. E.: Senear-Usher Syndrome and Internal Malignancy. Brit. J. Derm., *87*:1–5, 1972.
First report linking bronchogenic carcinoma and pemphigus erythematosus.

Jacobs, S. E.: Pemphigus Erythematosus and Ultraviolet Light. Arch. Derm., *91*:139–141, 1965.
Experimental induction of lesions of pemphigus erythematosus in normal skin by irradiation with filtered ultraviolet light (280–320 nm. band).

Cram, D. L., and Winkelmann, R. K.: Ultraviolet Induced Acantholysis in Pemphigus. Arch. Derm., *92*:7–13, 1965.
In 6 of 7 patients, ultraviolet light produced pemphigus erythematosus-like lesions, whereas friction, infrared irradiation, occlusive dressings and a rubefacient did not!

Chorzelski, T., Jablonska, S., Beutner, E. H., and Kowalska, M.: Can Pemphigus Be Provoked by a Burn? Brit. J. Derm., *85*:320–325, 1971.
Failure of thermal burn to heal was first sign of pemphigus erythematosus.

Kocsard, E.: Foudroyante Umwandlung eines Pemphigus seborrhoicus (Senear-Usher Pemphigus) in einen Pemphigus foliaceus nach Verabreichung einer Kapsel Terramycin. Derm. Wschr., *146*:58–67, 1962.
Terramycin produced explosive transition from local (pemphigus erythematosus) to generalized form (pemphigus foliaceus) with subsequent reversal.

Orfanos, C. E., Gartmann, H., and Mahrle, G.: Zur Pathogenese des Pemphigus erythematosus. Arch. Derm. Forsch., *240*:317–333, 1971.
Observed clinical and histologic conversion of discoid lupus erythematosus into pemphigus erythematosus.

Chorzelski, T., Jablonska, S., and Blaszczyk, M.: Immunopathological Investigations in the Senear-Usher Syndrome (Coexistence of Pemphigus and Lupus Erythematosus). Brit. J. Derm., *80*:211–217, 1968.
Autoimmune antibody stains typical for both pemphigus and lupus erythematosus, in 5 of 6 patients.

Beutner, E. H., Chorzelski, T. P., Hale, W. L., and Hausmanowa-Petrusewicz, I.: Auto-immunity in Concurrent Myasthenia Gravis and Pemphigus Erythematosus. J.A.M.A., *203*:845–849, 1968.
Five cases showing triad of thymoma, myasthenia gravis and pemphigus erythematosus; suggests presence of common immunologic defect.

Beutner, E. H., Chorzelski, T. P., and Jordon, R. E.: *Autosensitization in Pemphigus and Bullous Pemphigoid.* Charles C Thomas, Springfield, Illinois, 1970, pp. 82–90.
Details direct and indirect immunofluorescent intercellular staining, diagnostic for all forms of pemphigus including erythematosus.

Saikia, N. K.: Extraction of Pemphigus Antibodies from a Lymphoid Neoplasm and Its Possible Relationship to Pemphigus Vulgaris. Brit. J. Derm., *86*:411–414, 1972.
Tracks the source of IgG pemphigus antibodies to lymphoid tissue in one patient.

Wood, G. W., Beutner, E. H., and Chorzelski, T. P.: Studies in Immunodermatology. II. Production of Pemphigus-Like Lesions by Intradermal Injection of Monkeys with Brazilian Pemphigus Foliaceus Sera. Int. Arch. Allergy and Appl. Immunol., *42*:556–564, 1972.
Induction of micro-version of disease in primates by repeated intradermal injections of high-titer sera.

Tye, M. J., Blumenthal, G., and Lever, W. F.: Pemphigus Erythematosus Favorable Response to Topical Treatment. Arch. Derm., *90*:307–309, 1964.
Hot compresses followed by high-potency steroid cream.

Connor, B.: Herpetiform Pemphigus Foliaceus Responsive to Dapsone. Brit. J. Derm., *86*:99–101, 1972.
A variant of pemphigus erythematosus exhibiting the therapeutic response of dermatitis herpetiformis.

Jablonska, S., Chorzelski, T., and Blaszczyk, M.: Immunosuppressants in the Treatment of Pemphigus. Brit. J. Derm., *83*:315–323, 1970.
Methotrexate and azathioprine (Imuran) uniquely helpful in pemphigus erythematosus.

2

For the past three years this patient has experienced daily transient sites of swelling of her skin. Beginning as pruritus and flushing, local areas of edema suddenly appear in a seemingly random fashion. They gradually whiten and become asymptomatic, confluent, and stretched to the point of **follicular dimpling,** *as seen in this* **large geographic plaque of the abdomen.** *Persisting for hours, they slowly fade without a trace.*

She has learned that the ingestion of lobster, tuna fish or cheese or even the smell of a banana will trigger multiple lesions within minutes. Aspirin and penicillin are also known to have induced severe attacks many years ago. Furthermore, lesions can be made to appear simply by scratching.

There is no family history of this condition nor does she recognize any relationship to heat, cold, sweating, sunlight, emotional stress, climate or her general health.

Chronic Urticaria

This patient has hives in its most chronic, relentless and mysterious form. For over a thousand days and nights she has seen and felt her skin stretch and swell, in lumps, bumps and welts. And all with little rhyme or reason!

This is a problem that always calls for courage and patience on the part of both the victim and the doctor. It must not be dismissed as "due to nerves." Long, even repeated, hospitalization is the next step in any serious effort to identify the causes of her tribulation. No simple 5-day screening survey will do. Numerous tests, elimination routines, therapeutic trials and selected challenges are all indicated. None of these is an easy thing to do, no more than solving the problem of a fever of obscure origin. But it can and must be done! And in a methodical, scientific way. It requires the intelligent cooperation of the patient, her family and friends, as well as a full consultant and nursing staff, all sleuthing in a positive determined fashion.

This is not the easy casual puzzle of *acute* urticaria, which even if not understood can be treated with antihistaminics and will be but a memory in a few days. This is not one of the fascinating recurrent types due to

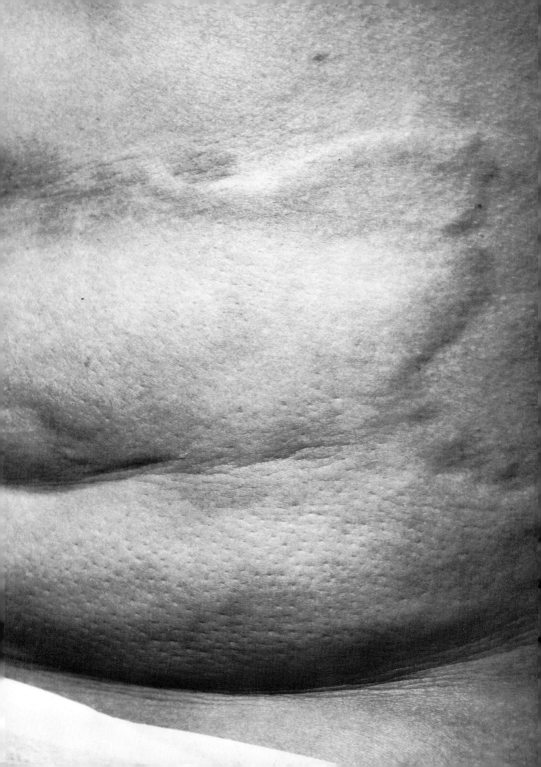

cold, heat, sunlight, or *ultraviolet* radiation. This is not the *cholinergic* hive of neural origin which is so characteristically tiny and over-shadowed by erythema. Nor is it the hive of mastocytosis, set in the fixed pigmented islands of mast cell overgrowth, and so aptly labeled *urticaria pigmentosa.* It is not the local hive produced by a specific external *contactant* such as food, water, fur or nettles. It is not the hereditary hive of *angio-edema,* classically exhibiting abdominal pain, and due to a familial deficit in the inhibitor to complement-induced vascular leakage. It is not the discrete *papular urticaria* of insect bites nor the hives of *serum sickness.* Nor is it the factitious hive of *dermographism,* although that phenomenon is present. No, this is the occult hive of true chronic urticaria. It is a challenge of the first rank, calling for a medical Sherlock Holmes.

Before attempting to search for the criminal, let us take a moment to reconstruct the crime. What is urticaria? Acute or chronic, it is still the same – a massive loss of fluid from the microvasculature into the dermis. The fluid shift temporarily far exceeds the capacity of the lymphatic drain even though the flow of lymph becomes greatly increased. With the local accumulation of extravascular fluid, the hive, i.e., circum-scribed edema, becomes clinically evident in a variety of shapes, sizes and locations.

The common denominator for the escape of fluid from the capil-laries or small vessels in the skin is a conjoint increase in capillary pres-sure *and* an increase in capillary permeability. And behind all this is a common chemical mediator, viz., histamine. Normally it is stored in the granules of perivascular mast cells in a concentration a thousand times that requisite for inducing a hive. Once released, it apparently works by selective contraction of a postcapillary or venular sphincter of smooth muscle, thereby creating capillary stasis, distention and cell separation in the endothelial wall.

Although numerous chemicals, the histamine liberators, are known to discharge these granules and initiate the primary protective inflam-matory event of exudation, an antigen-antibody reaction actually ex-plains the majority of hives experienced by patients. A clone of the pa-tient's B lymphocytes protectively responds to the presence of a foreign material by elaborating a specific immunoglobulin, IgE. This in turn selectively attaches to the cell surface of only the histaminocytes, i.e., the mast cells and basophil leukocytes. It is to this antibody that the circulat-ing antigen now joins. Such a union initiates secretion of the histamine-containing granules and the subsequent vascular leakage. Basopenia and degranulated mast cells remain as the major objective correlates of this histamine release. Thus, the hive of chronic urticaria is essentially an immediate or anaphylactic type of immune response. It is important to note that histamine release is not under neural control, and hence, except for the cholinergic version, hives are not psychogenic. In all this, histamine remains the sturdy central pathogenetic figure, although a spate of mediators such as complement, serotonin, kinins, slow-reacting substance and prostaglandins, as well as an induced form of histamine, have been proposed to replace it. This is underscored by the nettle, a plant prudent enough to synthesize histamine itself!

Our criminal is thus an antigen which returns daily to trigger attacks. But does he come from within or from without? The first step in identification is hospitalization, whereby the patient is placed in as strict environmental isolation as possible. The room must be devoid of flowers, wool rugs and drapes, fresh paint, and disinfectant odors, and as free from dust as possible. Special air-vent filters may be necessary. The pillow and mattress must be plastic covered or dustless. Upholstered furniture is to be removed, and even foam rubber is not above suspicion. The sheets must be cotton, not silk, and free of starch. The patient must not bring or use any sprays, personal toiletries, soaps, deodorants, antiperspirants, toothpaste, chewing gum, lozenges, pills, tablets, douches, suppositories, vitamins, mouthwash, eye drops, ear drops, nail polish, cigarettes, paints or garments other than the hospital robe. It is in this ascetic ambiance that the patient exists without food (save tea and water) for 48 hours.

During this retreat, the patient is repeatedly queried and instructed. She must be alerted to the fact that any inhalant, ingestant or injectant can be responsible for her hives. Build on her observation that fish, cheese and bananas are known culprits. Make her aware that these very food elements may still be hidden in her diet in trace amounts. She will have to learn to avoid eating the unknowns of restaurants, of friends and of canned and prepackaged foods. Make her realize that the cause may be a single organic chemical, but that it comes in many forms. Cite menthol urticaria, not cleared until cigarettes, toothpastes, candy, jelly, Noxzema, ice tea, room spray, hand cream and lozenges have *all* been eliminated. Acquaint her with the common threat of penicillin in milk, penicillium in blue cheese, and the fungi in moldy damp homes or basements. Reinforce her awareness of the insidious presence of urticariogenic aspirin in scores of medicines. Inform her of the hazards of tartrazine, the yellow food dye (FDC yellow #5), which produces hives in nearly all who are aspirin sensitive. It is not only in mayonnaise and vitamin C drinks, but it may also be used to dye vitamin pills, antibiotics and contraceptives. And instruct her to avoid benzoates.

Should the hives abate after two days, the vigorous environmental restrictions remain but a new food is added daily, the classic urticariogens, fish and nuts, as well as her known intolerances being avoided. Under the same routine of a challenge a day, necessities may be added later, and a strict log should be kept of what has passed the innocence test. It is this hospital baseline of safe foods which can be cautiously extended when the patient returns home. Nothing can be resumed casually or without notice, including contact with cats, perfume, saccharin, rugs or a mite-infested mattress. Re-education of the patient concerning the dozens of inapparent daily risks is all important. Once the hives have abated, consider a 6-hour pass for a critical home environmental challenge. The hive and antigen are never more than hours apart!

Should the hives remain indifferent to days of external antigen deprivation, internal sources must be explored extensively. Even if the history or physical examination does not point to a defect or suspect, full routine chemical, hematologic and radiologic monitoring is mandatory.

1. Specially sensitive areas: dental abscess, sinusitis, otitis media, pneumonitis, cholecystitis, cystitis and vaginitis. Have a periodontist survey for infection, since this can be a source of recurrent bacteremia and hives in the absence of any radiographic change.

2. Don't forget to examine stools for ova and parasites; blood for T3/T4, ANA, cryoglobulins, eosinophilia, basopenia; urine for bacteria; and vaginal specimens for Candida and Trichomonas.

3. Equally important are intradermal skin tests with fungal, bacterial and candidal antigens, as well as scrapings for fungal hyphae.

4. Still significant but less rewarding are a skin biopsy (angiitis?, amyloid?), x-rays of the upper and lower G.I. tract, a cholecystogram, and an I.V. pyelogram.

5. Scratch tests for inhalants as well as 20-minute patch tests are occasionally valuable, whereas little seems to stem from skin tests for food allergy.

6. If facilities exist for assessing the C'1 esterase-inhibitor, it should be done. Indirect basophil and mast cell degranulation tests remain as a research tool.

Be prepared for severe attacks in the hospital, necessitating epinephrine, intravenous antihistamines or steroids. As a general rule, however, supportive treatment should be avoided to prevent any masking effect during this essential testing and observational period. Topical preparations are without effect on the course of the hive, and since bland lotions and colloid baths do give symptomatic relief, they can be used.

Should laboratory results and diagnostic maneuvers fail and no serendipitous hospital insight develop, practical office therapeutic trials may be undertaken after hospitalization. Each may require one to two weeks.

1. Nystatin-candidiasis-orally and by vaginal suppository in association with a yeast-free diet.
2. Griseofulvin — tinea.
3. Tetracycline — occult infections.
4. Ampicillin — cystitis.
5. Diiodohydroxyquin — for amebic inhabitants.
6. Succinylsulfathiazole — bowel sterilization.
7. Chloroquine — autoimmunity, amebic infection.
8. Thiabendazole — helminths.
9. Gamma benzene hexachloride, topical — inapparent scabies.
10. Avlosulfon — urticarial dermatitis herpetiformis.
11. Metronidazole — trichomonal infection.

Finally, use the crutches of antihistaminics and steroids with caution. They can be crippling for both the patient and the physician.

Throughout all, have the confidence and the long-term mental and emotional commitments of a real sleuth. This patient's urticaria will yield to nothing less!

Miller, D. A., Freeman, G. L., and Akers, W. A.: Chronic Urticaria. A Clinical Study of Fifty Patients. Amer. J. Med., *44*:68-86, 1968.
Master review, emphasizing that nearly all patients appeared to have more than one demonstrable cause.

Tas, J.: Chronic Urticaria. A Survey of One Hundred Hospitalized Cases. Dermatologica, *135*:90-96, 1967.
Twenty-five known cures resulted from elimination of fungal and bacterial infection, discontinuance of specific drugs or foods and hyposensitization to house dust.

Champion, R. H., Roberts, S. O. B., Carpenter, R. G., and Roger, J. H.: Urticaria and Angio-oedema. A Review of 554 Patients. Brit. J. Derm., *81*:588-597, 1969.
Investigation of individual cases can be time-consuming and fruitless.

Zamm, A. V.: Chronic Urticaria: A Practical Approach. Cutis, *9*:27-37, 1972.
Investigation of individual cases can be time-consuming and fruitful.

Ebken, R. K., Bauschard, F. A., and Levine, M. I.: Dermographism: Its Definition, Demonstration and Prevalence. J. Allergy, *41*:338-343, 1968.
Elicitation of lesion by firm stroking seen in 7.5 per cent of chronic urticarias, only 1.5 per cent of controls.

Shelley, W. B., and Florence, R.: Chronic Urticaria Due to Mold Hypersensitivity. A Study in Cross Sensitization and Autoerythrocyte Sensitization. Arch. Derm., *83*:549-558, 1961.

A single basic cause, mold allergy, explained a jumble of otherwise erratic and inexplicable frequent episodes over a 5-year period.

Norman, P. S.: Antigens That Cause Atopic Disease.
In Samter, M. (Ed.): *Immunological Diseases,* 2nd ed. Little, Brown and Company, Boston, 1971, pp. 775-784.

Chlorogenic acid, an allergen in oranges responsible for urticaria, is also found in apples, pears, lettuce, cucumber, cabbage, plums, cherries, sweet potatoes, tobacco, as well as in castor bean and green coffee bean dust.

Papa, C. M., and Shelley, W. B.: Menthol Hypersensitivity. Diagnostic Basophil Response in a Patient with Chronic Urticaria, Flushing and Headaches. J.A.M.A., *189*:546-548, 1964.

Urtication unless she avoided peppermint-containing toothpastes, mouthwashes, cosmetics, medications, candy, chewing gum, jellies, ice creams, cigarettes and liqueurs.

Meyer de Schmid, J.-J., and Noble, J.-P.: Urticaire chronique par allergie a la "pilule" controlée et analysée par le T. T. L. Bull. Soc. Franc. Derm Syph., *77*:158-159, 1970.
Cherchez la contraceptive!

Aaronson, C. M.: Generalized Urticaria from Sensitivity to Nifuroxime. J.A.M.A., *210*:557-558, 1969.
Don't forget to check on vaginal suppositories (and intrauterine devices).

James, J., and Warin, R. P.: Sensitivity to Cyanocobalamin and Hydroxocobalamin. Brit. Med. J., *2*:262-262, 1971.
Chronic urticaria due to vitamin B_{12} cleared by substituting intrinsic factor.

Isaacs, N. J., and Ertel, N. H.: Urticaria and Pruritus: Uncommon Manifestations of Hyperthyroidism. J. Allerg. Clin. Immunol., *48*:73-81, 1971.
The T3 key to understanding chronic urticaria in four women.

Farah, F. S., and Shbaklu, Z.: Auto-immune Progesterone Urticaria. J. Allerg. Clin. Immunol., *48*:257-261, 1971.
Mid- and premenstrual urticaria suggests progesterone sensitivity; can be confirmed by challenge.

Shelley, W. B.: Urticaria of Nine Years' Duration Cleared Following Dental Extraction. Arch. Derm., *100*:324-325, 1969.
Invaluable help from the periodontist; nothing seen in radiograph.

Steck, W. D., and Byrd, R. B.: Urticaria Secondary to Pulmonary Melioidosis. Arch. Derm., *99*:80-81, 1969.
Sputa culture: Pseudomonas pseudomallei, a gram-negative rod. Urticaria gone after one week of tetracycline.

Weber, G., and Stetter, H.: Zur Frage: hautbeschrankte Ornithoseformen. Hautarzt, *20*:60-63, 1969.
Chronic urticaria due to psittacosis, also cured by tetracycline.

Singh, G., and Ojha, D.: Chronic Urticaria and Filariasis. Dermatologica, *136*:173-175, 1968.
Positive blood film at night; Hetrazan curative.

Shelley, W. B.: Case Report: An Analysis of a Case of Chronic Urticaria. Ann. Allerg., 24:421-425, 1966.
A detective story: the crime—four years of urticaria; the criminal—residual Pantopaque from myelography.

McKenzie, A. W., Aitken, C. V. E., and Ridsdill-Smith, R.: Urticaria after Insertion of Smith-Petersen Vitallium Nail. Brit. Med. J., 4:36-36, 1967.
Another iatrogenic urticaria, daily attacks for ten months, cure within 24 hours of removal of nail.

Flick, J. A.: Human Reagins: Appraisal of the Properties of the Antibody of Immediate-type Hypersensitivity. Bact. Rev., 36:311-360, 1972.
Master reference on these IgE antibodies which enable antigen to trigger histamine release in urticaria.

Haddad, Z. H., and Koratzer, J. L.: Immediate Hypersensitivity Reactions to Food Antigens. Detection of Human IgE Antibodies in Vitro and Exploration of Immunologic Mechanisms Using the Rat Mast Cell System. J. Allerg. Clin. Immunol., 49:210-218, 1972.
Mast cells, like basophils, used in specific IgE degranulation test for detecting urticariogens.

Rocha e Silva, M. (Ed.): Histamine, Its Chemistry Metabolism and Physiological and Pharmacological Actions. Eichler, O., and Farsh, A. (Eds.): *Handbook of Experimental Pharmacology,* Vol. 18, Part 1, 1966, pp. 1-991.
Histamine induces venular contraction, retrograde increase in pressure, vasodilation, capillary stasis and plasma leakage.

Kobinger, W., and Walland, A.: Die experimentelle Auslösung eines urtikariellen Exanthems an Hunden und seine Verwendung bei der Untersuchung von permeabilitätshemmenden Substanzen. Wien. Klin. Wschr., 78:420-424, 1966.
Experimental hives in dog elicited by histamine liberator, counteracted by I. V. calcium gluconate.

Juhlin, L., and Michaelsson, G.: Vascular Reactions in Urticaria. Brit. J. Derm., 82,Suppl. 5.:66-73, 1970.
Kinin release by peptidase (kallikrein) implicated in deep, persistent hive.

James, J., and Warin, R. P.: Chronic Urticaria: The Effect of Aspirin. Brit. J. Derm., 82:204-205, 1970.
Exacerbation of hives in 41 per cent.

Michaëlsson, G., and Juhlin, L.: Urticaria Induced by Preservatives and Dye Additives in Food and Drugs. Brit. J. Derm., 88:525-532, 1973.
Chronic urticaria often due to occult exposure to the yellow dye tartrazine, the preservative benzoate and the analgesic aspirin. Proved by challenge.

Weary, P. E., and Guerrant, J. L.: Chronic Urticaria in Association with Dermatophytosis. Response to the Administration of Griseofulvin. Arch. Derm., 95:400-401, 1967.
Griseofulvin-induced remissions; discontinuance relapses.

James, J., and Warin, R. P.: An Assessment of the Role of *Candida albicans* and Food Yeasts in Chronic Urticaria. Brit. J. Derm., 84:227-237, 1971.
One in every 4 sensitive to *C. albicans* **and responsive to nystatin** *and* **low yeast diet.**

3

These **inflammatory pustules** *appeared under the breasts two days ago. The patient has had diabetes mellitus for many years and has had other intertriginous eruptions in the past few months which have responded to topical gentian violet.*

Blood sugar level — 305 mg. per 100 ml.

KOH examination — yeast forms and pseudohyphae.

Culture — Candida albicans.

Candidiasis

Here are seen the three cardinal signs of a yeast infection: pustules, localization in moist intertriginous skin, and appearance in an uncontrolled diabetic. Diagnosis becomes the clinician's prerogative. Indeed, the microscopic examination of the scraping and a culture seem almost superfluous, although they do serve as laboratory monitors for our views. Although biopsy is rarely done, it requires the periodic acid-Schiff stain to reveal the causal spores and pseudohyphae in the outer horny layer. Otherwise, only the nonspecific intraepithelial pustule is seen.

The diagnosis is not always so simple, for candidiasis may present in a score of ways. The most common is as a simple intertrigo — raw, red, burning inflammatory areas at the sites of skin apposition and friction. Even here, however, there is frequently a telltale diagnostic fringe of satellite pustules or a collar-like scale. Folds of fat, the umbilicus, the inframammary, axillary, vulvar, scrotal, crural and perianal areas are all good host locales. Equally vulnerable are the angles of the mouth (perlèche), the interdigital spaces, areas under rings, and the webs of the fingers of people who perspire a great deal or do wet work (erosio interdigitalis blastomycetica). Particularly hazardous today is the occlusive plastic Saran Wrap, which if kept in place for long periods provides an ideal milieu for yeast growth. Prolonged wet dressings and continuous baths were similar hazards of yesteryear. The disease may also appear on the hands or feet as a nonspecific paronychia, representing a deeper, more purulent inflammatory change about the nails. More insidious and

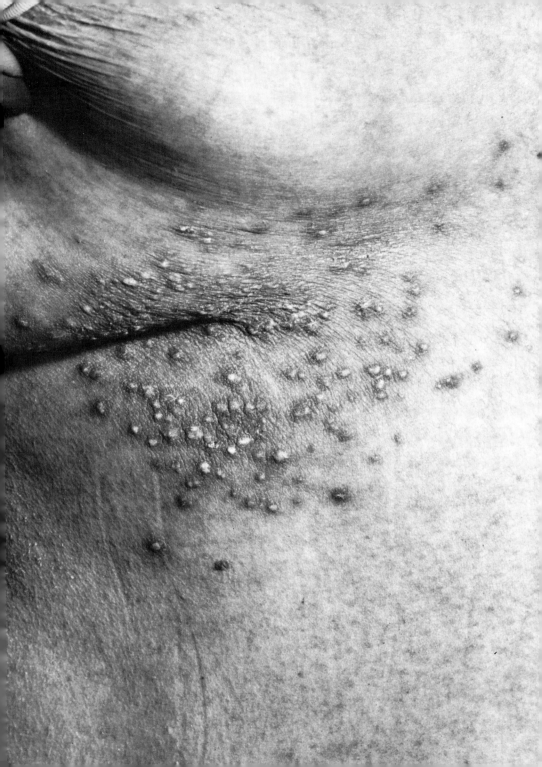

often unrecognized is the folliculitis of the face due to this yeast. It may present as a barber's itch or simply as a rosaceal or perioral dermatitis and is strangely indifferent to antibiotics.

Despite all these cutaneous signs, it is in the mucous membranes that candidiasis actually has its best known expression. For it is here that thrush, a condition recognized centuries ago, appears, with its distinctive white curdlike patches of adherent membrane overlying inflamed oral or vaginal mucosa. It may extend down the pharynx and into the respiratory tract as well as appear throughout the entire gastrointestinal tract, including the rectum. Lesser versions may occur as a balanoposthitis or a conjunctivitis.

Amazingly, essentially all this represents disease caused by just 1 of the 68 species which make up only one of the hundreds of genera of the immense yeast family, i.e., *Candida albicans*. In scrapings this organism is dimorphic, being present both as yeast cells (2 to 5 μ) and as filaments, the latter representing the pathogenic invasive form. Interestingly, an analogous yeast to filament transition is seen in tinea versicolor. Cultural characteristics of the Candida, i.e., chlamydospore formation and fermentation, allow identification of the common species. By contrast, serological and animal inoculation studies are ordinarily not valuable to the clinician.

Up to this point the story has been routine — yeast meets skin, skin becomes infected. But in the last few years this seemingly insignificant disease has become like a Rosetta stone in the deciphering of the body's immune defense systems.

It all began with an analysis of a rare, exquisitely chronic, extensive mucocutaneous form of candidiasis appearing in infancy and lasting for years. Why was *Candida albicans* such a virulent pathogen in these children? Normally it lived a pleasant commensal existence within the gut. Never did it appear on the skin except in the acute episodes of candidiasis that we have just delineated. Why?

The answer came with an awareness that these children suffered severe defects in the thymus-controlled lymphocyte defense system. Parallel developments in immunologic assessment made it possible to show that these children, parasitized with *C. albicans*, failed to show the normal delayed inflammation following a skin test to Candida antigens. Moreover, some of these children had lymphocytes which failed to show the expected proliferation or transformation in the presence of candidal antigen in vitro. Others failed to elaborate the macrophage inhibiting factor, regularly made in response to exposure to the Candida antigen. Conversely, phagocytosis of *Candida albicans* by their neutrophils was entirely normal. The humoral immune system, as measured by immediate type skin tests, agglutinins, precipitins and IgA, was showing an elevated response.

This resulted in the exciting proposition that patients with chronic mucocutaneous candidiasis are a model for the study of the *delayed* hypersensitivity defense system, each patient lacking one or more components. This entire system is under the control of the thymus and is composed of the so-called T lymphocytes, which proliferate and elaborate protective inflammatory substances. It is to be distinguished from the B lymphocytes and plasma cells which are under separate control and are programmed to elaborate the five immunoglobulins involved in immediate defense, as seen in urticaria.

Monthly the literature expands to record the triumphs of immunologic reconstitution in these children, previously barnacled with yeast and doomed to early death. Approaches include bone marrow grafts, fetal thymic transplants, lymphocyte/leukocyte transfusions, and injections of extracts of lymphocytes from normal individuals highly sensitive to Candida. This latter material is the transfer factor, which although nonantigenic and posing no risk of graft vs. host reaction, actually induces the patient's lymphocytes to react to the candidal organisms.

The problem of chronic candidiasis is not simple. Further sophistication in testing will no doubt divide it into a constellation of new laboratory diseases, each calling for a specific corrective factor. Such is the march of medicine.

But, back to today — and to our patient.

Her candidiasis reflects her elevated blood sugar level. Appropriate steps to return it toward normal will be accompanied by regression of the lesions. Meanwhile, much can be done locally by keeping the area dry. Sweating and maceration must be kept at a minimum. Wet clothing should be changed and only loose nonrubbing garments worn. A bra should not be worn.

A single painting of the inflamed area with Castellani paint would be helpful. Subsequently topical amphotericin B lotion should be applied three or four times daily. Alternate local remedies of value include those containing nystatin and haloprogin. As would be expected, the time-honored staining with gentian violet has yielded to these modern compounds. Oral nystatin (500,000 units t.i.d.) is also commonly employed to reduce the reservoir of gastrointestinal organisms. Also, it should be noted that the golden remedy for fungal infections, griseofulvin, has no effect on candidiasis.

Once rare, candidiasis will be seen with increasing frequency as medicine prolongs lives without restoring health. Day after day the ubiquitous saprophytic *Candida albicans* probes our patients' defenses. It assesses them one by one, establishing parasitic residence in those who lack any of the links in the chain of immunity and the barrier of a dry, healthy epidermis.

This is the disease of hyperhidrosis, burns, occupational exposure, diabetes mellitus, obesity and alcoholism. It is the disease of leukemia, lymphomas and cancer. It is the disease of catheterization of the veins or bladder and of the heroin addict. It is the disease of infants and old age, leukopenia, neutrophil defects and B and T lymphocyte deficits. It is the disease of endocrine disturbance and of iron deficiency. It is the disease of patients receiving long-term steroids, antibiotics or immunosuppressants. Can we wonder that it is increasing?

Winner, H. I., and Hurley, R.: Candida Albicans. Little, Brown and Company, Boston, 1964, 306 pp.
   The complete chronicle of candidiasis with an exquisite historical account and 87 pages of references.

Rhatigan, R. M.: Congenital Cutaneous Candidiasis. Amer. J. Dis. Children, *116*:545-546, 1968.
   Generalized and acquired in utero.

Ayres, S., Jr., and Mihan, R.: Wrist Watch Ringworm. Arch. Derm., *102*:235-235, 1970.
   Localized and hidden under a wrist watch, candidiasis simulating tinea.

Meinhof, W., Balda, B.-R., Vogel, H., and Braun-Falco, O.: Zum Krankheitsbild der Folliculitis barbae candidomycetica. Hautarzt, *21*:312-318, 1970.
   "Barber's itch" from Candida albicans.

Eyre, J., and Nally, F. F.: Oral Candidosis and Carcinoma. Brit. J. Derm., *85*:73-75, 1971.
   May mask underlying squamous cell carcinoma.

Eras, P., Goldstein, M. J., and Sherlock, P.: Candida Infection of the Gastrointestinal Tract. Medicine, *51*:367-379, 1972.
   What you see in the mouth may well extend into the esophagus and stomach.

Stankler, L., and Bewsher, P. D.: Chronic Mucocutaneous Candidiasis, Endocrine Deficiency and Alopecia Areata. Brit. J. Derm., *86*:238-245, 1972.
   Chronic form suggests parathyroid, thyroid, adrenal or other endocrine deficit, at times familial.

MacMillan, B. G., Law, E. J., and Holder, I. A.: Experience with Candida Infections in the Burn Patient. Arch. Surg., *104*:509-514, 1972.
Opportunistic invasion by Candida in over 60 per cent of 427 burn patients; associated in 5 per cent with positive blood cultures.

Fishman, L. S., Griffin, J. R., Sapico, F. L., and Hecht, R.: Hematogenous Candida Endophthalmitis. A Complication of Candidemia. New Eng. J. Med.,*286*:675-681, 1972.
A frightening complication of the dreaded blood stream dissemination of Candida albicans.

Balandran, L., Rothschild, H., Pugh, N., and Seabury, J.: A Cutaneous Manifestation of Systemic Candidiasis. Ann. Intern Med., *78*:400-403, 1973.
Papular rash in leukemics revealed spores on biopsy.

Portnoy, J., Wolf, P. L., Webb, M., and Remington, J. S.: Candida Blastospores and Pseudohyphae in Blood Smears. New Eng. J. Med., *285*:1010-1011, 1971.
Can find in blood smear even before culture.

Lehrer, R. I., and Cline, M. J.: Interaction of *Candida albicans* with Human Leukocytes and Serum. J. Bact., *98*:996-1004, 1969.
Immediate cellular defense centers on neutrophil; leukopenia favors candidemia.

Lehrer, R. I., and Cline, M. J.: Leukocyte Candidacidal Activity and Resistance to Systemic Candidiasis in Patients with Cancer. Cancer, *27*:1211-1217, 1971.
Lowered resistance associated with neutrophils that can phagocytose but not kill C. albicans.

Kirkpatrick, C. H., Rich, R. R., and Bennett, J. E.: Chronic Mucocutaneous Candidiasis: Model Building in Cellular Immunity. Ann. Intern. Med., *74*:955-978, 1971.
Delayed cellular defense centers on T lymphocytes: defective in 8 of 12 chronic candidiasis patients. A classic review.

Lehner, T., Buckley, H. R., and Murray, I. G.: The Relationship Between Fluorescent Agglutinating and Precipitating Antibodies to *Candida albicans* and Their Immunoglobulin Classes. J. Clin. Path., *25*:344-348, 1972.
Humoral defense includes IgG precipitins and IgM agglutinins to cell wall mannan.

Louria, D. B., Smith, J. K., Brayton, R. G., and Buse, M.: Anti-Candida Factors in Serum and Their Inhibitors. I. Clinical and Laboratory Observations. J. Infect. Dis., *125*:102-122, 1972.
Another defense, clumping of C. albicans by normal sera, absent in candidiasis.

Knight, L., and Fletcher, J.: Growth of *Candida albicans* in Saliva: Stimulation by Glucose Associated with Antibiotics, Corticosteroids and Diabetes Mellitus. J. Infect. Dis., *123*:371-377, 1971.
Diabetes, antibiotic or steroid therapy produces sharp rise in salivary glucose, favoring candidal growth.

Mackenzie, D. W.: Effect of Relative Humidity on Survival of *Candida albicans* and Other Yeasts. Appl. Microbiol., *22*:678-682, 1971.
Moisture favors candidiasis of skin.

Maibach, H. I., and Kligman, A. M.: The Biology of Experimental Human Moniliasis (*Candida albicans*). Arch. Derm., *85*:233-257, 1962.
Recipe: 100,000 organisms, dead or alive, under occlusive tape for 72 hours. Required reading.

Reynolds, I. M., Miner, P. W., and Smith, R. E.: Cutaneous Candidiasis in Swine. J. Amer. Vet. Med. Assoc., *152*:182-186, 1968.
Caused by lying around in hot, wet garbage.

Midgley, G., and Clayton, Y. M.: Distribution of Dermatophytes and Candida Spores in the Environment. Brit. J. Derm., *86(Suppl. 8)*:69-77, 1972.
Spore dispersion from candidiasis patient into air and bedding; may be source of cross infection in hospital.

Lynch, P. J., Minkin, W., and Smith, E. B.: Ecology of *Candida albicans* in Candidiasis of the Groin. Arch. Derm., *99*:154-160, 1969.
Source of organisms is rectal.

Krause, W., Matheis, H., and Wulf, K.: Fungaemia and Funguria After Oral Administration of *Candida albicans.* Lancet, *1*:598-599, 1969.
Heroic demonstration that C. albicans could pass through gut wall into blood stream — of senior author!

Montes, L. F., Ceballos, R., Cooper, M. D., Bradley, M. N., and Bockman, D. E.: Chronic Mucocutaneous Candidiasis, Myositis, and Thymoma. J.A.M.A., *222*:1619-1623, 1972.
Excision of thymoma without effect on candidiasis.

Toala, P., Schroeder, S. A., Daly, A. K., and Finland, M.: Candida at Boston City Hospital Clinical and Epidemiological Characteristics and Susceptibility to Eight Antimicrobial Agents. Arch. Intern. Med., *126*:983-989, 1970.
Only 1 of 151 cases required systemic antifungal therapy, since usually is simple colonization of susceptible or compromised host.

Witten, V. H., and Katz, S. I.: Nystatin. Med. Clin. N. Amer. *54*:1329-1337, 1970.
Anticandidal polyene compound from Streptomyces noursei useful orally and topically.

Bradford, L. G., and Montes, L. F.: Perioral Dermatitis and *Candida albicans.* Arch. Derm., *105*:892-895, 1972.
Cure with haloprogin cream.

Montes, L. F., Cooper, M. D., Bradford, L. G., Lauderdale, R. O., and Taylor, C. D.: Prolonged Oral Treatment of Chronic Mucocutaneous Candidiasis with Amphotericin B. Arch. Derm., *104*:45-56, 1971.
Despite unorthodox route for this standard candidicidal drug, some success.

Montes, L. F., Pittman, C. S., Moore, W. J., Taylor, C. D., and Cooper, M. D.: Chronic Mucocutaneous Candidiasis Influence of Thyroid Status. J.A.M.A., *221*:156-159, 1972.
Example of candidiasis, prodroming hypothyroidism, dramatically responsive to thyroid therapy.

Higgs, J. M., and Wells, R. S.: Chronic Muco-cutaneous Candidiasis: Associated Abnormalities of Iron Metabolism. Brit. J. Derm., *86(Suppl. 8)*:88-102, 1972.
Relates candidiasis to iron deficiency, affecting immune status and responding to iron therapy.

Levy, R. L., Huang, S. W., Bach, M. L., Bach, F. H., Hong, R., Ammann, A. J., Bortin, M., and Kay, H.E.M.: Thymic Transplantation in a case of Chronic Mucocutaneous Candidiasis. Lancet, *2*:898-900, 1971.
Improvement associated with appearance of T lymphocyte delayed hypersensitivity following fetal thymic transplants.

Valdimarsson, H., Moss, P. D., Holt, P. J. L., and Hobbs, J. R.: Treatment of Chronic Mucocutaneous Candidiasis with Leukocytes from HL-A Compatible Sibling. Lancet, *1*:469-472, 1972.

Immune defense restored by transfusion of white cells from his healthy brother.

Schulkind, M. L., Adler, W. H., III, Altemeier, W. A., III, and Ayoub, E. M.: Transfer Factor in the Treatment of a Case of Chronic Muco-cutaneous Candidiasis. Cell Immunol., *3*:606-615, 1972.

Growing literature attests to value of injections of transfer factor, i.e., lyophilized extract of leukocytes.

4

This rapidly growing, **dome-shaped nodule with central crater** *has arisen from normal skin in just the past three weeks. Regional lymphadenopathy is absent. The patient is 81 years old and has had actinic keratoses as well as a basal cell epithelioma previously removed from her face.*

Biopsy — prickle cell epithelioma — configuration of keratoacanthoma.

Keratoacanthoma

This lesion is the clinician's pride and joy. He exults in his awareness of the benign nature of this malignant-appearing tumor. Despite histologic evidence on biopsy of squamous cell epithelioma, the clinical story is that of a harmless growth which will disappear within months without any treatment. Failure to recognize that the keratoacanthoma is self-healing has been the basis for many a false claim for a cancer cure made by the professional and the quack alike.

This patient's lesion showed the phenomenal burst of growth which is so characteristic. That many full-grown tumors arise in such short periods of time excites disbelief. This is in keeping with the view that here we have a a tumor of the hair follicle, normally the most rapidly growing of all tissues. Further evidence of its follicular origins is the fact that the central mass beneath the crater is keratin; thus, it replicates the true function of the follicle. Its histogenesis within the hair follicle likewise is in keeping with its climactic surge in growth, followed by maturation, and later involution, albeit with scarring at times. All this recapitulates the hair cycle itself. This remarkable keratin-producing epithelioma thus has a well-defined, predictable life cycle of months. Its course is so regular and unvaried that any perturbations are alarming and call for review, with possible wide excision and lymph node resection. For in some few individuals the innocent keratoacanthoma converts into the true, awesome, metastasizing squamous cell epithelioma.

The singular solitary nature of this growth as well as its smooth

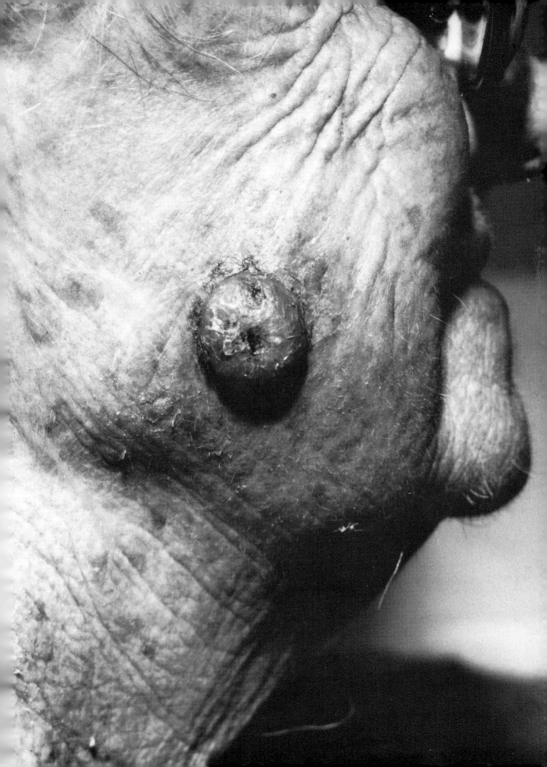

dome shape attests to its being a typically benign keratoacanthoma. It has the diagnostic crateriform opening into a central keratinous mass. It is not ulcerative or painful nor does it bleed, and adenopathy is absent. It is on the face and arises from essentially normal, although aged and actinically damaged, skin. It has neither the keratinous outgrowth of the cutaneous horn nor the low profile of actinic keratosis. It lacks the verrucous surface of the wart, and the solitary nature bespeaks against a giant molluscum contagiosum. All in all, it mimics well only the malignant squamous cell epithelioma.

A biopsy was mandatory and did demonstrate the signs of a keratoacanthoma: symmetry, well-differentiated follicular growths of squamous epithelium, keratinous plug, and absence of infiltrative growth below the zone of the follicular bulbs. The presence of numerous mitotic figures, essentially normal in appearance, was not interpreted as a sign of cancer, but rather of enhanced cell replication. To best sense the controlled nature of the entire process a deep central elliptical excision is preferable to a slice or curetting. Interestingly, the mere process of taking the biopsy specimen during the growth phase may accelerate regression, although occasionally it produces the very opposite yet temporary effect.

Incidentally, when keratoacanthomas are multiple, the prognosis is poor. This is virtually another disease, spreading widely at times, and showing a chronicity and recalcitrance to therapy. In these instances spontaneous healing is not to be anticipated as much as further spread with even involvement of skin grafts. Indeed, in these instances it is desirable to survey the patient. Has the immunosurveillance protective system been weakened by disease (Hodgkin's disease, lymphoma) or medicine (immunosuppressants)? Does the patient have an associated malignant tumor of the bowel? Equally indifferent to the physician are the rare widespread eruptive forms. Even the use of cytotoxic drugs externally and internally has been to no avail.

Why did our patient's lesion arise? One can only speculate that it is an abortive form of neoplasia, induced by a carcinogen. Despite its gross resemblance to the classic viral tumors, verrucae and molluscum contagiosum, no one has been able to isolate a virus to date. Sunlight remains a prime causal suspect, but some agents are even more precisely labelled as causative. Thus, in men working with tar, this keratoacanthoma was the "pitch wart" of old. In animals, keratoacanthomas are readily induced by simply painting the skin with the carcinogen dimethylbenz-anthracene (DMBA). At times the actual trigger factor is a cut, a bruise or a burn. None seem applicable to our patient's case, but certainly sunlight has taken its toll, for we see actinic keratoses, and she has a history of having had a basal cell epithelioma.

The question of treatment may sound rhetorical for a self-healing lesion. However, simple removal can often be the wisest procedure. It may be best to simply flush shave this patient's lesion, although curettage or even total excision is feasible. Chemotherapy with 5-fluorouracil is another successful yet slower approach. Some clinicians use cryotherapy with liquid nitrogen and a few employ x-ray. Our own recommendation here would be a superficial shave excision. Close followup for a year is essential, remembering that recurrence may occur and require re-treatment. A gentle approach, with the avoidance of mutilating extensive surgery, grafting, and lymph node resection, comes from our awareness of the benignity of keratoacanthoma.

Ordinarily a therapeutic triumph, this lesion can be the clinician's shame and sorrow should he fail to follow and treat any supervening squamous cell epithelioma. Remember, an absolute diagnosis of keratoacanthoma is always a retrospective one, made only after the lesion and the physician's responsibility for followup are completely gone.

Ghadially, F. N.: Keratoacanthoma. *In* Fitzpatrick, T. B. (Ed.): *Dermatology in General Medicine*. McGraw-Hill Book Co., New York, 1971, pp. 425-436.
Scholarly introduction to a growth that looks malignant but acts benign.

Kopf, A. W.: Multiple Keratoacanthomas. Arch. Derm., *103*:543-544, 1971.
The not-so-benign multiple version, resistant to all forms of therapy.

Winkelmann, R. K., and Brown, J.: Generalized Eruptive Keratoacanthoma. Arch. Derm., *97*:615-623, 1968.
Small papular form, resembles pityriasis rubra pilaris, equally resistant to treatment.

Gwiezdzinski, Z., and Kozlowski, J.: Keratoakanthoma tubero-serpiginosum exulcerans. Derm. Monatsschr., *157*:432-437, 1971.
Rare, nodular, ulcerative, serpiginous type.

Shapiro, L., and Baraf, C. S.: Subungual Epidermoid Carcinoma and Keratoacanthoma. Cancer, *25*:141-152, 1970.
Unique localization produces bone destruction.

Kohn, M. W., and Eversole, L. R.: Keratoacanthoma of the Lower Lip: Report of Cases. J. Oral Surg., *30*:522-526, 1972.
Almost impossible to distinguish from squamous cell epithelioma.

Burge, K. M., and Winkelmann, R. K.: Keratoacanthoma Association with Basal and Squamous Cell Carcinoma. Arch. Derm., *100*:306-311, 1969.
Case of sequential evolution of keratoacanthoma, basal cell epithelioma, squamous cell epithelioma at same site.

Vickers, C. F., and Ghadially, F. N.: Keratoacanthoma Associated with Psoriasis. Brit. J. Derm., *73*:120-124, 1961.
Lesions appeared only on eruptive plaques of psoriasis.

Szyszymar, B., and Gwiezdzinski, Z.: Keratoacanthoma in Sebaceous Nevus in a Child. Przegl. Derm., *58*:467-471, 1971.
A disease of the pilosebaceous unit localized to a nevus of the sebaceous unit.

Stevanovic, D. V.: Keratoacanthoma in Xeroderma Pigmentosum. Arch. Derm., *84*:53-54, 1961.
Sunlight as the pathogen.

de Moragas, J. M.: Multiple Keratoacanthomas. Relation to Jamarsen Therapy of Pemphigus Foliaceus. Arch. Derm., *93*:679-683, 1966.
Induced by painting skin for months with coal tar preparation.

Lowry, W. S., Clark, D. A., and Hannemann, J. H.: Skin Cancer and Immunosuppression. Lancet, *1*:1290-1291, 1972.
Immunosuppression leads to appearance of keratoacanthomas: aggressive examples in Hodgkin's disease and kidney allograft patients.

Weber, G., Stetter, H., Pliess, G., and Stickl, H.: Assoziiertes Vorkommen von eruptiven Keratoacanthomen Tubercarcinom und Paramyeloblastenleukämie. Arch. Klin. Exp. Derm., *238*:107-119, 1970.
Keratoacanthomas occurring in association with leukemia and carcinoma.

Muir, E. G., Bell, A. J. Y., and Barlow, K. A.: Multiple Primary Carcinomata of the Colon, Duodenum and Larynx Associated with Keratoacanthomata of the Face. Brit. J. Surg., *54*:191-195, 1967.
The keratoacanthoma patient always deserves medical review.

Ghadially, F. N., Barton, B. W., and Kerridge, D. F.: The Etiology of Keratoacanthoma. Cancer, *16*:603-611, 1963.
Readily induced in animals by topical application of the carcinogen dimethylbenzanthracene.

Bullough, W. S.: The Control of Epidermal Thickness. Brit. J. Derm., *87*:347-354, 1972.
Tumors lack chalones, the normal inhibitor of cell division.

How, S., and Snell, K. C.: Skin Tumors Induced in Rats by the Dietary Administration of N,N[1]-2,7-Fluorenylenebisacetamide. J. Nat. Cancer Inst., *38*:407-434, 1967.
After nearly a year, one keratoacanthoma and many analogous sebaceous gland tumors.

Prutkin, L.: Modification of the Effect of Vitamin A Acid on the Skin Tumor Keratoacanthoma by Applications of Actinomycin D. Cancer Res., *31*:1080-1086, 1971.
Topical vitamin A acid causes experimental keratoacanthomas to exude a copious, viscous, foul-smelling exudate — the result of mucous metaplasia of the keratinocytes.

Fisher, E. R., McCoy, M. M., and Wechsler, H. L.: Analysis of Histopathologic and Electron Microscopic Determinants of Keratoacanthoma and Squamous Cell Carcinoma. Cancer, *29*:1387-1397, 1972.
Even the electron microscope can't tell these tumors apart.

Belisario, J. C.: Cancer of the Skin. Butterworth & Co., London, 1959, pp. 80-96.
Before and after photographs of keratoacanthomas spontaneously disappearing in 3 months.

Grupper, C.: Treatment of Keratoacanthomas by Local Applications of the 5-Fluorouracil (5-FU) Ointment. Dermatologica, *140(Suppl. I)*:127-132, 1970.
Good result in 12 of 15 cases.

Jackson, I. T.: Diagnostic Problem of Keratoacanthoma. Lancet, *1*:490-492, 1969.
Whether you treat by shaving, curetting, excising, coagulating, freezing, irradiating or ignoring it, you must follow it as though it were a squamous cell epithelioma. Be alert to invasion and metastasis.

5

For five years this patient has had **pruritic violaceous licheni-**
fied plaques *on her forearms as well as hyperkeratotic pitted
areas on her palms and soles. Onset was associated with the emotional trauma of being unemployed, and she relates flareups to tension as well as to sun exposure. She drinks 20 cups of coffee a day,
is addicted to nail biting and gives a family history of diabetes
mellitus. No mucosal lesions seen.*

Biopsies from forearm and palm — lichen planus.

Lichen Planus

A single papule makes the diagnosis in this disease! Hunt for it. It is
polygonal, plano-topped and purplish — so distinctive as to demand a
label. Looking closely you will see that its glistening surface is characteristically criss-crossed with faint gray lines, seen even better under min-
eral oil and lens. Such is the amazing topography, coloring and surface
signature of one of the most remarkable and consistent lesions in dermatology. Whether the gross patterning be disseminate or grouped, annular or linear, the finding of one characteristic papule can be worth a
thousand tests.

No less striking is the virtually diagnostic localization of the lesions
to sites of trauma. Scratches, scrapes or tears all may be followed by a
procession of papules. The flexural areas of the wrist are a classic site for
this so called Koebner phenomenon. Well known to have a low threshold to itch stimuli and responsive to the trauma of scratching, our patient's lesions have resulted from years of such incessant scratching.
They now mimic the clinical picture of hypertrophic localized neurodermatitis, similarly the result of precision scratching of a single area.

Significantly, lichen planus is not limited to the skin, but may evolve
on any mucous membrane. Trauma again appears to be an inductive
factor; for example, the buccal mucosa commonly develops white striae
and papules at points of injury from biting and mastication.

With a disease so precise in its geometry and distribution, one is not
surprised to find an equally satisfying and tidy histologic picture. Here
the primary change is regularly in the germinative layer of the epidermis. It is one of degeneration and destruction of the basal cell layer

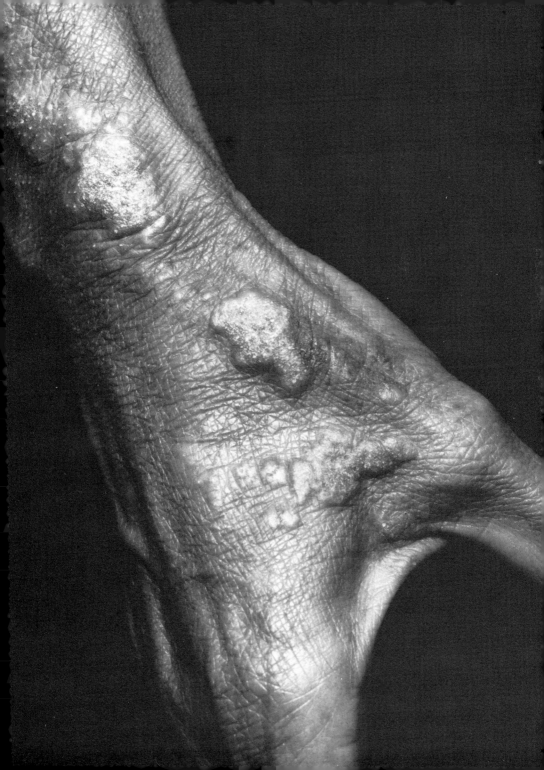

and its subjacent membrane. The overlying epidermis is healthy and indeed thickened, as though the daughter cells were released from a natural inhibitor or chalone. And just below the damaged basal cell layer is a reactive band of lymphocytes and histiocytes, many of the latter engulfing melanin released from the damaged melanocytes above.

It is this histologic picture which provides some raison d'être for the cardinal symptom of lichen planus, namely, pruritus. Since the itch organ consists of terminal fine nerve fibers ending within or just below the epidermis, the destructive inflammatory changes detailed would appear to initiate repetitive fine fiber stimulation associated with itch. Hence, finding lichen planus without an itch is like finding a sailboat without a sail.

Although lichen planus is ordinarily a benign pruritic and papular disease, it has within the seed of its histologic destructive nature a capability for gross clinical destructiveness. Thus, bullae may form if the basement membrane shearing occurs over a large area. Moreover, the sweat gland as well as the hair, and indeed the nails, may all be completely and permanently destroyed. Thus, heat intolerance, bald areas and permanent anonychia and mouth ulcers may all be seen.

Despite the satisfying consistency of this clinical and histologic portrait, little is known of how it comes to be painted. Yet there is one important clue. Lichen planus can be induced in some individuals by drugs or chemicals. Although this had been known for many years, it was first dramatized by the large number of soldiers in World War II who developed a lichen planus eruption. This was soon shown to be due to Atabrine. It is important to realize that, although Atabrine had been given to virtually millions as a routine prophylaxis against malaria, only hundreds developed lichen planus. Why?

Recent research would suggest that these were the susceptibles, identified by mass screening with Atabrine. These were the ones specifically born with a deficiency in the critical glucose-6-phosphate dehydrogenase (G-6-PDH) enzyme. It is the deficiency in this enzyme which is responsible for the hemolysis induced by antimalarials and other drugs. It would seem now that this same deficiency may be responsible for an analogous necrosis in the basal epidermis when these individuals are confronted with antimalarials. It is a burgeoning field as is that of the drug-induced hemolytic crises in the G-6-PDH-deficient individual. The Atabrine story has been repeated in miniature with many other drugs as well as organic paraphenylenediamine derivatives used in color film processing.

Thus, a cornerstone of therapy is elimination of all but truly life-maintenance drugs. The primary suspects include the phenothiazines paradoxically used to allay the stress long known to be associated with attacks of lichen planus. Equally suspect are the trio of thiazide diuretics, quinidine, and methyldopa used in helping the cardiac patient. The chloroquine and gold treatments of the arthritis patient and the para-aminosalicylate and streptomycin of the tuberculosis patient are also known offenders. Special occupational hazards of concern are those in the chemical industry or photographic developing. Here the search is for exposure to amino-diethyl aniline derivatives. It is now apparent that food additives must come under closer surveillance for these patients. We must be aware that one man's additive may be another man's poison. Always the search for drugs should be widened and intensified if the following two correlates of classic drug-induced lichen planus are present: the clinical finding of a normal buccal mucosa and the histologic finding of eosinophilia in the infiltrate in the papillary dermis. In any case, view, review and re-review. The art of taking a history is the art of making the unobvious obvious.

Although the cause may remain unknown, and the course would appear immutable, much can be done for our patient. She should be sympathetically instructed and guided toward a less turbulent life. The coffee pot must gradually be turned off. She must find a balance of productive work and relaxation for herself. The trauma of digging, rubbing and clawing her skin during tension crises serves only to perpetuate the disease. Psychotherapy, whether it springs from within or from without, whether it is personal or professional, may be really helpful.

But the ordered life is not enough to roll back the cutaneous changes of five years. For this, repeated intralesional injections of triamcinolone acetonide are best. Topically a powerful fluorinated steroid cream is advisable and some patients are helped by covering the area with steroid impregnated tape. Liquid nitrogen cryotherapy and salicylic acid ointment are two standard modalities also used for shrinking this hypertrophic form of lichen planus. More recently, topical vitamin A acid has been employed with help as an antikeratotic agent. The itching may be modulated by an antihistamine, but recall that phenothiazines and drugs in general are to be eschewed. Although systemic steroids may be used on a short-term basis to allay severe widespread inflammatory change seen in acute eruptive lichen planus, they are not indicated for our patient at this time. Finally, reinforce the patient's awareness of the danger of excessive sun exposure, long known to be a trigger for lichen planus.

These firm verrucous hypertrophic lesions are the most resistant form of lichen planus. Although it is true that lichen planus often spontaneously remits in a year or two, our patient's hypertrophic form may persist for decades. Furthermore, it can scar and even undergo malignant change. It is an undoubted therapeutic *locus majoris resistentiae* and must be treated as such.

Cram, D. L., and Muller, S. A.: Unusual Variations of Lichen Planus. Mayo Clin. Proc., *41*:677-688, 1966.
May be hypertrophic or atrophic, linear or annular, erythematous or bullous, follicular or onychal.

Siemens, H. W.: *General Diagnosis and Therapy of Skin Diseases.* University of Chicago Press, Illinois, 1958.
Two hundred of the most exciting pages on how really to see what you are looking at.

Almeyda, J., and Levantine, A.: Lichenoid Drug Eruptions. Brit. J. Derm., *85*:604-607, 1971.
Reviews drug-induced lichen planus indicating thiazines, phenothiazines, para-aminosalicylic acid, quinidine, methyldopa, chloroquine and gold.

Pillsbury, D. M., and Livingood, C. S.: Dermatology, pp. 543-675. *In* Anderson, R. S. (Ed.): *Internal Medicine in World War II.* Department of the Army, Washington, D.C., 1968.
The inside story on Army lichen planus induced by the antimalarial Atabrine.

de Graciansky, P., and Boulle, S.: Skin Disease from Colour Developers. Brit. J. Derm., *78*:297-298, 1966.
Authentic lichen planus may also be caused by paraphenylene diamine compounds used in color film developer.

Scarpa, C., and Ferrea, E.: Allergological Researches with Cadmium, Beryllium and Arsenic and a Case of Lichen Planus from Diazodiethylaniline. Panminerva Med. *10*: 93-96, 1968.
Lichen planus due to dust from blueprints containing analogue of color developer.

Frykholm, K. O., Frithiof, L., Fernstrom, A. B., Moberger, G., Blohm, S. G., and Bjorn, E.: Allergy to Copper Derived from Dental Alloys as a Possible Cause of Oral Lesions of Lichen Planus. Acta Dermatovener., *49*:268-281, 1969.
Cured by removing copper inlays.

Almeyda, J.: Lichen Planus Actinicus. Brit. J. Derm., *82*:426-427, 1970.
Sunlight induced.

Depaoli, M.: Lichen Ruber Planus Familiare. G. Ital. Derm., *45*:11-16, 1970.
Rare, but he found 12 intrafamily cases in series of 260 patients.

Shklar, G.: Lichen Planus as an Oral Ulcerative Disease. Oral Surg., *33*:376-388, 1972.
Definitive reviews; emphasizes stress as a cause.

Kronenberg, K., Fretzin, D., and Potter, B.: Malignant Degeneration of Lichen Planus. Arch. Derm., *104*:304-307, 1971.
Multiple squamous cell carcinomas developing at sites of chronic hypertrophic lichen planus.

Feuerman, E. J., and Sandbark, M.: Lichen Planus Pemphigoides with Extensive Melanosis Occurrence in a Patient with Malignant Lymphoma. Arch. Derm., *104*:61-67, 1971.
Extremely rare form associated with internal malignancy.

Stankler, L.: The Identity of Lichen Planus and Lichen Nitidus. Brit. J. Derm., *79*:125-126, 1967.
Lichen nitidus viewed as diminutive form of lichen planus.

Copeman, P. W. M., Schroeter, A. L., and Kierland, R. R.: An Unusual Variant of Lupus Erythematosus or Lichen Planus. Brit. J. Derm., *83*:269-272, 1970.
Four patients sharing features of both diseases.

Bologa, E. I., and Vaida, F.: In Rüchbildung begriffener Lichen ruber planus mit nachfolgender Dermatitis herpetiformis Duhring. Derm. Monatsschr., *157*:447-452, 1971.
Lichen planus evolving into dermatitis herpetiformis!

Summerly, R., and Wilson Jones, E.: The Microarchitecture of Wickham's Striae. Trans. St. Johns Hosp. Derm. Soc., *50*:157-161, 1964.
These grossly visible striae, diagnostic of lichen planus, result from focal thickening of epidermis.

Glickman, F., Rapp, Y., and Frank, L.: Capillary Microscopy in Inflammatory Dermatoses. Arch. Derm., *90*:500-505, 1964.
Capillaries appear in petalloid arrangement about the papule of lichen planus.

Sarkany, I., and Gaylarde, P. M.: Ultrastructural and Light Microscopic Changes of the Epidermo-Dermal Junction. Trans. St. Johns Hosp. Derm. Soc., *57*:139-142, 1971.
Primary event in lichen planus is liquefaction degeneration of basal cells.

Cotton, D. W. K., Van den Hurk, J. J. M. A., and Van der Staak, W. B. J. M.: Lichen Planus, an Inborn Error of Metabolism. Brit. J. Derm., *87*:341-346, 1972.
Evidence that lichen planus patients have a congenital deficiency in the epidermis of glucose-6-phosphate dehydrogenase, with attacks triggered by drugs, cf. favism.

Black, M. M., and Wilson-Jones, E.: The Role of the Epidermis in the Histopathogenesis of Lichen Planus. Arch. Derm., *105*:81-86, 1972.
Lichen planus is associated with diminished activity of many respiratory enzyme systems, the exact opposite of psoriasis.

Jolly, M.: Lichen Planus and Its Association with Diabetes Mellitus. Med. J. Aust., *1*:990-992, 1972.
Feels stress may elicit lichen planus and unmask latent diabetes.

Altman, J., and Perry, H. O.: The Variation and Course of Lichen Planus. Arch. Derm., *84*:179-191, 1961.
Two-thirds experienced spontaneous resolution after 15 months.

Emslie, E. S., and Hardman, F. G.: The Surgical Treatment of Oral Lichen Planus. Trans. St. Johns Hosp. Derm. Soc., *56*:43-44, 1970.
Advises excision of ulcerated areas.

Sehgal, V. N., Abraham, G. J. S., and Malik, G. B.: Griseofulvin Therapy in Lichen Planus. A Double-Blind Controlled Trial. Brit. J. Derm., *87*:383-385, 1972.
Associated with gradual improvement over period of weeks.

Boatwright, H.: Use of Flurandenolone Tape in Lupus Erythematosus and Other Diseases. J. S. C. Med. Assoc., *65*:173-175, 1969.
Occlusive steroid tape helpful in 87 of 124 cases of lichen planus.

Gunther, S.: Retinoic Acid in the Treatment of Lichen Planus. Dermatologica, *143*:315-318, 1971.
Hyperkeratotic lesions respond to 0.1 per cent retinoic acid ointment.

Welton, W. A.: How I Treat Lichen Planus. Postgrad. Med., *46*:196-197, July, 1969.
Hypertrophic lesions respond best to intralesional injection of triamcinolone acetonide suspension.

6

This 26-year-old man has had a **widespread pruritic vesicular eruption of the trunk** *for the past six months. Despite an initial response to prednisone therapy in dosage up to 100 mg. a day, the eruption is extending. His past history discloses diarrhea and bloody stools some nine years ago. Both his grandmothers died of malignancies of the gastrointestinal tract.*

Biopsy — dermatitis herpetiformis.

Dermatitis Herpetiformis

Here is a window to internal disease. Looking through it, you can be certain that this patient has both anatomic and physiologic defects in his small bowel. You can be confident that biopsies of his jejunum will show gross mucosal change, such as villous atrophy. You can suspect that he has intestinal malabsorption. Both oral lactose tolerance and d xylose absorption will be lowered. You can predict that secretion of intrinsic factor will be diminished and that intestinal disaccharidase levels are well below normal. You can anticipate that serum levels for iron, folate and vitamin B_{12} will be low. You can be aware that he may show protein loss, steatorrhea and diarrhea as a result of his enteropathy. You can know that he is sensitive to that insoluble yet elastic protein of wheat called gluten, and that a gluten-free diet will be immensely helpful in correcting his celiac syndrome. You can be alert to the fact that his spleen may show atrophy. You can advise that some of his relatives will have gross evidence of enteropathy. And most important, you can presage that he may develop a lymphoma or carcinoma of the gastrointestinal tract, as both his paternal and maternal grandmothers did. All this you see through his skin window, once you recognize that he has dermatitis herpetiformis.

And how do we recognize that he has dermatitis herpetiformis? We do it with ease, once we have grasped the remarkably consistent and characteristic symptom and sign of this disease. The symptom is a fiery pruritus. Dermatitis herpetiformis is the one disease with a fierce, burning, relentless itch, with paroxysms of excoriation and dug out skin, as well as postinflammatory hyper- and hypopigmentation. The sign is the

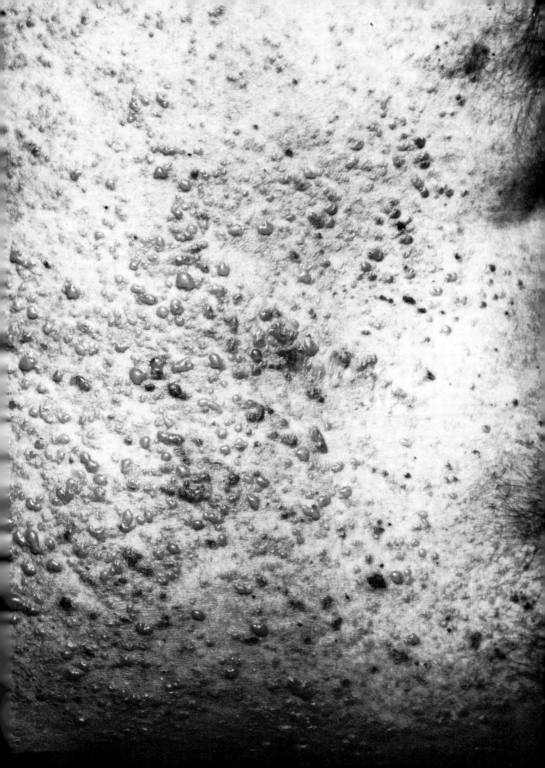

finding of small tense vesicles. Not only are they typically grouped, i.e., herpetic, but they erupt symmetrically at points of probable shearing trauma. It is this distribution which summons the diagnosis of dermatitis herpetiformis to mind: scalp, scapulae, sacrum, buttocks, elbows and knees. Without the telltale vesicle, dermatitis herpetiformis may be hard to sort out from atopic dermatitis, neurotic excoriations, insect bites or even scabies.

Auxiliary observations are simply confirmatory. The mucous membranes are not involved. The chronicity of this disease is legendary, many patients finding this not the 7-year itch, but rather closer to a 17-year itch. Ordinarily a disease of adult males, it may be flared by iodine, such as in seafood, treated water, medication or roentgen-contrast media. But most important of all, it is a disease singularly and regularly responsive to sulfone therapy. A rapid therapeutic response to dapsone is thus diagnostic.

Interestingly, our patient's itch points to the site of the critical histopathologic findings, viz., to the itch receptor organ area at the epidermal-dermal juncture. It is here that the intact epidermis simply separates from the dermis, first with a fibrin-filled cleft, later with an influx of neutrophils forming a subepidermal microabscess. The release of proteases from these disintegrating polymorphonuclear cells provides a strong, steady stimulus for the fine unmyelinated C fibers which subserve itch. Its intensity reaches beyond that of the basic urge to scratch, often giving rise to a virtually intolerable burning pain.

This is a "where the action is" disease. Not only have investigators in the past few years made this a window for internal illness, but they have made a startling advance in recognizing the immunologic nature of dermatitis herpetiformis. First it should be pointed out that these patients may have circulating antinuclear factors, as well as antibodies to thyroid microsomes, to gastric parietal cells and, most remarkably, to the reticulin found in the dermal papillae. Furthermore, there may be quantitative changes in the levels of serum immunoglobulin. All this is interesting, but the startling advance was finding by immunofluorescence the presence of deposits of IgA in the skin of these patients. Curiously IgA is not in the lesion being destroyed by the infiltrate of neutrophils. Rather, it is in the papillary dermis, just under the epidermis of widespread areas of normal-appearing skin. It is not to be compared to the antiepithelial antibody of pemphigus or the antibasement-membrane antibody of pemphigoid, two bullous diseases confused at times with dermatitis herpetiformis.

Dramatically, this IgA returns our attention to the gut. For it is the one immunoglobulin which is secreted by the immunocytes of the gastrointestinal tract. It serves as a first line of defense against such external antigens as viruses and foods. Thus, somehow the gut and the skin are immunologically intertwined. But how? Does the cutaneous change simply result from deposition of an antigen-IgA complex in the skin as in immune complex disease? Or, is the IgA reacting against some specific component of the dermis which shares structural antigenicity with gluten? Interestingly, although the gut rejects gluten, the skin is indifferent, as shown by patch-testing. More study is needed to learn how the skin and gut, the two great environmental interfaces of the body, interact in this intriguing disease of dermatitis herpetiformis.

From the standpoint of therapy, a good response of dermatitis herpetiformis to sulfones is so predictable as to make it practically a diagnostic test. For many years sulfapyridine was the bellwether therapeutic agent. An oral daily dose of several grams was followed by prompt resolution of pruritus and vesiculation. Although re-exacerbation quickly followed discontinuance, it was generally possible to find a maintenance level which provided essential relief but never cure. Today, dapsone or diaminodiphenylsulfone (DDS) is the therapy of choice, although it too must be continued for months and years at a maintenance level. Initial response can be expected in days when a single tablet of 100 mg. per day is prescribed. Derivates in the form of sulfoxone sodium (Diasone), 330 mg., and acetosulfone sodium (Promacetin), 500 mg., are similarly effective, but the mode of action is completely obscure. Other antibiotics as well as corticosteroids are without effect, and the sulfones remain the only consistently effective measure.

Dapsone therapy requires long-term monitoring because, although it is generally well tolerated, it can produce hematologic and renal damage. Neuropathy, hepatitis and exfoliative dermatitis are other adverse effects known to occur.

Adjuvant approaches include the elimination of iodine and iodides in foods as well as in medication. This stems from the fact that a significant number of these patients experience a flareup when given iodides and accounts for the injunction against seafood as well as iodine topically or as a radiopaque dye. From the dietary standpoint it is equally wise to eliminate wheat (gluten) and milk. Here the therapeutic results in terms of intestinal response are much more gratifying than those in the skin. However, in a few patients long-term avoidance of gluten has led to a reduction in the amount of dapsone required for control of the skin lesions.

In our present state of knowledge, this is a disease lingering for decades. It deserves long-term dapsone therapy and conjoint monitoring of the small bowel, not only for absorption defects but also for any late sequel of lymphoma. Dermatitis herpetiformis can be a window to internal disease only for those who would look into it!

Smith, E. L.: The Diagnosis of Dermatitis Herpetiformis. Trans. St. Johns Hosp. Derm. Soc., *52*:176-196, 1966.
A marvelously succulent review of Duhring's disease and its mad itch.

Lodin, A., and Stigell, P. O.: Dermatitis Herpetiformis Cases Observed at the Dermatologic Clinic, Karolinska Sjukhuset, 1954-1963. Acta Dermatovener., *45*:355-365, 1965.
Many of their 929 cases had been afflicted for over 15 years.

Ackerman, A. B., and Tolman, M. M.: Papular Dermatitis Herpetiformis in Childhood. Arch. Derm., *100*:286-290, 1969.
Has same severe pruritus, symmetry and localization to elbows, knees, scapulae, sacrum and buttocks as in adult.

Warner, J., Brooks, S. E. H., James, W. P. T., and Louisy, S.: Juvenile Dermatitis Herpetiformis in Jamaica: Clinical and Gastrointestinal Features. Brit. J. Derm., *86*:226-237, 1972.
Four cases showing flare when exposed to iodine-containing contrast media during jejunal biopsy.

Marks, J., May, S. B., and Roberts, D. F.: Dermatitis Herpetiformis Occurring in Monozygous Twins. Brit. J. Derm., *84*:417-419, 1971.
Identical dermatitis in identical twins.

Fry, L., and Johnson, F. R.: Electron Microscopic Study of Dermatitis Herpetiformis. Brit. J. Derm., *81*:44-50, 1969.
Key finding: areas of separation of normal epidermis from dermal papillae, filled with polymorphonuclear leukocytes.

Mustakallio, K. K., Blomquist, K., and Laiho, K.: Papillary Deposition of Fibrin, a Characteristic of Initial Lesions of Dermatitis Herpetiformis. Ann. Clin. Res., *2*:13-18, 1970.
An even earlier diagnostic sign.

Seah, P. P., Fry, L., Stewart, J. S., Chapman, B. L., Hoffbrand, A. V., and Holborow, E. J.: Immunoglobulins in the Skin in Dermatitis Herpetiformis and Coeliac Disease. Lancet, *1*:611-614, 1972.
All 18 D. H. patients showed IgA deposits in skin in dermal papillae.

Tomasi, T. B., and Grey, H. M.: Structure and Function of Immunoglobulin A. Progr. Allerg., *16*:81-213, 1972.
Formed by plasma cells in mucosa to limit absorption of potentially antigenic material.

Seah, P. P., Fry, L., Hoffbrand, A. V., and Holborow, E. J.: Tissue Antibodies in Dermatitis Herpetiformis and Adult Coeliac Disease. Lancet, *1*:834-836, 1971.
Demonstration of IgG antibody against reticulin in 1 in 5 cases of dermatitis herpetiformis.

Cormane, R. H., and Giannetti, A.: On the Occurrence of IgD in Dermatitis Herpetiformis and Pemphigoid. Brit. J. Derm., *84*:179-179, 1971.
Deposits of IgD found only in these two clinical cognates.

Fraser, N. G.: Auto-antibodies in Dermatitis Herpetiformis. Brit. J. Derm., *83*:609-613, 1970.
One in 5 has antibodies to thyroid.

Van der Meer, J. B.: Dermatitis Herpetiformis: A Specific (Immunopathological?) Entity. Batteljee and Terpstra, Leiden, 1972, 153 pp.
Monographic study suggests vesicles in skin result from neutrophil response to subepidermal deposit of an immune complex (antigen — IgA) originating from intestinal mucosa.

Jablonska, S., Chorzelski, T., Beutner, E. H., and Blaszczyk, M.: Juvenile Dermatitis Herpetiformis in the Light of Immunofluorescent Studies. Brit. J. Derm., *85*:307-313, 1971.
Pemphigoid readily distinguished by its specific immunofluorescent basement membrane antibodies.

Honeyman, J. F., Honeyman, A., Lobitz, W. C., and Storrs, F. J.: The Enigma of Bullous Pemphigoid and Dermatitis Herpetiformis. Arch. Derm., *106*:22-25, 1972.
Yet here are 5 patients sharing clinical, histopathological, immunofluorescent and therapeutic responses for both dermatitis herpetiformis and pemphigoid.

Brow, J. R., Parker, F., Weinstein, W. M., and Rubin, C. E.: The Small Intestinal Mucosa in Dermatitis Herpetiformis. Gastroenterology, *60*:355-369, 1971.
On repeated jejunal biopsy, all cases of dermatitis herpetiformis show at least patchy areas of atrophic mucosa or other abnormalities.

Johnson, D. P., and Alpert, M. E.: Dermatitis Herpetiformis — A Disease Associated with Intestinal Malabsorption. Amer. J. Gastroenterol., *55*:21-32, 1971.
Many show steatorrhea, diarrhea and associated low serum levels of folate, iron, B_{12}.

Marks, J., Birkett, D., Shuster, S., and Roberts, D. F.: Small Intestinal Mucosal Abnormalities in Relatives of Patients with Dermatitis Herpetiformis. Gut, *11*:493-497, 1970.
Seven of 19 kindred had had abnormally flat or convoluted mucosal pattern as seen in stereomicroscopy.

Andersson, H., Dotevall, G., and Mobacken, H.: Gastric Secretion of Acid and Intrinsic Factor in Dermatitis Herpetiformis. Scand. J. Gastroenterol., *6*:411-416, 1971.
Presence of gastropathy suggested by diminished secretion of intrinsic factor in 9 of 10.

Gjone, E., and Öyri, A.: Protein-losing Enteropathy in Dermatitis Herpetiformis. Scand. J. Gastroenterol., *5*:13-15, 1970.
May produce ankle edema.

Pettit, J. E., Hoffbrand, A. V., Seah, P. P., and Fry, L.: Splenic Atrophy in Dermatitis Herpetiformis. Brit. Med. J., *2*:438-440, 1972.
Scanning studies revealed 8 in 24 had splenic atrophy; also found in celiac disease.

Andersson, H., Dotevall, G., and Mobacken, H.: Malignant Mesenteric Lymphoma in a Patient with Dermatitis Herpetiformis, Hypochlorhydria and Small Bowel Abnormalities. Scand. J. Gastroenterol., *6*:397-399, 1971.
Lymphoma secondary to enteropathy of dermatitis herpetiformis.

Mansson, T.: Malignant Disease in Dermatitis Herpetiformis. Acta Dermatovener. (Stockholm), *51*:379-382, 1971.
Dermatitis herpetiformis, celiac disease and idiopathic steatorrhea are all associated with increased risk of lymphoma or carcinoma of G.I. tract.

Marks, R., and Whittle, M. W.: Results of Treatment of Dermatitis Herpetiformis with a Gluten-free Diet After One Year. Brit. Med. J., *4*:772-775, 1969.
Helps gut more than skin.

Fry, L., McMinn, R. M. H., Cowan, J. D., and Hoffbrand, A. V.: Gluten-free Diet and Reintroduction of Gluten in Dermatitis Herpetiformis. Arch. Derm., *100*:129-135, 1969.
Flare upon reintroduction.

Alexander, J. O.: The Treatment of Dermatitis Herpetiformis with Heparin. Brit. J. Derm., *75*:289-293, 1963.
Complete heparinization causes complete suppression.

Engquist, A., and Pock-Steen, O. C.: Dermatitis Herpetiformis and Milk-Free Diet. Lancet, *2*:438-439, 1971.
Removing the milk removed the rash.

Higdon, R. S., and Elgart, M. L.: How We Treat Dermatitis Herpetiformis. Postgrad. Med., *42*:A120-123, 1967.
Dapsone.

Scott, G. L., and Cream, J. J.: The Effects of Dapsone on Red Cells. Trans. St. Johns Hosp. Derm. Soc., *54*:137-140, 1968.
Methemoglobin, Heinz bodies and hemolysis.

Wyatt, E. H., and Stevens, J. C.: Dapsone-Induced Peripheral Neuropathy. Brit. J. Derm., *86*:521-523, 1972.
Motor weakness, numbness, paresthesias may last for a year and a half.

7

Prurigo

7

For 13 years this middle-aged woman has experienced **severe pruritus,** *especially of her arms and legs. The forearm shows the typical patterning of* **discrete excoriated papules,** *as well as the depigmented sites of previous lesions. She has had asthma for 28 years.*

Biopsy — nonspecific inflammatory changes, consistent with an itch-scratch cycle.

Prurigo

Know this disease for what it is: a terrible, tormenting, relentless itch. Know this disease for what it may be called: prurigo, neurotic excoriations, nodular neurodermatitis or compulsive picking of the skin. And know this disease for what it may portend: parasitosis, biliary cirrhosis, diabetes mellitus, uremia, lymphoma or any one of a number of internal medical derangements.

This is the disease of itch. Here we see the objective evidence of the purposive nature of scratching, the attempt to literally dig out the cause. For itching is that strange sensation primordially directed toward mechanical reflex removal of ectoparasites. Unlike pain, where the reflex action is to pull the skin away from the source of harm, itch demands the removal of the source of harm from the skin. To this end, itching is subserved by a primitive afferent network of unmyelinated C fibers which arise in the epidermis.

It is thus within nonspecialized nerve endings in the epidermis that the signals for itch arise, transduced by chemical mediators, in turn released by injury to the epidermis. Histamine was long the major substance known to be capable of arousing itch. Now we recognize equally powerful excitants in the proteases and, in particular, kallikrein. All these are present in the many inflammatory processes characteristically pruritic. No longer does the bite of the ectoparasite trigger the major share of our itches! Passing up the sensory nerves, the itch signals follow the anteriolateral cord tracts. From here they enter the mystery circuitry of the basal ganglia and thalamus, inducing reflex scratching, with or without cortical recognition.

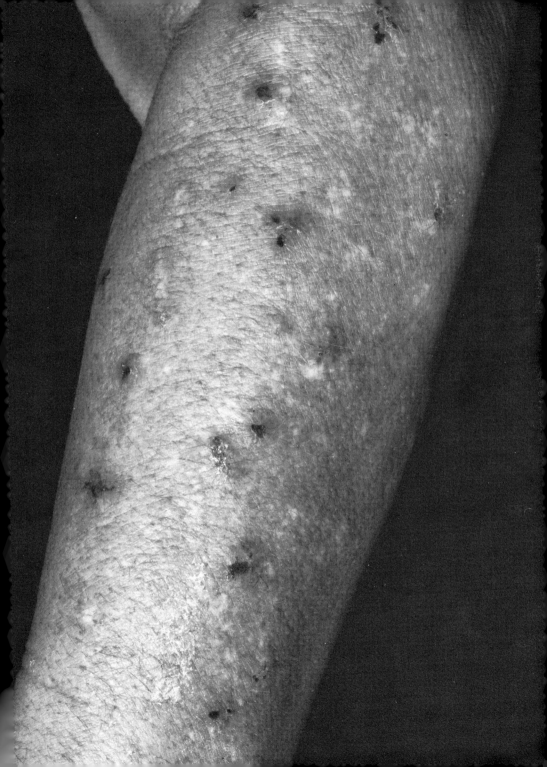

Our patient shows the graffiti of pruritus, a form of nail writing on her skin. And it appears as a special signature, well designated as prurigo. It does not take the form of long linear excoriations typical of the fierce scratching of Hodgkin's disease, nor of the scratch wheal of dermographism. Neither is it the thickened lichenified plaque resulting from the constant but modulated scratching of neurodermatitis. Rather it is a distinctive hyperkeratotic nodular eruption. Typically, it occurs on the extremities and in middle-aged women. One can see the discrete focal points where the itch crises occur. In an attempt to actually dig out the itch, the patient removes the epidermis, and obtains temporary gratification. This is followed by crusting, reactive epidermal overgrowth and the focal inflammatory papule or nodule. Regional lymphadenopathy is seen in some instances. Any given lesion remains for months, activated daily by picking, digging, excoriating finger nails. New lesions ensue, never grouped and never in large number. Gradually the old fade into no more than the scar of hypopigmentation.

The search for the cause of prurigo is the search for the cause of severe pruritus. It is not easy. It begins with a hunt for parasite contacts. Birds (a nest in the air conditioner?), dogs, cats, farm animals, even pruritic friends may carry an occult threat. Inanimate sources include clothing, cheese, straw, horse-hair mattresses, old office buildings and homes, as well as fields and streams. It extends, in our modern age, to an exploration for contact with that most pruriginous material, fiber glass, now incorporated in curtains, draperies and plastic furniture. A biopsy helps rule out such pruritic entities as dermatitis herpetiformis, hypertrophic lichen planus, eruptive keratoacanthoma, necrotizing vasculitis and insect bite — chitin granulomas.

Then the search turns within. Securing a complete blood count, urinalysis, blood urea nitrogen, sugar and thyroxin measurements, as well as chest x-ray, is the first step in forming a data base. Since the liver is the source of much pruritus, next look for evidence of cholestasis, even in the absence of jaundice, as well as biliary cirrhosis. Liver function tests and possibly a liver biopsy are valuable. Immunoelectrophoresis of serum proteins may alert one to an early lymphoma. Be sure the patient is not taking a contraceptive. It can produce the same prurigo as that of pregnancy. Indeed, medication of almost any type is suspect until assessed by a 2-week trial elimination. The vitamin B group, aspirin and diet pills are especially insidious offenders. Conversely, the lack of vitamin B_{12} has been associated with formication and delusions of parasitosis, promptly corrected by replacement therapy. The search may have to continue in the hospital with appropriate studies for the presence of a malignant lesion, a lymphoma, Hodgkin's disease, or even benign adenomatous tumors of the gastrointestinal tract or breast.

However, in our patient the most heuristic finding is in the concurrent history of prurigo and asthma for 13 years. This association alerts us to consider that our patient's problem could be a form of atopic dermatitis, long a full-fledged member of the eczema-asthma-hay fever axis. All this brings us squarely to a realization of the fact that allergens, such as house dust, which trigger her asthma may be equally responsible for her prurigo. The same immunoglobulin E, responsible for mediating her allergen-induced asthma, may be releasing histamine and proteases from the mast cells of her skin, as well as from those in her bronchi. Cooperative investigative studies by the allergist and dermatologist are clearly essential.

Despite the learned musings of the consultants, the terrible itch responsible for prurigo usually continues unabated. What can be done therapeutically? The single most effective agent in our experience is a systemic antibiotic such as erythromycin. This may have to be continued at a maintenance level for an unconscionably long time. Our means of controlling pain far excel those of subduing itch. Hydroxyzine (Atarax), cyproheptadine (Periactin) and promethazine (Phenergan) are among the popular so-called antipruritic drugs, but controlled studies in clinical practice often fail to distinguish them from placebos. A tranquilizer is occasionally of benefit, and in this case chlordiazepoxide (Librium) or diazepam (Valium) are worthy of trial.

The second major approach we have found helpful is the local injection of each lesion with triamcinolone acetonide suspension (5 to 10 mg. per ml.). This provides greater and more selective prolonged relief than the regular steroid ointments, creams, lotions or tapes. It is also more effective than the menthol-camphor lotion of yesteryear.

The patient must be encouraged to keep her nails short, her environment cool and her mind relieved of the fear that she has cancer. Such reassurance can be given effectively only after she has had the careful close medical study she deserves for a problem now in its second decade.

Greither, A.: On the Different Forms of Prurigo. *In* Mali, J. W. H.: *Current Problems in Dermatology*, Vol. 3, S. Karger, New York, 1970, pp. 1-30.
The distinctive yet idiopathic itch—dig reaction patterns of prurigo beautifully analyzed.

Aas, K.: The Biochemical and Immunological Basis of Bronchial Asthma. Charles C Thomas, Springfield, Illinois, 1972.
Absolutely engrossing account of the immunopathogenesis of our patient's asthma with much to teach of relevance to her prurigo.

Lyell, A.: Dermatitis Artefacta and Self-Inflicted Disease. Scott. Med. J., *17*:187-196, 1972.
Compulsive picking of the skin, nail biting, chain smoking, and problem drinking all show the common element of self-injury.

Cowan, M. A.: Neurohistological Changes in Prurigo Nodularis. Arch. Derm., *89*:754-758, 1964.
These discrete hyperkeratotic lesions represent marked proliferation of epidermis and neural tissue alike.

Thomsett, L. R.: Some Manifestations of Animal Disease Transmissible to Man: Pruritus. Proc. Roy. Soc. Med., *62*:1049-1050, 1969.
Migrant mites, fleas, lice or fungi may be cause of prurigo in patient exposed to pet given to rubbing, rolling, licking, nibbling, head shaking or feather picking.

Hetherington, G. W., Holder, W. R., and Smith, E. B.: Rat Mite Dermatitis. J.A.M.A., *215*:1499-1500, 1971.
Prurigo is another of the hazards of living with rats.

Lyell, A.: Diagnosis and Treatment of Scabies. Brit. Med. J., *2*:223-225, 1967.
Scabies should be considered first in every patient who complains of a persistent itch; shared with another member of the household or commune.

Eby, C. S., and Jetton, R. L.: School Desk Dermatitis. Primary Irritant Contact Dermatitis to Fiberglass. Arch. Derm., *105*:890-891, 1972.
Prurigo may mean exposure to fiber glass in plastic chairs, curtains or oven insulating material.

Pascher, F., Andrade, R., and Stolman, L.: Necrotizing Vasculitis. Arch. Derm., *98*:673-674, 1968.
Vasculitic nature of this form of prurigo revealed only on biopsy!

Hoischen, W., and Steigleder, G. K.: Überempfindlichkeit gegen Progesteron bei Prurigo mit prämenstrueller Exazerbation. Deutsch Med. Wschr., *91*:398-399, 1966.
Prurigo showing premenstrual exacerbation and demonstrated to be due to sensitivity to progesterone.

Kreek, M. J., and Sleisenger, M. H.: Estrogen-Induced Cholestasis Due to Endogenous and Exogenous Hormones. Scand. J. Gastroenterol., *5 (Suppl. 7)*:123-131, 1970.
A common cause of pruritus during contraceptive therapy or pregnancy.

Nurse, D. S.: Prurigo of Pregnancy. Aust. J. Derm., *9*:258-267, 1968.
Clears promptly at parturition.

Caravati, C. M., Jr., and Richardson, D. R.: Pruritus as a Symptom of Systemic Disease. Va. Med. Mon., *96*:656-658, 1969.
Think of Hodgkin's disease, diabetes mellitus, uremia.

Caravati, C. M., Jr., Richardson, D. R., and Wood, B. T.: Pruritus and Excoriation in Hyperthyroidism. Southern Med. J., *62*:217-219, 1969.
Only in 4 per cent.

Cormia, F.: Pruritus, an Uncommon but Important Symptom of Systemic Carcinoma. Arch. Derm., *92*:36-39, 1965.
Four examples of what the patient secretly fears.

Battle, J. D., Jr.: Bath Pruritus. New Eng. J. Med., *286*:845-845, 1972.
Pruritus triggered by bathing suggests polycythemia vera.

Zelicovici, A., Lahav, M., Cahane, P., and Bianu, G.: Pruritus as a Possible Early Sign of Paraproteinemia. Isr. J. Med. Sci., *5*:1079-1081, 1969.
Underscores need for comprehensive study of patient with prurigo.

Keele, C. A., and Armstrong, D.: Substances Producing Pain and Itch. Williams & Wilkins Co., Baltimore, 1964, 399 pp.
A scholarly summary of the role of histamine and proteolytic enzymes in the chemical mediation of itch.

Winkelmann, R. K., and Muller, S. A.: Pruritus. Ann. Rev. Med., *15*:53-64, 1964.
Skin stripped of its epidermis cannot itch.

Burnet, M., and White, D. O.: *Natural History of Infectious Disease,* 4th ed. University Press, Cambridge, 1972, 278 pp.
Much can be construed from realizing that a slow virus infection in sheep, scrapie, causes a most intense long-term pruritus.

Beare, J. M.: Antipruritics. Practitioner, *202*:55-61, 1969.
Comprehensive with special emphasis on phenol, menthol, camphor and tar topically.

Fischer, R. W.: Comparison of Antipruritic Agents Administered Orally. A Double-Blind Study. J.A.M.A., *203*:418-419, 1968.
Trimeprazine tartrate (Temaril), cyproheptadine hydrochloride (Periactin), or placebo: each effective in study of 43 patients.

Swanbeck, G., and Rajka, G.: Antipruritic Effect of Urea Solutions. Acta Dermatovener., *50*:225-227, 1970.
Twenty per cent solution may act as topical anesthetic.

Saint-André, P., Revil, H., Nosny, P., and Signoret, R.: Disparition rapide d'un prurigo feroce chez un vieillard après gastrectomie pour polypose gastrique. Bull. Soc. Franc. Derm. Syph., *75*:496-496, 1968.
Prurigo gone 4 days after gastrectomy for polyposis.

Massry, S. G., Popovtzer, M. M., Coburn, J. W., Makoff, D. L., Maxwell, M. H., and Kleeman, C. R.: Intractable Pruritus as a Manifestation of Secondary Hyperparathyroidism in Uremia. New Eng. J. Med., *279*:697-700, 1968.
Seven cases cured by parathyroidectomy.

Yatzidis, H., Digenis, P., and Tountas, C.: Heparin Treatment of Uremic Itching. J.A.M.A., *222*:1183-1183, 1972.
Treatment with 100 mg. I. V. every 12 hours — very helpful.

Datta, D. V., and Sherlock, S.: Cholestyramine for Long-Term Relief of the Pruritus Complicating Intrahepatic Cholestasis. Gastroenterology, *50*:323-332, 1966.
Details on oral anion exchange resin therapy for prurigo of hepatic origin.

Alarcon-Segovia, D., Mayorga-Cortes, A., and Wolpert, E.: Primary Biliary Cirrhosis. Prompt Relief of Pruritus with Azathioprine Treatment. J.A.M.A., *214*:367-368, 1970.
Imuran helpful in 5 cases refractory to anion exchange resin.

Mali, J. W. H.: Prurigo Simplex Subacuta. Acta Dermatovener., *47*:304-308, 1967.
Six of 23 patients responded dramatically to broad-spectrum antibiotic.

8

Eight months ago this young man noted separation of his right index finger nail. This was followed by **progressive inflammatory swelling,** *reduction in motion of that distal interphalangeal joint and* **loss of only that one nail.** *Other than a few isolated, guttate, scaling lesions seen on his legs, he has had no prior skin or joint disease. Systemic antibiotic and antifungal therapy has been without effect.*

Roentgenogram revealed marked swelling of soft tissue and erosive changes about distal joint space. Evidence of ankylosing spondylitis seen in the right sacroiliac joint. Serum rheumatoid factor absent. Uric acid normal, L. E. test negative. KOH exam of nail bed scales was negative. Repeated deep biopsy and synovial fluid cultures for aerobic, anaerobic organisms, deep fungi and acid-fast bacteria negative.

Biopsy — chronic nonspecific inflammation.

Psoriatic Arthritis

This is the "sausage finger" of psoriatic arthropathy. Although dramatic and significant, this man's problem is not readily recognized as psoriatic in nature, since his skin findings are so diminutive. Only the history of onycholysis and later nail loss, as well as some paltry psoriasiform papulosquamous lesions on the legs, alerts us to think of psoriasis. Yet, after an avalanche of negative general medical, surgical and roentgenologic studies it is increasingly evident that we were dealing not with osteomyelitis, not with some obscure chronic infectious process, but rather with true psoriatic arthropathy.

Psoriatic arthritis has had a troubled nosologic history. For want of a diagnostic sign, this form of arthropathy has languished, supported mainly by the fact that individuals with psoriasis of the fingers and nails often show an associated distal interphalangeal inflammatory joint change. Still the correlation between psoriasis and arthropathy is not precise, at times the joint changes appearing in one who has never had psoriasis. Furthermore, the severity of the changes in the two organs shows no true parallelism.

Actually the histologic, serologic and radiologic constellation of

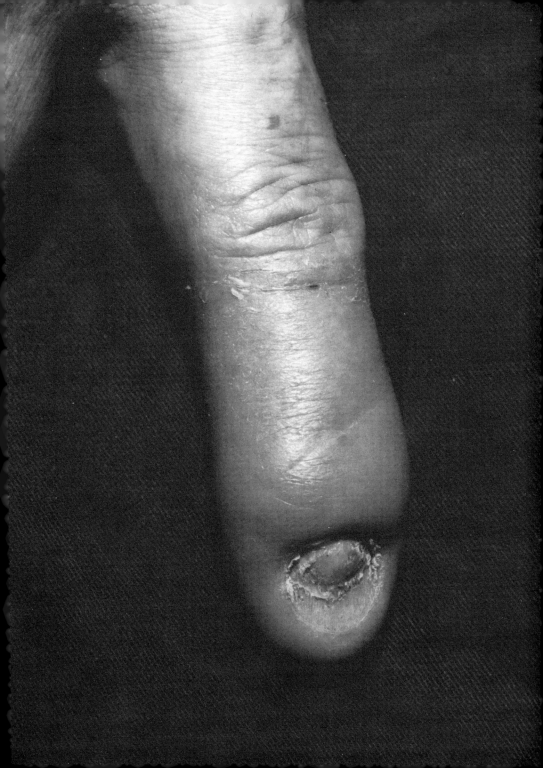

findings in psoriatic arthropathy is not as distinctive as the fact that the patient has psoriasis. But note the negatives. The early morning stiffness, the symmetrical involvement, the fusiform joint swelling of the proximal finger joints and the late deformity of ulnar deviation, all pathognomonic of rheumatoid arthritis, are not to be seen. Rheumatoid factors and rheumatoid nodules long associated with rheumatoid arthritis are also missing in these patients. Likewise, the absence of bony Heberden's nodes, the acute onset, the inflammatory changes and the young age of the patient speak against a diagnosis of osteoarthritis.

The concept of psoriatic arthropathy has thus taken hold and even gradually widened to include polyarthritis, and especially spondylitis. It is a concept that stresses incidence in young adults and an asymmetry of involvement. Radiologically, the process may be inapparent but basically it is osteolytic, with erosion and resorption of bone, widened joint spaces and later disabling ankylosis with limitation of motion. Clinically, it can vary from the swollen finger of our patient to an extremely mutilating disease that destroys joint and bone. Its chronicity is that of psoriasis, measured in years, with some of the changes being the irreversible ones of a lifetime.

The involved joint shows an inflamed thickened synovial membrane, with the same polymorphonuclear cell invasion as the epidermis. It is felt that lysozymes released by these cells have a lytic effect on the synovium, leading to effusion, erythema and pain. Accordingly, on aspiration the synovial fluid shows a nonspecific inflammatory exudate. The pathogenesis of the osteolytic changes appears to be of an equally obscure inflammatory nature.

In this patient, a proud display of our laboratory technology has led to a diagnostic denouement but not to a therapeutically appealing position. It is true that his friends' undoubted remedial recommendations of aspirin, heat and passive-active motion exercises can be endorsed professionally. Nonetheless, we lack a drug with specific promise. Perhaps the best approach is the injection of triamcinolone hexacetonide (Aristospan S), both intra-articularly and into the soft tissue. This should give prolonged symptomatic relief and may be repeated in six weeks. The extent and significance of his arthropathy at this time does not justify systemic steroids, methotrexate or gold, each of which is of some use in the more extensive crippling forms of psoriatic arthritis.

In this disease we can still but play grace notes in therapy. The thematic melody of a cure has not yet been written.

van der Korst, J. K.: Psoriasis and Arthritis. A Review of Recent Literature. Folia Med. Neerl., 12:181-189, 1969.
An acute onset of diffuse swelling of a single terminal phalanx points to psoriatic arthritis.

Ginsburg, J.: Clubbing of the Fingers. In Handbook of Physiology, Vol. 3, Section 2, American Physiological Society, Washington, D. C., 1965, pp. 2377-2390.
Drumstick fingers, sign of pulmonary disease, result of increased vascularity of nail bed.

Lassus, A., Mustakallio, K. K., and Laine, V.: Psoriasis Arthropathy and Rheumatoid Arthritis. Acta Rheum. Scand., 10:62-68, 1964.
Psoriatic skin or nail lesions, fine corroborative evidence, but in 23 per cent psoriatic arthropathy precedes skin change.

Wright, V., and Moll, J. M. H.: Psoriatic Arthritis. Bull. Rheum. Dis., 21:627-632, 1971.
Distinction from rheumatoid arthritis difficult but favored if sheep cell or latex agglutination tests for rheumatoid factor negative.

Baker, H.: Epidemiological Aspects of Psoriasis and Arthritis. Brit. J. Derm., 78:249-261, 1966.
If patient has polyarthritis, but no rheumatoid factor, chances are 1 in 5 that he has psoriatic skin lesions.

Tapanes, F. J., Rawson, A. J., and Hollander, J. L.: Serum Anti-immunoglobulins in Psoriatic Arthritis as Compared with Rheumatoid Arthritis. Arth. Rheum., 15:153-156, 1972.
Diagnosis of psoriatic arthritis further strengthened by finding IgG anti-immunoglobulin levels normal.

Avila, R., Pugh, D. G., Slocumb, C. H., and Winkelmann, R. K.: Psoriatic Arthritis: A Roentgenologic Study. Radiology, 75:691-702, 1960.
Anticipate erosive resorption, widened joint space, proliferation and ankylosis.

Wolf, P. L., and Farber, E. M.: Serologic Studies in Psoriasis and Arthritis. In Farber, E. G., and Cox, A. J. (Eds.): *Psoriasis, Proceedings of the International Symposium.* Stanford University Press. Stanford, California, 1971, pp. 141-148.
Yet recall that psoriatics may develop rheumatoid, infectious, or osteoarthritis as well as psoriatic arthritis.

Howell, F. A., Chamberlain, M. A., Perry, R. A., Torrigiani, G., and Roitt, I. M.: IgG Antiglobulin Levels in Patients with Psoriatic Arthropathy, Ankylosing Spondylitis and Gout. Ann. Rheum. Dis., 31:129-131, 1972.
No laboratory test, not even the IgG antiglobulin levels, can differentiate arthritis of psoriatic arthropathy from that of rheumatoid disease.

Sigler, J. W.: Psoriatic Arthritis. In Hollander, J. L. (Ed.): *Arthritis and Allied Conditions*, 8th ed., Lea & Febiger, Philadelphia, 1972, pp. 724-735.
Fundamental change is synovitis with synovial thickening, effusion, erythema and warmth.

Hirohata, K., and Morimoto, K.: Ultrastructure of Bone and Joint Diseases. Grune & Stratton, New York, 1971, p. 103.
An aggregation of plasma cells around venules prominent feature of psoriatic arthropathy.

Miller, J. L., Soltani, K., and Tourtellotte, C. D.: Psoriatic Acro-osteolysis without Arthritis. J. Bone Joint Surg., 53A:371-374, 1971.
Showed extensive distal phalangeal resorption but no articular change.

Langeland, N., and Roaas, A.: Spondylitis Psoriatica. Acta Orthop. Scand., *42*:391-396, 1971.
Think of this in psoriatic patient complaining of back pain.

McEwen, C., DiTata, D., Lingg, C., Porini, A., Good, A., and Rankin, T.: Ankylosing Spondylitis and Spondylitis Accompanying Ulcerative Colitis, Regional Enteritis, Psoriasis and Reiter's Disease. Arth. Rheum., *14*:291-318, 1971.
Asymmetry of sacroiliac changes and concurrent involvement of distal joints typical in psoriatic spondylitis.

Giuliano, V. J., and Scully, T. J.: Atlanto-axial Subluxation in Psoriatic Arthropathy. Arch. Derm., *105*:247-248, 1972.
Potentially fatal.

Bork, K., and Holzmann, H.: Psoriasis Arthropathica und Amyloidose. Arch. Derm. Forsch., *242*:191-201, 1972.
Late complication.

Lewin, K., DeWit, S., and Ferrington, R. A.: Pathology of the Fingernail in Psoriasis. Brit. J. Derm., *86*:555-563, 1972.
Nail plate may be pitted, dystrophic or absent; nail bed shows splinter hemorrhages, hyperkeratosis and separation from plate.

Mom, A. M., Polak, M., Fabeiro, J. L., and Garibaldi, I. B.: The Psoriatic Myopathy. Dermatologica, *140*:214-218, 1970.
Further suggestive histologic, electromyographic and enzymatic evidence that psoriasis may be more than skin deep.

Black, R. L.: Psoriatic Arthritis. *In* Fitzpatrick, T. B. (Ed.): *Dermatology in General Medicine,* McGraw-Hill Book Co., New York, 1971, pp. 231-236.
Advises treatment with salicylates, heat and physical therapy.

Hunter, G. A., and Millazzo, S. C.: Response of Psoriatic Arthropathy to Methotrexate. Aust. J. Derm., *8*:137-141, 1965.
Helpful.

Wessinghage, D., and Denk, R.: Zur operativen Behandlung der Psoriasis Arthropathica. Der Hautarzt, *22*:125-127, 1971.
Dramatic operative joint reconstruction changing hand from pathetic uselessness to functional level.

9

Discoid Lupus Erythematosus

9

*For the past year this 61-year-old man has had sharply margin-ated, **inflammatory plaques on the sides of his face.** The borders, slightly raised and hyperpigmented, show **follicular plugging** and the centers are slightly **atrophic and depig-mented.** In the scalp a few areas of scaling with scarring can be found. He has always been in excellent health, and there are no ab-normalities on physical and routine laboratory examination.*

Biopsy—characteristics of discoid lupus erythematosus: liquefac-tion of the epidermis, degeneration of the basal cell layer and the subjacent collagen, as well as a patchy lymphocytic infiltrate.

Discoid Lupus Erythematosus

This is one of those times when the clinician stands ten foot tall. He towers above the mere facts of laboratory data, histologic study, medical findings and skin tests. He sees only that this is chronic discoid lupus erythematosus in its undeniable form.

Look again at what he sees:
— sharply circumscribed, chronic inflammatory plaques
— with borders, swollen, erythematous and telangiectatic
— with centers, at a scarred, atrophic white end-stage
— with scaling that strangely fills and distends pits and follicles
— and all this limited to the head and neck.

Any differential dissolves and disappears in the certainty of in-stant recognition. He is secure in knowing that this is a benign yet dis-figuring affliction, limited to the skin and posing little threat to the pa-tient's health or longevity.

But it is a short-lived confidence, for the next case of cutaneous lupus erythematosus may present as but an insignificant yet persistent flush across the cheek and bridge of the nose — a red butterfly. It may ap-pear to be only a prolonged sunburn, and early rosacea, or unexplained hair loss. Or it may present more vividly as urticaria, petechiae, purpura or seborrheic dermatitis. Or it may loom as a threatening erosive or ul-cerative process anywhere on the skin. All this can be cutaneous lupus, nondiagnostic, nonspecific and nonedifying to the clinician. Now, it is the clinician's confidence and not his differential which disap-

56

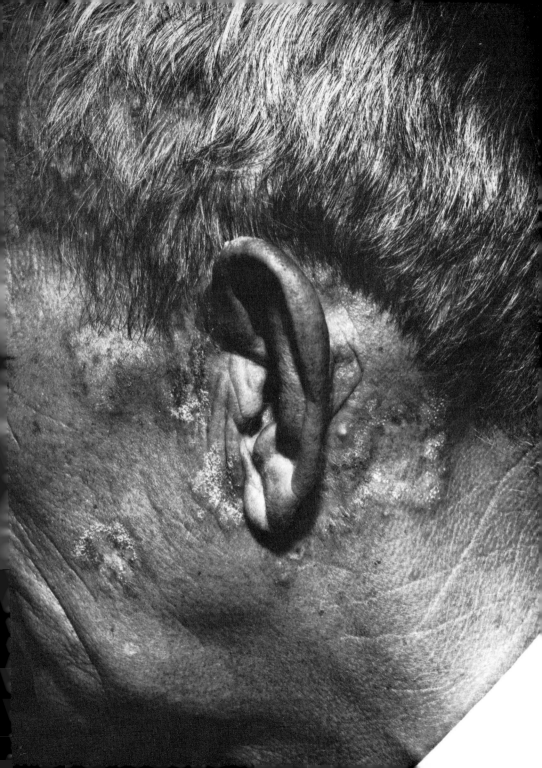

pears, for any one of these vague inflammatory changes can be the cutaneous clue to a potentially fatal multisystem lupus erythematosus.

It is disconcerting that the clinician, although able to identify with certainty the benign discoid form of lupus, is not able to diagnose the fatal rash of systemic lupus. This paradox reflects the fact that the benign form is highly patterned and specific. The initiating cause is external, sunlight and trauma triggering most cases. In contrast, the cutaneous sign of systemic lupus is commonly vague and nonspecific. It is much the same as a persistent reactive hyperemia from simple pressure or windburn. But it is a complex host immune response triggered more often from within than from without. Viruses and drugs are the known initiators. The vasculature is the target organ, and indeed the best clinical clue is presence of linear telangiectasia of the periungual skin as well as macular and papular telangiectatic lesions of the palms and fingers. But more important than any skin sign, the patient with systemic lupus feels poorly. He is sick.

Although it seems that the more serious the rash the less assured the clinician, the important role of any nonspecific vascular rash is to initiate the general medical study systemic lupus demands. Is our patient sick? Does he have a fever or show weight loss? Does he complain of asthenia, arthralgia, myalgia, or pleurisy? Are there renal, cardiac or neurologic signs of disorder? Is there enlargement of the liver, spleen or lymph nodes? Is there anemia, leukopenia, thrombocytopenia, increased gamma globulins? Positive findings direct one toward a diagnosis of systemic lupus, but it is the modern serologic tests which are decisive. The diagnosis of active systemic lupus erythematosus is on firm ground with the demonstration of a positive L.E. cell preparation as well as antinuclear antibodies. An increase in serum antibodies to native DNA is considered to be an even more specific sign of systemic L.E.

We have proudly separated the discoid lupus erythematosus of our patient's skin from a host of nonspecific erythemas and vasculitides which are the external markers of internal systemic L.E. But is there a fundamental difference? This has been debated now for an entire century, and it would seem now to be ended. Surely there is only a practical clinical difference between discoid L.E. and systemic L.E., and none of a fundamental nature. How can the debate continue

— when we know that both discoid and systemic L.E. show a familial incidence.

— when we know that mothers with systemic L.E. may give birth to infants with discoid L.E.

—when we know that discoid L.E. may later evolve into systemic L.E.

—when we find serologic evidence of systemic L.E. such as elevated anti-native DNA antibodies in patients with discoid L.E.

—when we see the same deposition of immunoglobulins at the dermal epidermal junction in discoid L.E. as in systemic L.E.

—when we see in electron microscopy the same tubular paramyxovirus-like structures in the skin lesions of discoid L.E. as in the kidney of systemic L.E.

Thus, discoid L.E. is the mild benign end of the spectrum of systemic L.E. It is the autoimmune, the collagen, the connective tissue disease occurring in the one organ, exposed to the trauma of sunlight. In view of the current theories of systemic L.E. it is attractive to assume that the sunburned skin releases a UVL-altered DNA which serves as the antigen causing the locally destructive lesion. But much remains to be learned especially about those rare occasions when discoid L.E. converts into the malevolent systemic form.

But to return to our patient, treatment begins with an uncommon attention to his health, his aches and pains, with solicitude rather than alarm. A complete medical and laboratory workup enables us to distinguish his problem, not as the tip of an iceberg, but rather as the tip of an ice cube. He must clearly understand the practical dichotomy between his diagnosis and that of systemic L.E. He must equally be aware of the hazard of sunburning and the indiscriminate use of systemic medication, as well as the threat of specific injuries to his skin. As a matter of principle, he must be enjoined to practice the rules of good hygiene.

As for the lesions, Lidex cream or one of the other topical fluorinated steroids should be applied sparingly but regularly four or five times a day. Occlusion with Saran Wrap is difficult from a practical standpoint, but if used at night does enhance the effectiveness of topical steroids. The steroid cream should be used until the signs of inflammation have abated and then should be discontinued. If progress is slow, triamcinolone acetonide (5 mg. per ml.) may be injected intralesionally. The alopecia areas on the scalp probably will not show hair regrowth because of scarring, but they should be treated also to the point at which inflammation disappears, which may take months.

Should the patient be by necessity exposed to sun or ultraviolet light, a sun screen must be employed. This should be applied prior to exposure and reapplied if washed off. Examples are para-aminobenzoic acid in alcohol (Presun), 2 hydroxy-4-methoxybenzophenone-5-sulfonic acid in a suitable base (UVAL), digalloyl trioleate 3 per cent in cream (Neo-A-Fil) and red veterinary petrolatum (RVP). A-Fil sun stick is also available for lip protection. Much can be achieved by avoiding golfing, boating, fishing, swimming, gardening and hunting, except in the early hours of the day. Wearing a wide-brimmed hat, long sleeves and gloves and using a parasol are equally valuable. One of our patients had a leather face mask made which he wore with benefit when riding to the hounds.

Older remedies used to combat discoid lupus erythematosus include freezing with dry ice or liquid nitrogen, light electrodesiccation and excision. Each may be rewarding in selected instances. Topically, 30 per cent sulfur in petrolatum was a standby before the steroids.

Most patients, including this one, do not require systemic therapy. However, in those with disfiguring widespread lesions who do need more than local help, the antimalarials of the 4-amino-quinoline group are dramatically effective at times. Unfortunately, the specter of ophthalmic problems is associated with such an approach. Our current preference is to use a mixture of chloroquine (65 mg.), hydroxychloroquine (50 mg.) and quinacrine (25 mg.) in one capsule daily. Ophthalmologic consultation is obtained prior to initiating treatment and every four months during therapy. Decreased accommodation, halos, photophobia, corneal deposits, keratitis and retinopathy are among the known complications. The rare possibility of irreversible blindness due to such retinopathy makes monitoring mandatory.

To sum up, this patient must not be overstudied or overtreated, yet we as physicians must ever remain cognizant of the life-long medical significance of his skin changes. Perhaps this can be done by considering that "no discoid lesion is an island; entire of itself," and therefore, never send to know for whom the bell tolls, it tolls for systemic L.E.

Tuffanelli, D. L.: Lupus Erythematosus. Arch. Derm., 106:553–566, 1972.
   The whole story beautifully told, 315 references on this genetically predetermined host immune response.

Dubois, E. L. (Ed.): *Lupus Erythematosus. A Review of the Current Status of Discoid and Systemic Lupus Erythematosus and the Variants.* McGraw-Hill Book Co., New York, 1966, 479 pp.
   Classic monograph on a disease that has replaced syphilis as the "great imitator." Therapy section excellent. 1453 references.

Haim, S., and Shafrir, A.: The Nature of Discoid Lupus Erythematosus. Acta Dermatovener. *50*:86–88, 1970.

Ten of 37 cases of systemic L.E. presented discoid lesions 2 to 28 years earlier!

Findlay, G. H., and Lups, J. G. H.: The Incidence and Pathogenesis of Chronic Discoid Lupus Erythematosus. An Analysis of 191 Consecutive Cases from the Transvaal. S.A. Med. J., *41*:694–698, 1967.

None of the 191 developed acute systemic form of L.E.

Burch, P. R. J., and Rowell, N. R.: Lupus Erythematosus. Analysis of the Sex and Age Distribution of the Discoid and Systemic Forms of the Disease in Different Countries. Acta Dermatovener., *50*:293–301, 1970.

Complex mathematics to indicate both discoid and systemic L.E. as coming from genetic fabric but as separate threads.

Winkelmann, R. K.: Chronic Discoid Lupus Erythematosus in Children. J.A.M.A., *205*:675–678, 1968; *206*:2319–2319, 1968.

More support for viewing discoid L.E. as part of systemic L.E. syndrome.

Kern, A. B., and Schiff, B. L.: Discoid Lupus Erythematosus Following Trauma. Arch. Derm, *75*:685–688, 1957.

Sweep of literature reveals wide variety of antecedent injuries, e.g., sunburn, frostbite, laceration, injection, vaccination, x-ray.

Chowdhury, D. S. R., and Banerjee, A. K.: Development of Discoid Lupus Erythematosus in Vitiligo. Bull. Calcutta Sch. Trop. Med., *16*:111–112, 1968.

Twelve examples to indicate triggering effect of damage from ultraviolet light.

Fields, J. P., Little, W. D., Jr., and Watson, P. E.: Discoid Lupus Erythematosus in Red Tattoos. Arch. Derm., *98*:667–669, 1968.

Again, selective localization due to mercuric sulfide sensitizing skin to ultraviolet light; lesions induced experimentally.

Schmitt, C. L., and Silverman, A.: Discoid Lupus Erythematosus in an Arc Welder. Cutis, *8*:476–477, 1971.

Occupational ultraviolet irradiation from discoid L.E. as result of gas tungsten arc welding of aluminum.

Hetherington, G. W., Jetton, R. L., and Knox, J. M.: The Association of Lupus Erythematosus and Porphyria. Brit. J. Derm., *82*:118–124, 1970.

Examples of these two diseases of photosensitivity occurring in same patient.

Freeman, R. G., Knox, J. M., and Owens, D. W.: Cutaneous Lesions of Lupus Erythematosus Induced by Monochromatic Light. Arch. Derm., *100*:677–682, 1969.

Repeated exposures (300 nm.) reproduced lesions clinically and histologically in 3 of 8 discoid L.E. patients.

Mladick, R. A., Pickrell, K. L., Thorne, F. L., and Hall, J. H.: Squamous Cell Cancer in Discoid Lupus Erythematosus. Plast. Reconstr. Surg., *42*:497–499, 1968.

Rare, but another sign of patient's radiation intolerance.

de la Faille-Kuyper, E. H. B., and Cormane, R. H.: The Occurrence of Certain Serum Factors in the Dermal-Epidermal Junction and Vessel Walls of the Skin in Lupus Erythematosus and Other (Skin) Disease. Acta Dermatovener., *48*:578–588, 1968.

Immunoglobulins strictly limited to lesions in discoid L.E., but present in clinically uninvolved skin in systemic L.E.

Hashimoto, K., and Thompson, D. F.: Discoid Lupus Erythematosus Electron Microscopic Studies of Paramyxovirus-like Structures. Arch. Derm., *101*:565–577, 1970.

Tubular structures similar to paramyxoviruses in blood vessels of skin lesions of 10 consecutive patients with discoid L.E.

Strejcek, J., Malina, L., and Bielicky, T.: Antinuclear Factors, Rheumatoid Factors and Bordet-Wassermann Reaction in Chronic and Systemic Lupus Erythematosus. Acta Dermatovener., *48*:198–202, 1968.
Rarely find antinuclear antibody in discoid L.E. patient, in contrast to systemic L.E., in which it is a sine qua non.

Mandel, M. J., Carr, R. I., Weston, W. L., Sams, W. M., Jr., Harbeck, R. J., and Krueger, G. G.: Anti-native DNA Antibodies in Discoid Lupus Erythematosus. Arch. Derm., *106*:668–670, 1972.
If elevated, watch for progression into S.L.E.

Cormane, R. H., and Bruinsma, W.: Exchange Autografts of Skin in Lupus Erythematosus. Ann. Clin. Res., *2*:22–27, 1970.
Normal skin rejects autograft of discoid L.E. skin within one week.

Schaller, J.: Illness Resembling Lupus Erythematosus in Mothers of Boys with Chronic Granulomatous Disease. Ann. Intern. Med., *76*:747–750, 1972.
Indirect evidence that patients with discoid L.E. may have defective leukocytes.

Molin, L., and Rajka, G.: Phagocytic Activity of Neutrophil Leukocytes in Pustulosis Palmo-Plantaris, Chronic Discoid Lupus Erythematosus and Erysipelas. Acta Dermatovener., *51*:138–140, 1971.
Direct evidence that leukocytes from 14 discoid L.E. patients showed diminished ability to phagocytize yeast.

Perry, H. O.: Discoid Lupus Erythematosus and Photosensitive Eruptions. Mod. Treat., *2*:908–915, 1965.
Avoid sunlight and drugs; apply sun screen and steroids.

Steffen, J.: Die Behandlung des Lupus erythematodes chronicus discoides mit Triamcinolon-Acetonid-Tinktur in Occlusiverband-technik. Hautarzt, *21*:474–477, 1970.
Occlusive dressing, although awkward, potentiates good effect of steroid creams.

Kraak, J. H., van Ketel, W. G., Prakken, J. R., and van Zwet, W. R.: The Value of Hydroxychloroquine (Plaquenil) for the Treatment of Chronic Discoid Lupus Erythematosus: A Double Blind Trial. Dermatologica, *130*:293–305, 1965.
Valuable, but remember—retinopathy could have made this study a triple blind one!

Messner, K. R.: Discoid Lupus Erythematosus. Arch. Derm., *105*:768–770, 1972.
If antimalarials used, ophthalmologic consultation prior to therapy and every 4 months; if chloroquine used, keep lifetime dose below 500 grams, if possible.

Jansen, G. T., Dillaha, C. J., and Honeycutt, W. M.: Discoid Lupus Erythematosus. Is Systemic Treatment Necessary? Arch. Derm., *92*:283–285, 1965.
The answer is no, in 4 out of every 5 patients.

10

Granuloma Annulare

10

*For the past 2 years, this 62-year-old woman has had asymptomatic **infiltrated plaques** over her arms, legs and trunk. Slightly reddish-brown in color, the lesions have a **rolled edge,** are of varying size and are an ill defined or distorted **ring shape.***

No personal or familial history of diabetes mellitus. Blood count, urinalysis and tests for antinuclear and antithyroid antibodies negative.

Biopsy—focal necrobiosis of the dermis, palisading histiocytes.

Treatment with systemic corticosteroids, cephalexin, griseofulvin, mycostatin and chloroquine without benefit. Grenz ray irradiation produced partial local involution.

Granuloma Annulare

Here are lesions literally embossed in the leather of her skin. Not as elegantly annular as the localized form seen in youth, they still display arcs, discs and rings of papules to those who would look for form. The diagnostic bas-relief sculpturing is best seen, as are many lesions, by empirically varying the lighting, the positioning, the distance and the skin tension during inspection.

This is generalized granuloma annulare, and a surprising change accounts for these surface designs, namely, actual tissue death. It is obviously not gross necrosis but rather a subclinical gangrene. To sense this we must turn to the microscope and use low power. The epidermis is normal, but in the dermis we see islands of acellular collagen which fail to stain well. This is the necrobiosis, the death of cells in the midst of living tissue, which is so characteristic of granuloma annulare. In its minimal form, only the nuclear dust of dead cells is seen between normal collagen bundles. At the other end of the spectrum, the collagen as well as the small vessels and sweat ducts is necrotic. Only the redoubtable elastic tissue remains! The swelling and peripheral reparative cell infiltrate crowding around the necrotic zone account for the pushing out or embossing of the skin.

But why does the dermis die? We don't know. Indeed the whole picture of such necrobiosis is ill defined and understudied. It has never

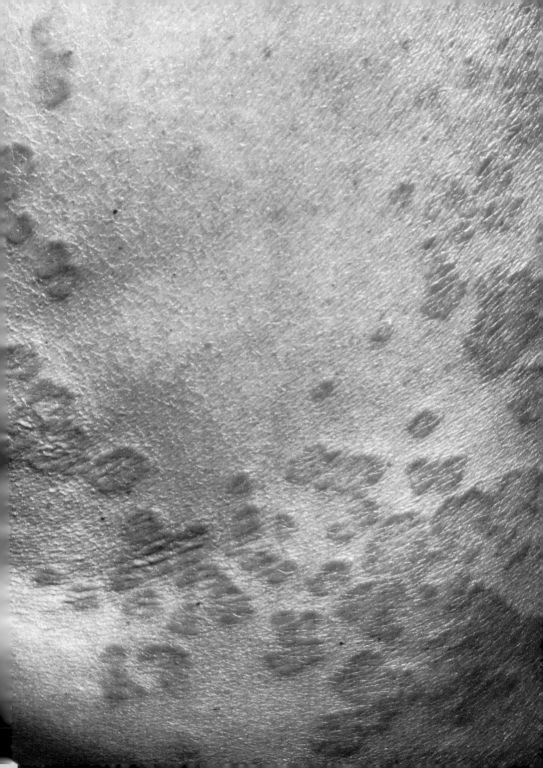

been reproduced experimentally. But there are some interesting observations. This distinctive asymptomatic process is perfectly benign, appearing at any age and only rarely in siblings. In children it is more localized, occurring and recurring on the hands and feet, at times as a solitary papule but more often as one or more perfect rings of confluent papules. In the middle-aged, granuloma annulare is florid and widespread. It appears typically on the trunk, is more chronic, and diplays a more muted ring structure.

But it is the difference in response to therapeutic maneuvers in these two age groups which is most instructive. In young children granuloma annulare reminds us of the viral wart, in that it can be charmed or threatened away. As simple a procedure as a small biopsy may be followed by complete involution. Equally apposite is the observation that the serious threat of biopsy may erase the lesions. We have found adults regularly indifferent to this and to thaumaturgic remedies successful in treating both warts and granuloma annulare in the young age group. Actually, little is gleaned from reviewing the annals of therapeutic frustration experienced by clinicians for the 70 years during which the disease has been identifiable. As dermatologists acquired facility with each new magic bullet, they regularly turned for a shot at granuloma annulare. But there were no hits, despite plenty of rounds of bismuth, gold, x-ray, steroids, antibiotics and antihistaminics.

More instructive are the few notes which have been made on factors which trigger lesions. Insect bites as well as physical injury to a specific site may initiate granuloma annulare in children. The disseminate adult form seems to begin at times as a local photosensitivity reaction, spreading gradually to areas not exposed. And strangely parallel, the use of the sunlight vitamin, calciferol, has been charged with flaring generalized granuloma annulare in adults. Conversely, the one systemic drug helpful in alleviating the adult form has been chloroquine, well known for its specific effect in allaying photosensitivity.

Interestingly, the gross differential diagnosis of granuloma annulare may include

sarcoidosis	papular mucinosis
annular lichen planus	gout
basal cell epithelioma	reactive collagenosis
creeping eruption	tertiary syphilis

However, it is the histologic differential which really gives us further clues as to the possible nature of this disease. The characteristic ball of necrotic tissue can be seen in bacterial immune responses prototypically observed in the papulonecrotic tuberculid. Such necrobiosis is furthermore an essential of the autoimmune rheumatoid nodule. In fact, granuloma annulare developing in the fat can be misconstrued, even histologically, as a rheumatoid nodule. The similarity is compounded by the fact that arthritis is the complaint of some patients with granuloma annulare. Further evidence of autoimmunity is the fact that two of our patients had thyroid auto-antibodies. Fascinating also is the histologic similarity to necrobiosis lipoidica diabeticorum. Yet, despite a great deal of study, it is not possible to view granuloma annulare as a disease of the diabetic.

To us, another challenging histologic identity is with cat-scratch disease, purportedly a viral disease. It is noteworthy that not only the skin and lymph node lesion but also the positive skin test response to the antigen reproduces the same picture of necrobiosis. Thus, we see immune responses to bacterial, viral and autoimmune antigens, as well as diabetic vascular damage, all of which can produce the same type of histologic picture as that of granuloma annulare.

With all this, what can be done for our patient? The previous therapists have left little to suggest for this patient that is rational or federally approved. Unfortunately, the use of intralesional steroids, cryotherapy and excision, so helpful in selected local lesions, is without avail in this instance. As the great therapist John H. Stokes used to advise, there is a time to pull on the oar and a time to rest. Perhaps this is the time to rest. Reassure the patient as to the benign nature of her problem. Point out that it is not a sign of cancer. Stress that it is a self-limited entity and that one day her skin will return to health again.

Although granuloma annulare may be only a curiosity to the physician, to this patient it is a real disease. We need to know more, to do more.

Dicken, C. H., Carrington, S. G., and Winkelmann, R. K.: Generalized Granuloma Annulare. Arch Derm., *99*:556-563, 1969.
Introduction to 26 patients with this disease. All healthy!

Stankler, L., and Leslie, G.: Generalized Granuloma Annulare. A Report of a Case and Review of the Literature. Arch. Derm., *95*:509-513, 1967.
Differential diagnosis includes sarcoidosis, annular lichen planus and papular mucinosis. 47 cases.

Frenken, J. H., and Ten Thije, O. J.: A Really Generalized Granuloma Annulare. Dermatologica, *134*:73-83, 1967.
Even though thousands are present, primary lesion is still a flesh-colored papule.

Selmanowitz, V. J., Vandow, J. E., and Director, W.: Atypical Granuloma Annulare. Arch. Derm., *93*:454-456, 1966.
Erythematous, nodular, subcutaneous, nonannular forms.

Owens, D. W., and Freeman, R. G.: Perforating Granuloma Annulare. Arch. Derm., *103*:64-67, 1971.
Necrobiotic collagen quietly extruded transepithelially.

Leppard, B., and Black, M. M.: Disseminated Granuloma Annulare. A Variant in Which the Lesions Involve the Sun-Exposed Areas. Trans. St. Johns Hosp. Derm. Soc., *58*:186-190, 1972.
But did not follow sun exposure and could not be elicited by irradiation.

Zangel, V.: Granuloma Annulare den Mundschleimhaut. Derm. Wschr., *148*:581-584, 1963.
May appear on oral mucosa.

Arner, S., and Aspergren, N.: Familial Granuloma Annulare. Acta Dermatovener., *48*: 253-254, 1968.
Occasional concurrent familial incidence.

Rubin, M., and Lynch, F. W.: Subcutaneous Granuloma Annulare. Arch. Derm., *93*:416-420, 1966.
Views vascular insufficiency as cause of necrobiosis.

Moyer, D. G.: Papular Granuloma Annulare. Arch. Derm., *89*:41-45, 1964.
Gnat bite induced histologic picture of granuloma annulare.

Pinkus, H., and Mehregan, A. H.: A Guide to Dermatohistopathology. Appleton-Century-Crofts, New York, 1969, pp. 257-260.
Granuloma annulare and papulonecrotic tuberculid are histologic twins.

Wood, M. G., and Beerman, H.: Necrobiosis Lipoidica, Granuloma Annulare and Rheumatoid Nodule. J. Invest. Derm., *34*:139-147, 1960.
All three are basically focal areas of connective tissue degeneration.

Johnson, W. T., and Helwig, E. B.: Cat-Scratch Disease. Histopathologic Changes in Skin. Arch. Derm., *100*:148-154, 1969.
And here is another disease showing the same control acellular zone of necrosis, surrounded by histiocytes, giant cells and a mantle of lymphocytes.

Bucci, T. J.: Intradermal Granuloma Associated with Collagen Degeneration in Three Cats. J. Amer. Vet. Med. Assoc., *148*:794-800, 1966.
Cherchez le chat! Might not granuloma annulare be another form of cat-scratch disease?

Feldman, F. F.: Granuloma Annulare and Necrobiosis Lipoidica in the Same Patient. Arch. Derm., *98*:677-678, 1968.
Rare, but could diabetes mellitus be the underlying common denominator?

Haim, S., Friedman-Birnbaum, R., and Shafrir, A.: Generalized Granuloma Annulare: Relationship to Diabetes Mellitus as Revealed in 8 Cases. Brit. J. Derm., *83*:302-305, 1970.
Latent diabetes discovered in 7 of 8.

Meier-Ewert, H., and Allenby, C. F.: Granuloma Annulare and Diabetes Mellitus. Arch. Derm. Forsch., *241*:194-198, 1971.
Finds no relationship: granuloma annulare not seen in 368 diabetics followed over 7 years; 25 cases granuloma annulare show normal glucose tolerance.

Gross, P. R., and Shelley, W. B.: The Association of Generalized Granuloma Annulare with Antithyroid Antibodies. Acta Dermatovener., *51*:59-62, 1971.
An association seen in two patients, both responding clinically to chloroquine.

Cramer, J. E.: Intra-lesional Injection of Triamcinolone. Aust. J. Derm., *7*:140-147, 1964.
Helpful in localized form.

Ravits, H. G.: How I Treat Granuloma Annulare. Postgrad. Med., *48*:176-177, 1970.
Biopsy, cryotherapy, grenz rays, local steroids.

Wells, R. S., and Smith, M. A.: The Natural History of Granuloma Annulare. Brit. J. Derm., *75*:199-205, 1963.
Over half of 208 patients cleared spontaneously within two years.

11

This **black necrotic** *area appeared on the glans penis one week ago.* **Indurated areas** *have been palpable along the shaft for 6 years, and on erection the penis is curved and painful. A biopsy of an indurated area 6 years ago showed dense fibrosis with some calcification and a diagnosis of Peyronie's disease was made.*

The indurated areas failed to respond to intralesional and systemic steroids, systemic antibiotics, vitamin D_2, as well as E, thyroid, POTABA and radiation (1000 rads). The pain of frequent nocturnal erections became more severe, and now at age 29 he has progressive dysuria, hesitancy and frequency, requiring urethral dilatation.

Chest roentgenogram — nodular densities.

Urethrogram — narrowing due to compression.

Biopsy of indurated area — epithelioid sarcoma: fibrosis with nodules of epithelioid cells showing pleomorphism and abnormal mitoses. Review of former biopsy revealed early signs of the same type of tumor.

Epithelioid Sarcoma

This is gangrene, but behind it is an amazing story. It is the story of a newly minted (1970) malignancy, epithelioid sarcoma, completely simulating a very old (1743) benign process, Peyronie's disease.

For six long years this malignant sarcoma remained completely covert. It behaved as a model Peyronie's disease: palpable plaques producing the diagnostic pain and bowing of the penis on erection. And the initial biopsy was not at variance in showing dense fibrosis and some calcification. Virtually indifferent to a barrage of therapy, growing at an imperceptible rate, producing neither skin nor surface contour change, it again appeared to come from the first template of de La Peyronie. It had neither the shape nor the form of a tumor. Moreover, none of the signs of cancer was there — hematuria, bound-down skin, lymphadenopathy. Its simulation of benign induration of the penis was complete.

And yet there were signals that, in retrospective analysis, might have

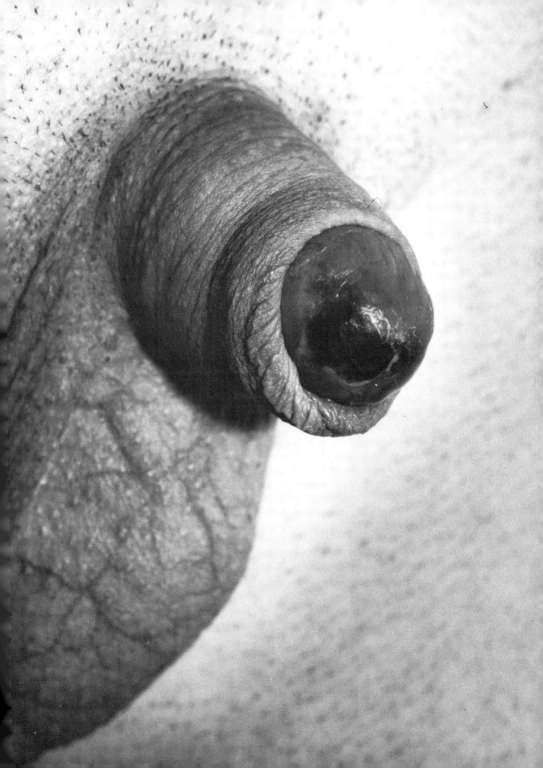

awakened diagnostic doubt. One was the pain. It was inordinately severe, causing the patient to seek out medical help constantly. Another was the increasing frequency of nocturnal erections. This is not the simple characteristic painful intercourse of Peyronie's disease. And a third signal was the interference with urinary outflow. Although reported in Peyronie's disease, it is distinctly unusual.

None of these findings called for the critical second biopsy. After all, the penis is a privileged organ, not subject to casual and serial surgical maneuvers which threaten to alter its erectile potential. The differential diagnostic list for Peyronie's disease is slender. There was no clinical evidence of lymphogranuloma venereum, no history of trauma or abscess, and no histologic finding of tumor. The current texts express a comfortable diagnostic confidence which comes from having a medical acquaintance of over 240 years. Only in the reviews on penile tumors do we find at least one case of undifferentiated sarcoma, which was originally diagnosed Peyronie's disease. Furthermore, in the 3000 reported cases there has never been an example of Peyronie's disease cited as becoming malignant. Finally, once a diagnosis is established, physicians properly become preoccupied with therapy.

Not until the day of the gangrene was the diagnosis really challenged. Gangrene is not a sign of Peyronie's, nor its fibrotic congeners, Dupuytren's contracture and knuckle pads. Could it be from vascular obstruction associated with urinary obstruction? Or cryoagglutinemia? Could it be necrotizing angiitis or of diabetic origin? Had he taken coumarin, or received an intra-arterial injection? Even a factitial origin or Loxosceles spider bite had to be considered. The answer was in the second biopsy—epithelioid sarcoma.

What is this epithelioid sarcoma? We have long recognized sarcomas as malignant tumors of the mesenchyme, but it was only a short time ago that Enzinger perceived a significant subset of this group. Having the riches of the Armed Forces Institute of Pathology material, he described 62 cases in which epithelioid cell nests uniformly appeared in the matrix of malignant spindle cells. Most importantly, his identification of this tumor purely on histologic criteria alone has led to a remarkable, uniform clinical story. This is a growth of young adults, usually male. It is one associated with the fascia and tendons. Virtually limited to the extremities, it grows with a slowness belying its lethal potential. Relentlessly and inexorably, it progresses to widespread metastases, often to the lungs, sometimes to the scalp. It may invade bone or ulcerate the overlying skin.

Confusion in the past over this strange deceptive entity has been both clinical and histologic. It has come in the guise of a ganglion, a granuloma, a tenosynovitis, as well as a nodular fasciitis, this latter being called pseudosarcomatous. It has come as the hybrid synovial sarcoma, as well as in a sprinkling of cases with a variety of adjectival phrases. And now it has appeared for the first time as Peyronie's disease — but having the constellation of the remarkable characteristics Enzinger discovered. It has appeared in a young adult male, along a fascial sheath, on an extremity, if you will. It has been growing at an unbelievably slow rate, and now finally after 6 years has metastasized apparently to the lungs. The pain, penile deviation and reduction in urinary stream are changes induced by this epithelioid sarcoma but uniquely related to the functions of this organ. The gangrene reflects thrombosis which in an inapparent form may have accounted for both the pain and the epithelioid patterning of the tumor.

What can be done for our patient? Amputation of the penis is mandatory. This malignant tumor has compromised the blood supply to his penis and must be removed in toto. It is not radiosensitive, nor are the chemotherapeutic agents a primary weapon. Such agents, however, do need to be considered in any program directed against the presumed inoperable pulmonary metastases. For this the patient may best be directed to a tumor center or the National Institutes of Health for the special expertise required.

In conclusion, this patient has introduced us to a new disease, a new view of what penile induration can mean and a new respect for the serial biopsy. Only a few consultations are as instructive.

Enzinger, F. M.: Epithelioid Sarcoma. A Sarcoma Simulating a Granuloma or a Carcinoma. Cancer, 26:1029-1041, 1970.
   Definitive delineation of 62 cases of a new class of sarcomas: insidious, invading fascial planes and tendons, involving extremities of males, and imitating Peyronie's disease in our patient.

Dehner, L. P., and Smith, B. H.: Soft Tissue Tumors of the Penis. A Clinicopathologic Study of 46 Cases. Cancer, 25:1431-1447, 1970.
   One, an undifferentiated sarcoma, originally diagnosed as Peyronie's disease. Excellent review.

Abeshouse, B. S., Abeshouse, G. A., and Goldstein, A. E.: Sarcoma of the Penis. A Review of the Literature and a Report of a New Case; and a Brief Consideration of Melanoma of the Penis. Urol. Int., *13*:273-293, 1962.
Biopsy early.

Nelson, F. R., and Crawford, B. E.: Epithelioid Sarcoma. A Case Report. J. Bone Joint Surg., *54A*:798-801, 1972.
Lethal tumor, easily misdiagnosed as benign, i.e, as a granuloma, tenosynovitis or a pseudosarcomatous nodular fasciitis.

Heppenstall, R. B., Yvars, M. F., and Chung, S. M. K.: Epithelioid Sarcoma. Two Case Reports. J. Bone Joint Surg., *54A*:802-806, 1972.
Color photos of the distinctive nests of epithelioid cells surrounded by spindle cells.

Males, J. L., and Lain, K. C.: Epithelioid Sarcoma in XO/XX Turner's Syndrome. Arch. Path., *94*:214-216, 1972.
Be alert to the association of neoplasia and chromosomal abnormalities.

McRoberts, J. W.: Peyronie's Disease. Surg. Gynec. Obstet., *129*:1291-1294, 1969.
The study of benign induration of the penis, with curvature and pain on erection. 42 references.

Smith, B. H.: Peyronie's Disease. Amer. J. Clin. Path., *45*:670-678, 1966.
A closer look at the fibrotic plaques responsible for the chordee Peyronie.

Tubiana, R., and Hueston, J. T. (Eds.): *La Maladie de Dupuytren,* 2nd ed., Expansion Scientifique Française, Paris, 1972.
Details on the palmar analogue of Peyronie's disease.

Thomas, M. L., and Rose, D. H.: Peyronie's Disease Demonstrated by Cavernosography. Acta Radiol., *12*:221-224, 1972.
Plaques seen as filling defects of smooth contour of corpus cavernosus.

Frank, I. N., and Scott, W. W.: The Ultrasonic Treatment of Peyronie's Disease. J. Urol., *106*:883-887, 1971.
Summary of modern management including intralesional steroids, radiation and, now, ultrasonics.

Poutasse, E. F.: Peyronie's Disease. J. Urol., *107*:419-422, 1972.
Thirty-six cases to prove excision beneficial and no threat to erectile function.

Bystrom, J., Johansson, B., Edsmyr, F., Korlof, B., and Nylen, B.: Induratio Penis Plastica (Peyronie's Disease). Scand. J. Urol. Nephrol., *6*:1-5, 1972.
Good review, poor therapeutic results; cytotoxic drugs have promise.

Williams, J. L., and Thomas, G. G.: The Natural History of Peyronie's Disease. J. Urol., *103*:75-76, 1970.
Six of 21 disappeared spontaneously after average period of 4 years.

Markland, C., and Merrill, D.: Accidental Penile Gangrene. J. Urol., *108*:494-495, 1972.
Painless dry gangrene of glans from self-applied rubber band.

Beathard, G. A., and Guckian, J. C.: Necrotizing Fasciitis Due to Group A Beta Hemolytic Streptococci. Arch. Intern. Med., *120*:63-67, 1967.
Rare gangrene of subcutaneous fascia due to toxins; demands surgery.

Burpee, J. F., and Edwards, P.: Fournier's Gangrene. J. Urol., *107*:812-814, 1972.
Scrotal, not penile, sudden onset, massive, like Loxosceles spider bite.

Hodgins, T. E., and Hancock, R. A.: Hemangio-endothelial Sarcoma of the Penis: Report of a Case and Review of the Literature. J. Urol., *104*:867-870, 1970.
Penile sarcomas are rare, are radioresistant and require amputation.

12

Since age 9, this woman of 24 has had **chronically swollen legs.** *Beginning at her ankles, the swelling gradually extended up her legs and onto her lower abdomen, over a period of 5 years. A lymphangioma showed hypoplastic lymphatic vessels. Prolonged bed rest and diuretics both reduce the edema, and penicillin controls her recurrent attacks of streptococci cellulitis. Surgical excision of the subcutaneous tissue of the left leg was not dramatically helpful.*

For the past 3 years, she has had extensive verrucae of the vulva, fingers and sole, proved by biopsy and refractory to treatment. Two years ago, a smallpox vaccination produced a marked locally destructive reaction. Recently, she has had a prolonged unexplained febrile pulmonary illness.

Primary Lymphedema

This is not the leg of obesity but a problem in lymphodynamics. It is a circulatory disorder but not one of arterial delivery or venous return. It is rather a failure of lymphatic return. Normally, the lymphatic system continuously aliquots protein-rich fluid through the lymph nodes for immunologic surveillance and action, subsequently returning it to the central venous system for recirculation. In our patient the lymphatic vasculature is inadequate for this mission. Rarely seen in this degree, this condition appears in milder forms in a number of women. In this instance there is a demonstrable congenital hypoplasia and aplasia of the lymphatic trunks of her legs. Her water-clogged skin and subcutaneous tissue are thus like a marshland for which there is no river drainage.

Her lymphatic defect is probably not limited to the legs, but we are still largely blind to this lymphatic system. Lymphatic vessels remain virtually invisible in histologic section, evading stains. Lymph, from the Latin word for water, is well named. Similarly, visualization of the larger trunks by angiography is difficult and can be hazardous. Thus, we sense her lymphatic deficiency best clinically. It is her legs where massive amounts of tissue fluid awaiting lymphatic transport distend her legs to elephantiasic proportions.

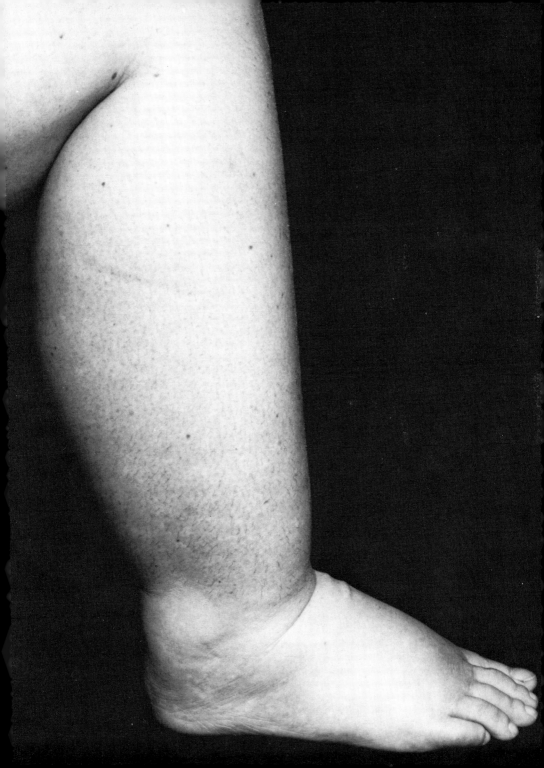

It is in the legs that woman is closest to lymphatic decompensation, and note well that primary lymphedema is essentially a disease of women. It is in the legs that we first sense the edema of cardiac failure, renal disease or hypoproteinia. The normal system of capillary filtration and reabsorption, coupled with the lymphatic siphon, is just narrowly in balance in the legs, stressed as it is by the force of gravity in our upright stance. It is apparent that our patient with a reduced number of lymph trunks has always been in jeopardy. Although she exhibited no fluid retention in childhood, at the first hormonal murmurings of puberty the lymphedema became evident. Thus, hers is *lymphedema praecox* in contrast to that with its onset at birth (congenita) or at menopause (tarda). Presumably her lymphedema resulted from an added load on the lymphatics initiated by estrogen, noted for its capacity to induce fluid retention even in normal women.

All this produces an evil cycle. The presence of stagnant protein-rich fluid serves as a tissue culture stimulating fibroblast proliferation. The consequent fibrosis occludes many of the fine lymphatic termini. Fissures as well as impaired resistance of the swollen limb lead to recurrent bacterial cellulitis, with endolymphangiitis initiating additional obstructive change. The lymphatics can be further compromised by trivial trauma, such as a sprain, which aggravates the lymphostasis. Such irreversible cycles continue for decades, eventually producing gargantuan limbs, indifferent to all but the mutilating scalpel of the surgeon. And in some few, there develops the ultimate evil—a highly malignant lymphangiosarcoma, analogous to that seen in the Stewart-Treves syndrome of postmastectomy lymphedema.

The fact that congenital disorders cluster alerts us to suspect that our patient may have other disorders, such as cardiovascular or skeletal abnormalities. Interestingly these may be as insignificant as fusion of the metacarpals, or as important as a lymphaticovenous anastomosis, which in some patients completely exempts one leg from the lymphedema. The wide range of reported correlates extends to include eyelid defects, blue sclerae, absent fingers, dislocated hips and urachal fistulas. More searching study will surely reveal others, and certainly our attention should be focused on occult pathologic change which could stem from inadequate lymphatic supply to other areas and organs. Here, the lung, liver, intestine and kidney are of special concern, with cases of pleurisy, cholestasis and malabsorption already having been recorded.

Our patient directs us to an additional area of concern—

immunity. The lymphoid nodal tissue of the lymphatic system is charged with a major role in defense against infection. The experiences which this patient has had suggest that not only is the vasculature of her lymphatic trunk hypoplastic, but her immune capabilities may be equally stunted. Certainly she has inadequate defense against the verruca virus, as manifested by the extensive verrucae vulgaris of the fingers and vulva and a large mosaic wart of the sole. This has been seen but, to our knowledge, not commented upon in other patients with primary lymphedema. It is important to stress that these are true viral warts, not the warty hyperkeratosis which develops over the toes in long-standing secondary lymphedema, nor the xanthomas of extravasated chylomicra. Moreover, she failed to show the normal immunity to the smallpox vaccine, suffering a rather severe local necrosis. Awareness that patients with congenital lymphedema may suffer an immune deficit deserves additional study and recognition.

The history and findings are so characteristic of nonfamilial primary lymphedema that the secondary forms are given but scant attention. Nonetheless, we should double check that she has no history of surgery, irradiation or tropical exposure to filariasis nor any evidence of retroperitoneal fibrosis (methysergide) or malignant disease. Moreover, cardiac, renal, hypoproteinemic and venous stasis edema must be excluded as contributing causes. A biopsy specimen obtained by a small circular knife excision would also be helpful in a confirmative sense, ruling out mucinoses and other infiltrates.

Treatment rests squarely on our knowledge of lymphodynamics. Bed rest for 10 days will remove the burden of gravity and greatly reduce swelling. After this, regular daily periods of gravity drainage are required, preferably with good centripetal massage. Regular exercise is valuable, and quiet standing is always hazardous, for it is the external muscular movement which aids the climb of fluid in these valued lymph vessels—even as in the veins. Support in the form of a Jobst leotard is more often prescribed than used, but without question external pressure support aids lymphatic flow. Specifically, it prevents disruption and tearing of the lymphatics which occur when the skin is extremely distended. Such a leotard must be put on before rising, since two hours of standing without support will fill her legs with an amount of fluid that would require 10 days in bed to drain!

Diuretics and the low-salt diet are medical adjuvants of proved value. The patient must be carefully instructed to avoid specific salty foods, which must be viewed as poisonous. Furosemide in a daily dose of 40 mg. and supplemental with potassium should be considered and monitored as usual. Estrogens, conjugated or otherwise, should be scrupulously avoided because they promote fluid retention.

Foot hygiene and care are as essential as the use of a small prophylactic daily dose of penicillin to prevent future attacks of streptococcal cellulitis. The interdigital spaces must be carefully dried and powdered after showering. Fissures are best painted with Castellani paint. Caution is advised against any well-intentioned but potentially disastrous surgery such as venous ligation, lymph node biopsy and sympathectomy. Our patient's lymphatic drain lines must be protected against any assault.

A direct surgical attack on her problem is an extreme measure to be considered when all else fails. The approach which has stood the test of time is excision of all the tissue of the lower leg superficial to the deep fascia. This is followed by covering the entire defect with split-thickness grafts. More recently, deep dermal flaps have been buried into the skin in an attempt to unite the normally separate deep and superficial lymphatic trunks. Experimental procedures of promise attempt either to create a major lymphaticovenous shunt in the leg or to transplant part of the omentum into the leg, thereby gaining a new, unusually rich lymphatic vasculature.

This patient has a complex progressive disease which is not only an esthetic liability but physically incapacitating and carries the continual threat of cellulitis. She deserves serious life-long medical attention.

Kinmonth, J. B., Taylor, G. W., Tracy, G. D., and Marsh, J. D.: Primary Lymphoedema. Clinical and Lymphangiographic Studies of a Series of 107 Patients in Which the Lower Limbs Were Affected. Brit. J. Surg., 45:1-10, 1957.
   A tour de force in the analysis of lymphostasis due to maldeveloped lymphatics.

Gates, G. F., and Dore, E. K.: Primary Congenital Lymphedema in Infancy Evaluated by Isotope Lymphangiography. J. Nucl. Med., 12:315-317, 1971.
   New way that shows lymphatic aplasia is basic defect: inject colloidal gold, ^{198}Au, subcutaneously; scan for nuclide.

Calnan, J.: Lymphoedema: The Case for Doubt. Brit. J. Plast. Surg., 21:32-44, 1968.
   And the need for more research! Tantalizing questions like "Why are the lymphatic vessels adequate until puberty?"

Maisels, D. O.: Anonychia in Association with Lymphoedema. Brit. J. Plast. Surg., 19:37-42, 1966.
   Nails may be yellow, dystrophic or even absent.

Hiller, E., Rosenow, E. C., III, and Olsen, A. M.: Pulmonary Manifestations of the Yellow Nail Syndrome. Chest, 61:452-458, 1972.

With yellow nails of lymphedema, look for pleural effusion due to underdeveloped lymphatics, and be alert for neoplasms.

Sigstad, H., Aagenaes, ϕ., Bjorn-Hansen, R. W., and Rootwelt, K.: Primary Lymphoedema Combined with Hereditary Recurrent Intrahepatic Cholestasis. Acta Med. Scand., *188*:213-219, 1970.
Five cases of itching and jaundice – evidence that lymphatic maldevelopment involved liver as well as legs.

Tabbara, K. F., and Baghdassarian, S. A.: Chronic Hereditary Lymphedema of the Legs with Congenital Conjunctival Lymphedema. Amer. J. Ophthal., *73*:531-532, 1972.
Defective lymph drainage everywhere – you look.

Beninson, J., Jacobson, H. S., Eyler, W. R., and DuSault, L. A.: Additional Observations on Genetic Lymphedema as Studied by Venography, Lymphangiography and Radio-Isotopic Tracers Na$_{22}$ and RISA. Vasc. Surg., *1*:43-52, 1967.
Even in the kidney.

Mishkel, M. A.: Xanthomatosis and Chylous Lymphedema. Arch. Derm., *106*:601-602, 1972.
Result of connection of intestinal lacteals and incompetent leg lymphatics: chylomicron extravasation into tissue.

Alvin, A., Diehl, J., Lindsten, J., and Lodin, A.: Lymph Vessel Hypoplasia and Chromosome Aberrations in Six Patients with Turner's Syndrome. Acta Dermatovener., *47*:25-33, 1967.
Primary lymphedema demands search for other developmental defects.

Jackson, B. T., and Kinmonth, J. B.: Pes Cavus and Lymphoedema. An Unusual Familial Syndrome. J. Bone Joint Surg., *52B*:518-520, 1970.
This combination in 3 persons of two generations favors genetically linked association.

Woodward, A. H., Ivins, J. C., and Soule, E. H.: Lymphangiosarcoma Arising in Chronic Lymphedematous Extremities. Cancer, *30*:562-572, 1972.
Whether it be primary or postmastectomy, lymphedema can lead to this fatal tumor, on rare occasions. 24 cases.

Messen, H.: *Lymph Vessel System. Handbuch der Allgemeinen Pathologie,* Vol. 3, Part 6, Springer Verlag, Berlin, 1972, pp. 1-708.
Encyclopedic: structure, function, pharmacology, chemistry and immunology in English; embryology, physiology and pathology in German.

Rusznyak, I., Foldi, M., and Szaba, G.: *Lymphatics and Lymph Circulation Physiology and Pathology,* 2nd ed., Pergamon Press, New York, 1967, 971 pp.
Another exciting reference on the system that maintains fluid balance by carrying away the protein the blood capillary can't reabsorb.

Leak, L. V.: The Fine Structure and Function of the Lymphatic Vascular System. *In* Messen, H.: *Lymph Vessel System. Handbuch der Allgemeinen Pathologie,* Vol. 3, Part 6, Springer Verlag, New York, 1972, pp. 148-196.
Anchoring filaments automatically pull open lymphatics when tissue fluid increases.

Fison, L., and Awdry, P.: Leber's Lymphangiectasia Hemorrhagica Conjunctivae. Arch. Ophthal., *81*:278-279, 1969.
Exquisite clinical photographs of lymphatics filled with blood; result of lymphaticovenous anastomoses.

Van Haeften, F. F.: The Value of Foot-to-Throat Circulation Time in Chronic Venous Insufficiency and Lymphedema of the Leg. Vasc. Surg., *2*:174-181, 1968.
Venous blood moves faster than normal in lymphedematous limb.

Abramowitz, I.: Lymphangiography and Phlebography in Obscure Limb Oedema. S. Afr. J. Surg., *9*:65-76, 1971.
Full investigation of chronically swollen limb requires lymphography as well as venography.

Munro, D. D., Craig, O., and Feiwel, M.: Lymphangiography in Dermatology. Brit. J. Derm., *81*:652-660, 1968.
Complications include death, pulmonary infarct, wound infection, lymphangiitis and lymphatic rupture.

Neviaser, R. J., Butterfield, W. C., and Wieche, D. R.: The Puffy Hand of Drug Addiction. A Study of the Pathogenesis. J. Bone Joint Surg., *54*:629-633, 1972.
This is nonpitting edema due to obliteration of lymphatics by fibrosis. Cannot do lymphangiogram.

Luginbühl, H., Chacko, S. K., Patterson, D. F., and Medway, W.: Congenital Hereditary Lymphoedema in the Dog. Part II. Pathological Studies. J. Med. Genet., *4*:153-165, 1967.
Due to failure of lymph vessels to anatomically connect with central lymphatic system in a family of 17 dogs!

Pflug, J. J., and Calnan, J. S.: The Experimental Production of Chronic Lymphoedema. Brit. J. Plast. Surg., *24*:1-9, 1971.
Due to neoprene latex injections to produce blockage of both deep and superficial lymphatics.

Cattell, W. R., Taylor, G. W., and Aitken, D.: Diuretic Therapy of Primary Lymphoedema. Lancet, *2*:312-315, 1965.
Helpful in one-third of their 25 patients.

Babb, R. R., Spittell, J. A., Jr., Martin, W. J., and Schirger, A.: Prophylaxis of Recurrent Lymphangitis Complicating Lymphedema. J.A.M.A., *195*:871-873, 1966.
Daily penicillin for one week of each month.

Hugo, N. E.: Recent Advances in the Treatment of Lymphedema. Surg. Clin. N. Amer., *51*:111-123, 1971.
Excellent survey of the ways in which the modern surgeon heroically excises and grafts.

Kinmonth, J. B.: *The Lymphatics; Diseases, Lymphography and Surgery*. Williams & Wilkins Co., Baltimore, 1973.
The last word!

13

Pityriasis Rubra Pilaris

13

This 67-year-old man presents a **fissured hyperkeratotic thickening of his palms and soles** *as a part of a virtually generalized erythroderma. The eruption began 9 months ago as a seborrheic scaling of the chest. Gradually it extended to cover his body with a salmon-colored, scaling, erythematous process, but peculiarly it has left islands of unaffected skin.*

The surface is rough, being studded with fine keratotic follicular papules best seen on the dorsa of the fingers, on the arms and on the trunk, even in the islands of uninflamed skin. Topical and systemic steroids have been without effect.

Health, excellent; family history, noncontributory; general medical studies, normal; serum vitamin A level, 108 μg. per ml.

Biopsy — keratotic plugging of hair follicles, mild inflammatory infiltrate.

Pityriasis Rubra Pilaris

This is a rare patchwork quilt of dermatitides.

This man's palms and soles remind one of *psoriasis*, fissured and hyperkeratotic. But note that unlike psoriasis the fissures are filled with keratin. Moreover, the scaling has a skin line patterning, a dermatoglyphic scale, as it were. Closer inspection of the middle finger also shows a distinctive keratinous plugging of the sweat pores.

The initial lesions were suggestive of a *seborrheic dermatitis*. They appeared in the sternal area, and later facial lesions developed, accompanied by a thick cradle-cap scaling of the scalp. They then extended to involve his entire face, head and neck in an exfoliative process. However, as the process became erythrodermic and generalized there was a remarkable exemption of small islands of skin. And most important, his skin acquired a unique salmon coloring.

The skin has the roughness of *keratosis pilaris*, or of the vitamin A deficiency, phrynoderma. We can both see and feel keratotic plugs in the hair follicles. It is a change present even in the islands of spared skin and is best perceived on the backs of his fingers.

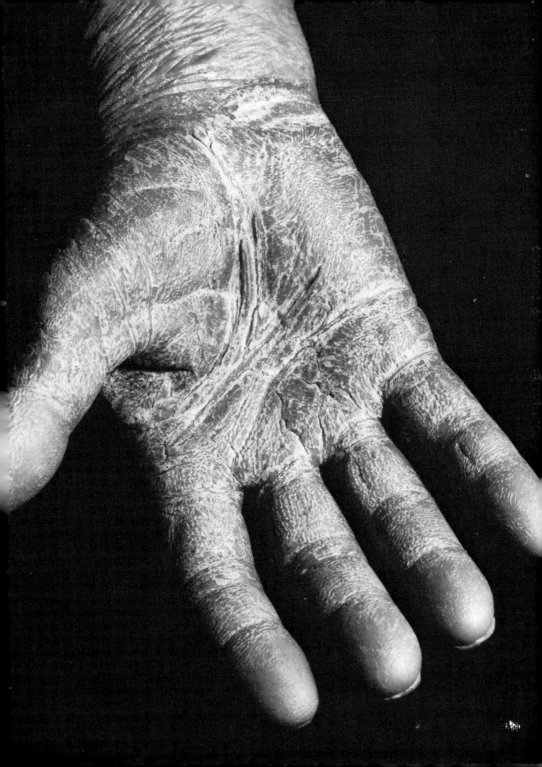

The legs show a scaling characteristic of *lamellar ichthyosis* — thin flat sheets. But all this is on top of a reticulate erythroderma and has been present for only months. And finally, although the oral mucosa is normal, it could show dramatic white streaks similar to *lichen planus.*

All the bits and pieces add up to one and only one diagnosis, pityriasis rubra pilaris. And such a diagnosis is marvelously mnemonic — it scales, it's red and it affects the hair follicle. It is a clinical diagnosis but an indisputable one, not to be challenged by any laboratory test. Even the biopsy is one of assent.

What's happening here? We know that the epidermis is producing keratin at a very rapid rate, again resembling psoriasis. Large areas of the body are exfoliating daily, and a virtual keratodermic or tylotic sandal may form on the soles. And yet, fundamentally the process is a *focal* hyperkeratosis, for it is the hair follicles which bulge with keratin to form the diagnostic conical, acuminate papules.

We don't know the why of this disease, but there is a haunting idea that, like psoriasis, it may be hereditary in nature. Some familial cases have been described, but the usual finding is that of this patient, who knows of no one else with his affliction.

We do know that ingestion of chlornaphthalenes or their analogues can induce widespread follicular hyperkeratosis as well as hyperkeratosis of the palms and soles. The concept of occult poisoning by an organic chemical of the type excreted by the oil gland is supported by the acute onset, the relentless course, the disappearance of the sebaceous gland and the fact that some patients describe neuromuscular weakness and others photosensitivity. It is imperative to secure a most detailed history concerning the possibility of accidental ingestion or exposure to oils, greases or timber preservatives. A single chance exposure could have a trail of change that lasts for as many years as are necessary to degrade the chemical stimulant.

Treatment at this stage in our knowledge means suppression of the hyperkeratinization while the disease runs its course. We have powerful tools for this in the form of the modern antimetabolites. But they must be used only in a patient with a severely disabling and generalized process. With all of them, effects are seen after weeks, *not* days, of therapy, again calling for a special perseverance on the part of the patient and physician. The first to be recommended is vitamin A. In a pharmacologic dosage of 300,000 to 500,000 U daily, water-soluble vitamin A

(Aquasol A) is helpful in a significant number of patients. It is not acting as a vitamin, and this is not a disease of vitamin A deficiency, serum levels being unrelated to the disease. Vitamin A may be continued for months, with appropriate supervision. Topically, the new vitamin A acid is worthy of local trial, but data are not yet available concerning its value.

Two stronger antimetabolites, methotrexate and azathioprine, have distinguished themselves in the treatment of pityriasis rubra pilaris. Indeed, until their use, it could be argued that not a single one of the score of agents employed in treating pityriasis rubra pilaris was consistently effective. Still, they act slowly, and improvement is not obvious until after several months. Furthermore, prolonged treatment may be necessary before they can be stopped without the danger of relapse again slowly ensuing. Both these agents are antineoplastic compounds and are thus nonspecific inhibitors of the overgrowth of epidermis. It is equally important that they are immunosuppressive and that their prolonged administration carries an element of risk, as yet not completely assessable. As a rule, they are not suitable for children or pregnant women, nor anyone who cannot be carefully and repeatedly investigated from the general medical standpoint. Methotrexate is used in a daily oral dose of 5 mg. per day and azathioprine in an oral dose of 100 mg. per day.

Other members of this rapidly enlarging class of antimetabolites which deserve consideration in the therapy of pityriasis rubra pilaris include Hydrea and topical nitrogen mustard (mechlorethamine). Both have been used with success in suppressing the scaling of psoriasis and offer promise in pityriasis rubra pilaris. Strangely, systemic steroids do not produce the striking improvement in pityriasis rubra pilaris that they do in psoriasis.

As for local treatment, this is an exfoliative erythroderma and as such deserves tender loving care. Harsh, irritant or sensitizing types of treatment are to be avoided. Frequent baths followed by Aqua-Aquaphor or other bland lubricants are among the most agreeable approaches, since our patient does not elaborate sebum. Nor does he sweat in the affected areas. He thus must be cautioned to avoid high environmental temperature, since his serious yet inapparent deficit in heat regulation makes him liable to fever, asthenia and collapse.

Pityriasis rubra pilaris remains an enigma. It is a disease for which there is no internal concomitant, no laboratory test, no specific therapy and no rational explanation. As we grope toward understanding, we have only the lodestar of clinical knowledge that this is a disease of excessive production of keratin within the orifices of both the hair follicles and the sweat pores. It is truly a keratoderma enigmatum.

Gross, D. A., Landau, J. W., and Newcomer, V. D.: Pityriasis Rubra Pilaris. Report of a Case and Analysis of the Literature. Arch. Derm., 99:710-716, 1969.
Concise IBM computer analysis of all you ever wanted to know about the 300 cases of PRP in the literature.

Stanoeva, L., Konstantinov, D., and Ristov, R.: Clinical Aspect of Pityriasis Rubra Pilaris in Childhood. Dermatologica, 142:1-6, 1971.
Acute erythroderma, islands of normal skin, keratotic follicular papules, fissured thickened palms and soles.

Baden, H. P., and Roth, S. I.: Oral Lesions in Pityriasis Rubra Pilaris. Oral Surg., 25:691-694, 1968.
Looks like lichen planus.

Braun, W., Petter, O., and Wildführ, G.: Akute eworbene Toxoplasmose unter dem Bild einer Pityriasis rubra pilaris. Arch. Klin. Exp. Derm., 232:295-311, 1968.
Acute toxoplasmosis presenting as pityriasis rubra pilaris.

Bergeron, J. R., and Stone, O. J.: Follicular Occlusion Triad in a Follicular Blocking Disease (Pityriasis Rubra Pilaris). Dermatologica, 136:362-367, 1968.
Pityriasis rubra pilaris patient developed hidradenitis suppurativa, acne conglobata and dissecting cellulitis.

Crow, K. D.: Chloracne. Trans. St. Johns Hosp. Derm. Soc., 56:79-99, 1970.
References showing that widespread follicular hyperkeratosis as well as palmar and plantar keratoderma can result from ingestion of chlornaphthalenes.

Porter, D., and Shuster, S.: Epidermal Renewal and Amino Acids in Psoriasis and Pityriasis Rubra Pilaris. Arch. Derm., 98:339-343, 1968.
Epidermal turnover accelerated in both.

Pinkus, H., and Mehregan, A. H.: *A Guide to Dermatohistopathology.* Appleton-Century-Crofts, New York, 1969, pp. 343-345.
Remarkable hypertrophy of arrectores muscle, atrophy of sebaceous gland and follicular keratotic plug characteristic of pityriasis rubra pilaris.

Knowles, W. R., and Chernosky, M. E.: Pityriasis Rubra Pilaris Prolonged Treatment with Methotrexate. Arch. Derm., 102:603-612, 1970.
Careful documentation of reversible anhidrosis found in pityriasis rubra pilaris.

Watt, T. L., and Jillson, O. F.: Pityriasis Rubra Pilaris. Penicillin and Antituberculosis Drugs as Possible Therapeutic Agents. Arch. Derm., 92:428-430, 1965.
Lists two dozen remedies but favors penicillin.

Waldorf, D. S., and Hambrick, G. W., Jr.: Vitamin A Responsive Pityriasis Rubra Pilaris with Myasthenia Gravis. Arch. Derm., 92:424-427, 1965.
Vitamin A effective, both systemically and topically, in some patients.

Parish, L. C., and Woo, T. H.: Pityriasis Rubra Pilaris in Korea. Treatment with Methotrexate. Dermatologica, 139:399-403, 1969.
Powerful, reserved for chronic disabling forms.

Hunter, G. A., and Forbes, I. J.: Treatment of Pityriasis Rubra Pilaris with Azathioprine. Brit. J. Derm., *87*:42-45, 1972.
Another antimetabolite, Imuran, distinctly helpful in 5 patients.

Reilly, M. J. (Ed.): *American Hospital Formulary Service*, Vols. 1 and 2, American Society of Hospital Pharmacists, Washington, D. C., 1973.
Our office Bible! See practical summaries on methotrexate, azathioprine, Hydrea and mechlorethamine.

Davidson, C. L., Winkelmann, R. K., and Kierland, R. R.: Pityriasis Rubra Pilaris. A Followup Study of 57 Patients. Arch. Derm., *100*:175-178, 1969.
No matter what the treatment, half these Mayo Clinic patients were well, on the average, in 2.3 years.

14

For many years this woman in her fifties has noted discrete bright red areas on the mucosal surface of her lips. Frankly **angiomatous**, *these* **macules and papules** *blanch on diascopy.*

She gives a lifelong history of frequent nosebleeds, but no hematemesis or melena. Her son has similar telangiectatic vascular lesions.

Treatment with estinyl estradiol, 0.05 mg. t.i.d., as well as tetracycline has not been effective.

Hereditary Hemorrhagic Telangiectasia

These lesions are your diagnostic friend. Whether on the tongue, in the nasal or buccal mucosa, on the fingers, or here on the vermilion border of the lips, they guide you. Whether they are flat or raised, punctate, stellate or linear, they assist you in the care of this patient and other members of her family. They aid you in understanding her recurrent epistaxis. They alert you to possible causes of future illness which could range from simple fatigue, through obscure neurologic disease, to sudden collapse and shock.

These are the lesions of vessels without walls. These are congenital, focal areas of vascular flaw. The small venules here fail to form a normal elastic contractile wall. At these sites even the ensheathing connective tissue is inadequate. Early childhood and youth pass without this becoming evident, but at puberty a focal macular telangiectasia appears. The venular channel becomes grossly dilated. With the circulatory pressure changes and dermal atrophy of aging, the lesions may become raised, papular, and even nodular. All this would excite little comment, if it were not for the remarkable highly penetrant dominant mendelian transmission that such telangiectasia exhibits.

However, this is not a microangiopathy just of the lips, but one that may extend through the entire length of the gastrointestinal tract, and

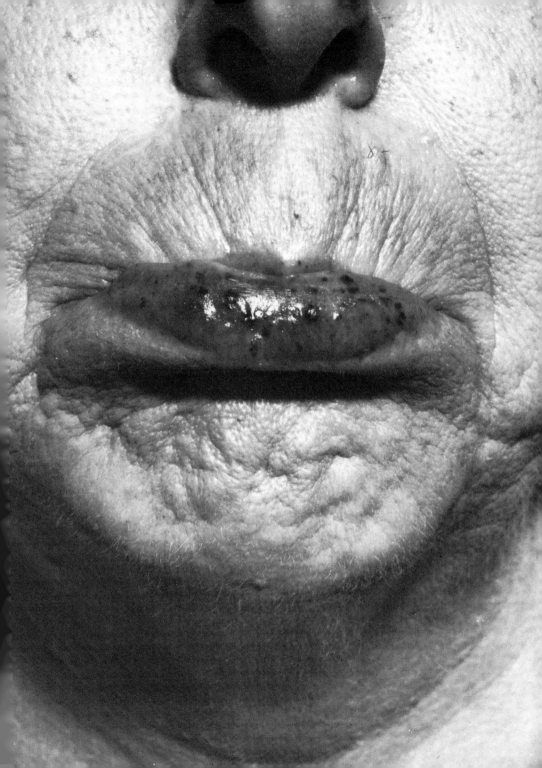

one which may affect any organ of the body. We see it on the palms and soles, on the fingers, even under the nails. We see it in the nasal mucosa, in the eye, and, at operation, spotting the surface of the liver and the kidneys. It would still be a curiosity except for the fact that it bleeds. Even in childhood when upper respiratory infections or dry air erode the thin epithelial coating, dramatic nosebleeds may ensue. With aging, there is further dilatation of the vessel, as well as thinning of both the epithelial and dermal sheaths, so that trauma can be the cause of major bleeding. Thromboses also occur, resulting in ulceration. Repeated hemorrhagic episodes of an emergency nature may ensue, requiring in some patients transfusions by the dozens over the years. As much as one thousand milliliters of blood may be lost in an hour or two. This is truly a bleeder's disease, and fatalities do occur. A comb and a toothbrush have each been recorded as accounting for deaths in the pre-transfusion days.

Thus, it is evident that this lip sign is critical in the diagnostic study of any patient who has unexplained bleeding or blood-loss type anemia. We look for it in any patient with melena, hematuria, hematobilia, hemothorax, hemoptysis, hematemesis or even bloody tears. If the patient is a child, we must not forget to look and inquire for it in the older relatives or siblings! Likewise, if the patient is in acute circulatory shock, this sign may vanish and, again, only the study of relatives or a history will be helpful. Remember, though, that 20 per cent of these patients give a negative family history. We are looking for the sign of the vessel that cannot contract but continues to bleed profusely once traumatized, despite the fact that all the bleeding and clotting factors are entirely normal. This is the bleeding of hereditary hemorrhagic telangiectasis so carefully worked out by eponymic Osler, Rendu and Weber.

But the lip lesions are indicative even beyond the bleeding. They indicate not only a weakened vessel fabric in the tiny venules but defects in the walls of major arteries as well. Modern angiography has confirmed that these patients may have not only microangiopathy of the telangiectasia but also focal angiopathy in the form of aneurysms. Additionally, they have arteriovenous shunts and fistulas. As many as 15 per cent of these patients have pulmonary A. V. shunts with a host of sequential events, including dyspnea, cyanosis and clubbing of the fingers. Significantly neurologic disorders ranging from seizures to paralysis may also be a consequence. It is the lip sign that cautions us not to overlook the bruit and the thrills in any area during the physical examination. Our patient thus has a universal angiectasia and could present peculiar hemodynamic and cardiovascular problems.

With a diagnostic sign as valuable as this, it is important that there be no confusion in identifying the sign itself. It has a marvelously mnemonic label, that is to say, unless it is familial, unless it bleeds and unless it is telangiectatic, it is not the authentic Osler's sign. Actually the appearance in adult life and the clustering of lesions on the lips and hands and in the nasal and buccal mucosa sharply eliminate many of the other random or generalized telangiectasias. Thus the facial telangiectasia of scleroderma or lupus erythematosus or the spider nevi of the chest in patients with cirrhosis pose no difficulty in recognition if one does not fall into the habit of lumping together all forms of telangiectasia. Venous lakes and rubber bleb nevi, much larger and more bluish than red, do not bleed except under unusual circumstances. Vascular nevi do not have symmetry, the telangiectasis of radiodermatitis presents with a distinctive background, and essential telangiectasis is far more widespread and progressive than what we see in this patient.

Routine blood counts to detect any anemia resulting either from her nosebleeds or from occult gastrointestinal bleeding are required for this patient. Appropriate iron replacement therapy can then be undertaken. She should be instructed regarding the hazards of abrasive tooth brushing and warned to avoid aspirin in view of its erosive and anticoagulant properties when taken into the stomach in large quantities. Her diet should tend to be low in potential roughage. Should she have acute abdominal pain, it is important for her to know that it may call for immediate medical review, since it could signal a thrombotic episode in the gut, in turn to be followed several hours later by gross or occult bleeding!

Specifically, with regard to the nosebleeds, she must see that her room air is humidified in the winter months. Noting that pregnancy ameliorates the severity and frequency of attacks, some authorities recommend estinyl estradiol, 1 mg. per day. This dose, higher than that in contraceptives, may induce a protective metaplasia of the nasal mucosa. This therapy is not universally acclaimed, since it may induce feminization in men and can substitute menstrual for nasal bleeding in postmenopausal women. During epistaxis, pressure is the sine qua non of first aid. It may be necessary to use packing and electrodesiccation at the medical level. In a few patients with life-threatening repeated attacks major surgical approaches are employed, including submucous resection, septectomy, ligation of vessels and skin grafting.

With regard to the possibility of large vessel abnormalities, there is no need to cross a bridge that may never have been built. Simple examination for bruit and thrill and the continued diagnostic awareness that our patient could have an arterial aneurysm, a pulmonary arteriovenous fistula or angiodysplasia elsewhere should suffice. Angiography and specialized vascular studies are indicated in times of trouble rather than in the asymptomatic present.

Medicine is always a dimly lighted room, and we can be grateful for the small flickering flame provided by the telangiectasia that this patient exhibits.

Bean, W. B.: *Vascular Spiders and Related Lesions of the Skin.* Charles C Thomas, Springfield, Illinois, 1958, pp. 132-157.
A scholar's adventures with Osler's disease, hereditary hemorrhagic telangiectasia — enjoy it by the fireside!

Quick, A. J.: Telangiectasia: Its Relationship to Minot-von Willebrand Syndrome. Amer. J. Med. Sci., *254*:585-601, 1967.
Luminous account of the paradox of Osler's bleeders: hemorrhage in the presence of a normal coagulogram.

Wolper, J., and Laibson, P. R.: Hereditary Hemorrhagic Telangiectasis (Rendu-Osler-Weber Disease) with Filamentary Keratitis. Arch. Ophthal., *81*:272-277, 1969.
Examine the eye as well as the skin and mucosa.

Davis, D. G., and Smith, J. L.: Retinal Involvement in Hereditary Hemorrhagic Telangiectasia. Arch. Ophthal., *85*:618-623, 1971.
Look for (1) tortuosity and segmental dilatations of retinal veins and (2) vitreous and retinal hemorrhages. Color photos.

Sweeting, J. G.: Fiberoptic Examination of the Small Intestine in a Case of Familial Telangiectasia. Gastrointes. Endosc. *14*:152-153, 1968.
Telangiectatic vessels, potential bleeding sites, seen throughout entire length.

Stocks, L. O., Halpern, M., and Turner, A. F.: Spontaneous Closure·of an Arteriovenous Fistula. Report of a Case in Hereditary Hemorrhagic Telangiectasia. Radiology, *92*:1499-1500, 1969.
Etiology of gastrointestinal bleeding is thrombosis of dysplastic vessels distal to the vascular arcades, thus causing mucosal ulcerations!

Halpern, M., Turner, A. F., and Citron, B. P.: Hereditary Hemorrhagic Telangiectasia. An Angiographic Study of Abdominal Visceral Angiodysplasias Associated with Gastrointestinal Hemorrhage. Radiology, *90*:1143-1149, 1968.
Selective celiac and superior mesenteric arteriography indicated in patients with bleeding of obscure etiology.

Michaeli, D., Ben-Bassat, I., Miller, H. I., and Deutsch, V.: Hepatic Telangiectases and Portosystemic Encephalopathy in Osler-Weber-Rendu Disease. Gastroenterology, *54*:929-932, 1968.
Unexplained systolic bruit in left epigastrium proved to be due to aneurysm of hepatic artery.

Razi, B., Beller, B. M., Ghidoni, J., Linhart, J. W., Talley, R. C., and Urban, E.: Hyperdynamic Circulatory State Due to Intrahepatic Fistula in Osler-Weber-Rendu Disease. Amer. J. Med., *50*:809-815, 1971.
Massive blood flow from hepatic artery to hepatic vein, with strain on heart.

Trell, E., Johansson, B. W., Linell, F., and Ripa, J.: Familial Pulmonary Hypertension and Multiple Abnormalities of Large Systemic Arteries in Osler's Disease. Amer. J. Med., *53*:50-63, 1972.
A variety of vascular shunts produce unbelievable sets of hemodynamic change. 115 references.

Gomes, M. R., Bernatz, P. E., and Denis, D. E.: Pulmonary Arteriovenous Fistulas. Ann. Thorac. Surg., *7*:582-593, 1969.
Complaint of dyspnea; may have cyanosis and clubbing of fingers; over half have hereditary hemorrhagic telangiectasia!

Dyer, N. H.: Cerebral Abscess in Hereditary Hemorrhagic Telangiectasia: Report of Two Cases in a Family. J. Neurol. Neurosurg. Psych., *30*:563-567, 1967.
Pathogenesis: presence of pulmonary arteriovenous fistula allows bacteria to bypass lung, reach brain.

Reagan, T. J., and Bloom, W. H.: The Brain in Hereditary Hemorrhagic Telangiectasia. Stroke, *2*:361-368, 1971.
Neurologic symptoms more likely due to pulmonary A. V. fistula (embolism, abscess, polycythemia) than cerebrovascular malformation.

Heffner, R. R., Jr., and Solitare, G. B.: Hereditary Hemorrhagic Telangiectasia; Neuropathological Observations. J. Neurol. Neurosurg. Psych., *32*:604-608, 1969.
Central nervous system telangiectasia, angiomas and arteriovenous malformations.

Myles, S. T., Needham, C. W., and LeBlanc, F. E.: Alternating Hemiparesis Associated with Hereditary Hemorrhagic Telangiectasia. Canad. Med. Assoc. J., *103*:509-511, 1970.
Another reason for examining patient's skin.

Davidson, P., and Robertson, D. M.: A True Mycotic (Aspergillus) Aneurysm Leading to Fatal Subarachnoid Hemorrhage in a Patient with Hereditary Hemorrhagic Telangiectasia. J. Neurosurg., *35*:71-76, 1971.
At autopsy mucocutaneous lesions so obvious in life were not discernible!

Hashimoto, K., and Pritzker, M. S.: Hereditary Hemorrhagic Telangiectasia. Oral Surg., *34*:751-768, 1972.
Electronmicroscopy: dilated vessels are venules — but without wall of smooth muscle, elastic tissue or pericytes, and without normal perivascular connective tissue support.

Rappaport, I., and Shiffman, M. A.: Multiple Phlebectasia Involving Jejunum, Oral Cavity and Scrotum. J.A.M.A., *185*:437-440, 1963.
Not hereditary hemorrhagic telangiectasia, but dilatation of venule which has lost connective tissue support because of aging.

Shelley, W. B.: Essential Progressive Telangiectasia: Successful Treatment with Tetracycline. J.A.M.A., *216*:1343-1344, 1971.
All that is telangiectasia is not Osler's disease. Lists 18 conditions in differential.

Cockayne, E. A.: Inherited Abnormalities of the Skin and Its Appendages. Oxford University Press, Oxford, 1933.
Osler's disease in horses.

Killey, H. C., and Kay, L. W.: Hereditary Hemorrhagic Telangiectasia. Brit. J. Oral Surg., 7:161-167, 1970.

Advises care in oral hygiene; cites fatality in 1908 from brushing teeth.

Harrison, D. F. N.: Hereditary Hemorrhagic Telangiectasia and Oral Contraceptives. Lancet, 1:721-721, 1970.

Good results in 60 men and women treated with 1 mg. ethinyl estradiol daily.

Stecker, R. H., and Lake, C. F.: Hereditary Hemorrhagic Telangiectasia. Review of 102 Cases and Presentation of an Innovation to Septo-dermoplasty. Arch. Otolaryngol., 82:522-526, 1965.

Complete review of therapeutic maneuvers including lubricants, estrogens, pressure, electrodesiccation, vessel ligation, grafting and iron.

Kwaan, H. C., and Silverman, S.: Fibrinolytic Activity in Lesions of Hereditary Hemorrhagic Telangiectasia. Arch. Derm., 107:571-573, 1973.

Increased. Successful treatment of epistaxis with topical inhibitor, aminocaproic acid.

15

Peutz-Jeghers Syndrome

15

For years the patient has noted these **asymptomatic pigmented macules on her lips.** *Similar pigmented spots are found on the gums and labia, as well as in the perianal area. She gives no familial history of perioral pigmentation, nor has she experienced abdominal symptoms or surgery.*

Biopsy — lentigo — epithelial hyperplasia and hyperpigmentation.

Peutz-Jeghers Syndrome

These brown spots serve as entrance signs to tell us there are polyps within! They tell us that there are polyps in the jejunum and ileum and possibly in the stomach, duodenum and colon, or even in the esophagus. They tell us that these polyps may be large or small and may number from a few to thousands. They tell us that the polyps are benign, but in the colon or stomach they may on occasion undergo malignant change. They tell us that these polyps can cause recurrent intestinal intussusception, as evidenced by postprandial colicky pain, at times leading to obstruction, with nausea, vomiting and abdominal distention. They tell us that the polyps can produce melena, with its subsequent weakness and anemia. They tell us that both the pigment and the polyps are hereditary, due to a single dominant gene with pleiotrophic capabilities. We cannot ignore these little brown spots, for they have much to tell us.

These are periorificial signs, so not surprisingly we learn that mucosal polyposis is not limited to the gut, but may occur in the nose, the bronchus, the renal pelvis, the ureter and the urinary bladder. Surprising, however, is the new awareness that 10 per cent of the women with this Peutz-Jeghers sign have ovarian tumors. These tumors are of many types, usually not significant clinically, although occasionally they may be functional, accounting for precocious puberty, or they may be malignant. In contrast, testicular tumors have not been reported as yet.

What is so consistent about this pathognomonic sign of mucosal polyposis is its peculiar distribution. Although the lips and oral mucosa are almost invariant sites, it does occur on the perioral skin, on and

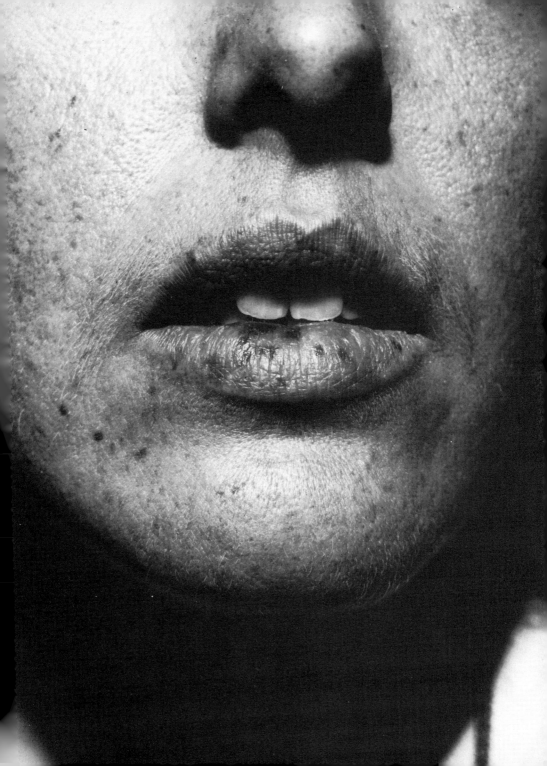

about the eyelids, on the labia and on the perianal skin as well. Presumably the adjacent mucosa is similarly pigmented, but few data are recorded concerning this point. Noteworthy is the essential absence of these macules within the gut itself. They simply appear as sentinel signs at both ends of the great long tube. The pigment loci may also appear on the palms and soles and under, as well as in, the nail plate itself. They do not appear elsewhere, and hence their distribution is not randomized. It is interesting to note the remarkable similarity of localization of these pigment spots of "hereditary pigmentary polyposis" to the mucocutaneous vascular lesions of hereditary hemorrhagic telangiectasia. They usually appear at birth or in childhood, so that this patient has a tardive variety.

What are these brown spots? Benign and harmless of themselves, they are simply areas of overproduction of melanin. They are not moles, because they show no nevus cells on biopsy, but rather the result of simple excess production of melanin. They are technically designated as lentigines, close relatives of the everyday freckles (ephelides).

What are the polyps? When first described they were felt to be malignant because they show spurts of growth and immense mitotic activity. Also, there is a tree-like growth of smooth muscle within the polyp which on an inverted view can be read as invasion of the mucosal tissue. Actually it is now agreed that the polyps are benign adenomatous hamartomas — genetically determined. They represent an overgrowth of not one cell type but the entire mucosal tissue. Apparently the pigment cells, the polyp anlage, as well as certain ovarian tissue have a common embryologic origin from the ganglionic crest.

What should be done? The marker lentigines are benign and require no treatment unless for cosmetic reasons. In that event, surface shave removal of some of the larger more prominent lentigines is adequate and gratifying. As to diagnostic studies, the nonsurgical ways to confirm the presence of the polyps are roentgenologic, using barium or air contrast, fiberoptic endoscopy and sigmoidoscopy. In the absence of symptoms, melena or iron deficiency anemia, such investigations would seem academic and at times can be misleading. Many times the polyps are numerous, yet so small as to defy roentgen visualization. Likewise, it is well to remember the possibility of polyps in the respiratory and genitourinary tracts but to explore for them only if relevant symptoms arise. Regular pelvic examinations are indicated with a special awareness of the possibility of ovarian tumors. The study of over 300 cases of Peutz-Jeghers syndrome reported in the literature since 1949 has led to this current, conservative view.

The Peutz-Jeghers sign is most valuable when one is confronted with the symptoms of unexplained abdominal colicky pain, an abdominal mass, melena or intestinal obstruction. It is here that the knowledge of polyps and the role they play in intussusception is so illuminating. It is not enough to look for the sign. In its absence we must inquire whether perioral lentigines occur in other members of the family, since this is a dominant gene affecting half of the offspring. In the older patient we must directly ask whether this condition may have been present at one time, only to have disappeared, since fading can occur. Such "lip reading" is not always easy in the rush of a surgical emergency, but it can be rewarding.

Conservative treatment remains the rule, since Peutz-Jeghers polyps are usually only in the small bowel, and removal of a large segment of the small bowel can be fatal. Polypectomy, when specifically indicated, remains preferable to resection. Although it is true that these polyps are benign hamartomas, their benignity is best demonstrated in their natural habitat, the small bowel. In the colon or in the stomach or the duodenum, they deserve the special attention accorded any potentially premalignant polyp, and it must be recognized that these patients do show a tendency to show gastrointestinal malignancy at a rate above that of the general population.

Remember the entrance sign when confronted with a patient with obscure recurrent abdominal pains. It helps to know there are polyps within.

Jeghers, H., McKusick, V. A., and Katz, K. H.: Generalized Intestinal Polyposis and Melanin Spots of the Oral Mucosa, Lips and Digits. New Eng. J. Med., *241*:993–1005, 1031–1036; 1949.
  A classic in clinical dermatology and gastroenterology.

Zegarelli, E. V., Kutscher, A. H., Mercadante, J., Kupferberg, N., and Piro, J. D.: Atlas of Oral Lesions Observed in the Syndrome of Oral Melanosis with Associated Intestinal Polyposis (Peutz-Jeghers Syndrome). Amer. J. Dig. Dis., *4*:479–489, 1959.
  Vary greatly in size, shape, color and intensity.

Godard, J. E., Dodds, W. J., Phillips, J. C., and Scanlon, G. T.: Peutz-Jeghers Syndrome: Clinical and Roentgenographic Features. Amer. J. Roentgenol. Radium Ther. Nucl. Med., *113*:316–324, 1971.
  Polyps easily overlooked on perfunctory roentgen examination.

Dozois, R. R., Judd, E. S., Dablin, D. C., and Bartholomew, L. G.: The Peutz-Jeghers Syndrome. Is There a Predisposition to the Development of Intestinal Malignancy. Arch. Surg., *98*:509–517, 1969.
Polyps are basically benign.

Dodds, W. J., Schulte, W. J., Hensley, G. T., and Hogan, W. J.: Peutz-Jeghers Syndrome and Gastrointestinal Malignancy. Amer. J. Roentgenol. Radium Ther. Nucl. Med., *115*:374–377, 1972.
Yet Peutz-Jeghers patients have greater tendency to develop carcinoma of colon or stomach than others.

Kieselstein, M., Herman, G., Wahrman, J., Voss, R., Gitelson, S., Feuchtwanger, M., and Kadar, S.: Mucocutaneous Pigmentation and Intestinal Polyposis (Peutz-Jeghers Syndrome) in a Family of Iraqi Jews with Polyceptic Kidney Disease with a Chromosome Study. Isr. J. Med. Sci., *5*:81–90, 1969.
Two years passed before anyone associated patient's vague abdominal pains with pigmentation of lips.

Sommerhaug, R. G., and Mason, T.: Peutz-Jeghers Syndrome and Ureteral Polyposis. J.A.M.A., *211*:120–122, 1970.
Polyps are found in nose, bronchi, renal pelvis, ureter and bladder, as well as G.I. tract.

Christian, C. D.: Ovarian Tumors: An Extension of the Peutz-Jeghers Syndrome. Amer. J. Obstet. Gynec., *111*:529–534, 1971.
Any woman with perioral lentigines is a candidate for a careful pelvic exam as well as a G.I. series.

Trodahl, J. N., and Sprague, W. G.: Benign and Malignant Melanocytic Lesions of the Oral Mucosa. An Analysis of 135 Cases. Cancer, *25*:812–823, 1970.
Advise biopsy, since 25 per cent of malignant melanomas were described by clinician as merely a pigmented spot on mucosa.

Dummett, C. O., and Barens, G.: Oromucosal Pigmentation: An Updated Literary Review. J. Periodont., *42*:726–736, 1971.
A refreshing thesaurus.

Crowe, F. W.: Axillary Freckling as a Diagnostic Aid in Neurofibromatosis. Ann. Intern. Med., *61*:1142–1143, 1964.
Macules on the lips — intestinal polyposis. Macules in the armpits — neurofibromatosis.

Gorlin, R. J., Anderson, R. C., and Moller, J. H.: The Leopard (Multiple Lentigines) Syndrome Revisited. Laryngoscope, *81*:1674–1681, 1971.
Macules everywhere — leopard syndrome! See a cardiologist, otologist and endocrinologist.

Bandler, M.: Hemangiomas of the Small Intestine Associated with Mucocutaneous Pigmentation. Gastroenterology, *38*:641–645, 1960.
Peutz-Jeghers pigmentation associated with multiple cavernous hemangiomas causing recurrent bleeding.

Kaltiala, E. H., Lenkkeri, H., and Larmi, T. K. I.: The Peutz-Jeghers Syndrome. Ann. Chir. Gynaec. Fenn., *61*:119–123, 1972.
Indications for surgery: intestinal obstruction, severe hemorrhage.

McKittrick, J. E., Lewis, W. M., Doane, W. A., and Gerwig, W. H.: The Peutz-Jeghers Syndrome. Report of Two Cases, One with 30-Year Followup. Arch. Surg., *103*:57–62, 1971.
Polypectomies preferable to bowel resection.

16

Urticarial and annular erythematous lesions have coursed over this 53-year-old patient's skin for the past six months. Repeated biopsies showed only nonspecific inflammatory change. Topical corticosteroids and systemic griseofulvin therapy were without effect. An intensive study during two weeks of hospitalization failed to disclose any cause. General physical examination blood studies, bone marrow and L. E. preparations, as well as roentgenograms of chest, kidney and gastrointestinal tract, were normal.

During the past few weeks she has developed this **ulcerative tumor of the sternum**, *as well as other rapidly growing tumors of the right breast and leg. Touch imprints reveal highly malignant lymphocytes, and biopsy shows presence of malignant lymphoma, possibly reticulum cell sarcoma type.*

Malignant Lymphoma

This is a fatal skin disease. It is not the surfacing tumor of a leukemia nor the outward spread of Hodgkin's disease. It is not the cutaneous metastasis of lymphosarcoma or reticulum cell sarcoma. Yet, it is related to all these, for it is a neoplastic malignant growth arising out of the primitive reticular tissue of the dermis. This is a primary cutaneous malignant lymphoma.

Originating as it has in the skin, we have been given an unparalleled daily clinical view of what is completely masked in systemic lymphomas. For a full six months we have been puzzled by the vast and, until now, unidentified panorama of her immunologic defense against these malignant cells. We have seen the strange immediate-type urticarial response and the delayed erythematous rings of reaction, but without understanding. Now the immune battle has been lost and the malignant cells take the field. Before this, their small number eluded histologic recognition, but now they come in diagnostic number.

We see these malignant lymphoma cells in the touch smears as well as in the biopsy specimen taken from this tumor. Yet classification is difficult. There is no marker cell. The neoplastic cell is ill defined, conceptual and variable in form. Even changing the tissue fixative used can

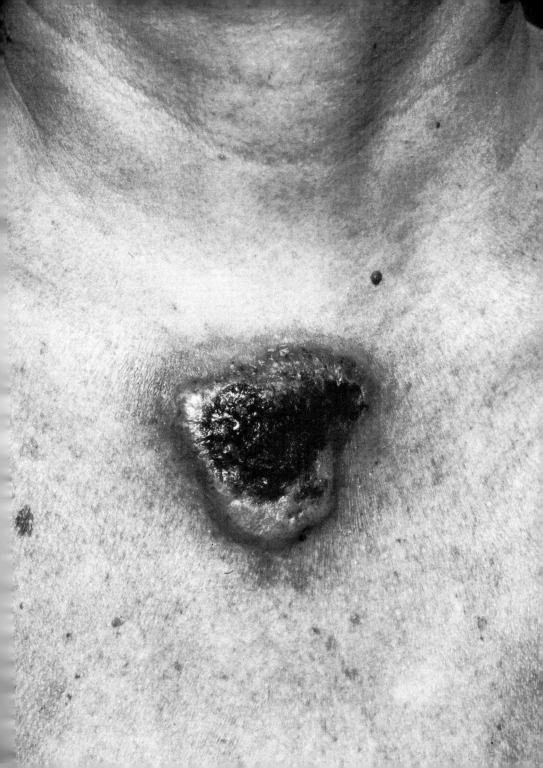

alter the histopathologic interpretation. The multicellular immune response further fogs the scene. Serial and multiple biopsies may provide even more confounding data. Add to this the semantic, synonymic and eponymic confusion which has arisen out of a century of struggling with this, the most complex of cancers. Little wonder that many pathologists are content to stop with the generic designate, malignant lymphoma. Nonetheless, it is possible to discern that at times the malignant cells may be in monomorphous array, appearing to reflect an origin from either the stromal reticulum cells (reticulum cell sarcoma) or from the lymphocytes (lymphosarcoma). In contrast they may be polymorphic, and here the Sternberg-Reed multinucleated malignant histiocyte, a reticular cell, is diagnostic. The only other grouping is the polymorphic malignant infiltrate associated with monocytic microabscesses in the epidermis (Pautrier). This is the distinctive histologic picture of mycosis fungoides. But these are matters for expert histopathologic discussion, debate and decision. The diagnosis is made by the pathologist, not the clinician.

Yet, there is one malignant cutaneous lymphoma that the clinician can identify. This is mycosis fungoides. Arising in the skin, it classically exhibits an exquisitely chronic course of sequential stages. In the first stage, which may extend for years, indeed decades, a nonspecific clinical and histopathologic pattern of rash appears. This is the premycotic chronic dermatitis, poikiloderma or pruritus. This is the immune struggle and the varying, ceaseless inflammatory response. We are unable to perceive the sequence and remain thwarted in our attempts to treat this. The patient remains in good health. In the second stage, with its large geographic infiltrative plaques over the body, the diagnosis becomes apparent "from the doorway." And now the characteristic polymorphous cell pattern confirms the diagnosis. Next, the third stage, fraught with tumors—fungating necrotic growths which eventually metastasize throughout the body, especially if life is prolonged and defenses reduced by modern immunosuppressive chemotherapy. An erythrodermic variant (Sézary's) is known but less common.

Our patient might well be considered to have an extremely malignant misshapen version of mycosis fungoides. She may have telescoped a lifetime of lymphoma into less than a year. With her immune defenses protecting her for a scant six months instead of 20 years, and with her infiltrative stage being one of days, instead of several years, we would presume that death would come in a few months. And yet, the histopathologic picture is not that of mycosis fungoides, and the clinical picture has raced by, blurred and unrecognizable. Thus, while recognizing a similarity between the nature of this condition and mycosis fungoides, we would prefer to label it as a cutaneous malignant lymphoma and keep the term mycosis fungoides for the more predictable protracted clinical picture.

Treatment of any neoplasm involves surgical removal or destruction. Our patient's growths are multiple and beyond the reach of the surgeon. We must turn to the radiologist, who has at his command teleroentgen therapy and electron-beam as well as conventional ortho-voltage x-ray. Temporary success or failure here depends on the radio-sensitivity of the tumor, which can be assessed only by trial. Chemotherapy is the other avenue of selective destruction. In this regard cyclophosphamide (Cytoxan) and amethopterin (methotrexate) have been widely used, as has mechlorethamine (nitrogen mustard). It is important to note that systemic corticosteroids are disappointing even in high dosage. The new antimitotic, bleomycin, has but limited success in temporarily suppressing a reticulum cell sarcoma, the effect being seen in the skin only.

The grim prognosis is for spread of this patient's malignant tumor from her skin to other organs throughout her body. She may have but a few months to live. Under these circumstances treatment must include full measures of palliation, support and comfort. And throughout all, we should never speak the language of despair, and never be the thief of hope.

Bluefarb, S. M.: *Cutaneous Manifestations of the Malignant Lymphomas.* Charles C Thomas, Springfield, Illinois, 1959, 534 pp.
   Think lymphoma when patient has pruritus, eczema, infiltrated plaques or tumors. Encyclopedic monograph.

Kim, R., Winkelmann, R. K., and Dockerty, M.: Reticulum Cell Sarcoma of the Skin. Cancer, *16*:646-655, 1963.
   The malignant lymphoma which arises from stromal reticulum cell: noninflammatory nodules and tumors.

Rosenberg, S. A., Diamond, H. D., Jaslowitz, B., and Craver, L. F.: Lymphosarcoma: A Review of 1269 Cases. Medicine, *40*:31-84, 1961.
   The malignant lymphoma which arises from lymphocyte: noninflammatory nodules and tumors.

Ultmann, J. E.: Clinical Features and Diagnosis of Hodgkin's Disease. Cancer, *19*:297-307, 1966.
   The malignant lymphoma, with pathognomonic multinucleated Sternberg-Reed cells and polymorphic infiltrate: noninflammatory nodules and tumors.

Epstein, E. H., Jr., Levin, D. L., Croft, J. D., Jr., and Lutzner, M. A.: Mycosis Fungoides Survival, Prognostic Features, Response to Therapy and Autopsy Findings. Medicine, 51:61-72, 1972.
The malignant lymphoma of dermatology, primary in the skin: sequence of nonspecific premycotic dermatitis, infiltrative plaques and finally ulcerative tumors.

Clendenning, W. E.: Mycosis Fungoides. *In* Borrie, P. (Ed.): *Modern Trends in Dermatology*, Vol. 4, Appleton-Century-Crofts, New York, 1971, pp. 214-237.
Checklist of 26 critical studies for evaluation of cutaneous lymphoma suspects.

Helwig, E. B.: Malignant Lymphomas and Reactive Lymphoid Hyperplasias. *In* Graham, J. H. (Ed.): *Dermal Pathology*. Harper & Row, New York, 1972, pp. 683-713.
Diagnosis is always histopathologic — rarely clinical.

Graham, J. H., and Urbach, F.: Cytodiagnosis of Cutaneous Tumors. *In* Graham, J. H. (Ed.): *Dermal Pathology,* Vol. 5, Harper & Row, New York, 1972, pp. 675-681.
Tissue imprints show that malignant cells have large size, mitotic figures, bizarre hyperchromatic nuclei. Valuable adjunct to biopsy.

Musso, L. A.: Histological Problems in the Early Diagnosis of Malignant Lymphomata of the Skin. Aust. J. Derm., 13:20-26, 1972.
Early nonspecific dermatitic changes baffle pathologist.

Gall, E. A.: Enigmas in Lymphoma Reticulum Cell Sarcoma and Mycosis Fungoides. Minn. Med., 38:674-681, 1955.
Frolicsome essay on the ambiguities of nomenclature.

Muller, S. A., and Schulze, T. W.: Mucha-Haberman Disease Mistaken for Reticulum Cell Sarcoma. Arch. Derm., 103:423-427, 1971.
Absence of malignant cells in touch imprint is major clue to correct diagnosis.

Benninghoff, D. L., Medina, A., Alexander, L. L., and Camiel, M. R.: The Mode of Spread of Hodgkin's Disease to the Skin. Cancer, 26:1135-1140, 1970.
By retrograde lymphatic flow.

Fichtelius, K. E., Groth, O., and Liden, S.: The Skin, a First Level Lymphoid Organ? Int. Arch. Allerg., 37:607-620, 1970.
Miniaturized lymph nodes in skin — could be origin of malignant lymphomas arising in skin.

Doak, P. B., Montgomerie, J. Z., North, J. D. K., and Smith, F.: Reticulum Cell Sarcoma After Renal Homotransplantation and Azathioprine and Prednisone Therapy. Brit. Med. J., 4:746-748, 1968.
Immunosuppression — the cause?

Waldman, T. A.: Immunodeficiency Disease and Malignancy. Various Immunologic Deficiencies of Man and the Role of Immune Processes in the Control of Malignant Disease. Ann. Intern. Med., 77:605-628, 1972.
Marked increase in incidence of malignant lymphomas in patients with impaired immunity.

Peckham, M. J., and Steel, G. G.: Cell Kinetics in Reticulum Cell Sarcoma. Cancer, 29:1724-1728, 1972.
Volume doubling time of tumor may be less than ten days!

Trujillo, J. M., Drewinko, B., and Ahearn, M. J.: The Ability of Tumour Cells of the Lymphoreticular System to Grow in Vitro. Cancer Res., 32:1057-1065, 1972.
In cell culture, malignant lymphoma cells grow for much longer periods, but not a diagnostic test.

Lowenbraun, S., Sutherland, J. C., Feldman, M. J., and Serpick, A. A.: Transformation of Reticulum Cell Sarcoma to Acute Leukemia. Cancer, 27:579-585, 1971.
Rare, but common for lymphosarcoma.

Reilly, C. J., Han, T., Stutzman, L., Slack, N. H., and Webster, J.: Reticulum Cell Sarcoma. A Review of Radio-Therapeutic Experience. Cancer, 29:1314-1320, 1972.
Treatment of choice for localized form.

Aaron, H.: The Choice of Therapy in the Treatment of Malignancy. Medical Letter on Drugs and Therapeutics, 15:9-16, 1973.
The latest compendium of chemotherapeutic agents.

Ribeiro, G. G.: Primary Lymphosarcoma and Reticulum Cell Sarcoma of Skin. A Review of Thirty-Two Cases. Clin. Radiol., 23:279-285, 1972.
Mean survival time — 21.8 months.

17

For years this 25-year-old black juvenile diabetic has felt a gradu-ally enlarging mass on the back of his neck. At times the area is tender, especially after a haircut. Inspection reveals a well-defined zone of **firm, confluent papules and nodules** *which is just with-in the occipital hairline. The area is virtually alopecic, with some residual atrophic hairs growing out of orifices which define the very summit of these domelike papules.*

Bacterial culture—heavy growth of Staphylococcus aureus; *moderate growth of* Corynebacterium acnes; *scanty growth of coagulase-negative micrococci.*

Folliculitis Keloidalis

This is one of the unmistakables. A firm, pebbly surfaced lesion on the back of the neck in a black male makes for an "Augenblick" diag-nosis. Closer inspection proves comfortably confirmatory as we see that many of the domed lesions are truly follicular, a small atrophic hair wav-ing from their very centers. Even later comes the awareness that this lesion is really alopecic. On probing, we sense that some of the follicular papules have a pustular, cystic, inflammatory element. Superficial in-cision with a #11 Bard-Parker blade may uncover long coiled ingrown hairs in the nonfollicular nodules. A biopsy would show the solid fibrous hyperplasia of keloidal stroma, embedded dead hairs and occasional patches of chronic inflammation. This is unmistakably keloidal follicu-litis.

Over the past 100 years it has gathered its share of the moss of synonymy. It was christened dermatitis papillaris capillitii, a label still used by those with an assured orthography. The French confirmed it with the euphonious acne keloid, and now its adult name of follicu-litis keloidalis reflects a growing awareness that it is truly a follicular infection. An alternate designation, sycosis nuchae, also firmly places it in the follicular pyoderma class. But none of this makes for ease in searching or, for that matter, in preparing indices.

Folliculitis keloidalis displays a chronicity which discourages most clinical investigators, and as a result it is not one of the best understood diseases. Despite its glacier pace of extension up the back of the head, we

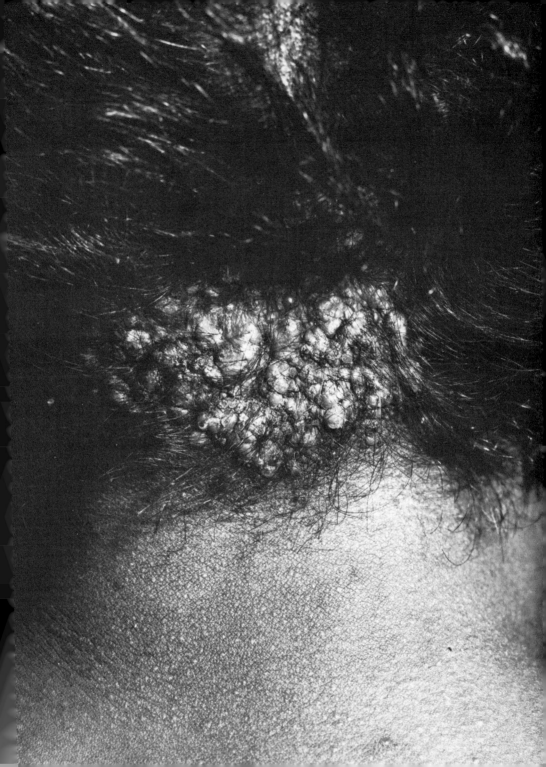

do know that it is a follicular disease of bacterial origin. Regularly, cultures show pathogenic staphylococci, as did those from this patient. In this instance a background diabetes mellitus which contributes to the chronicity and recalcitrance of the folliculitis is of importance. Equally significant in others may be the recognition of nephritis, hypogammaglobulinemia or dysgammaglobulinemia, but often no known defect is disclosed.

We also recognize that fundamentally this process is a perifollicular keloid. It is a scar that throttles the pilosebaceous apparatus, destroying the sebaceous gland, the follicular capacity to produce hair and eventually the follicle itself. As such, it is not surprising that the process is almost limited to the blacks, the race with a dermis most responsive to injury and most capable of producing the hypertrophic scar and keloid.

Yet another factor peculiar to the black race is operating here. That is the tendency of the black's hair to curve, so that follicular inflammation and breakdown can and does lead to ingrown hairs. This is most dramatically seen in two related diseases in the black male, the common pseudofolliculitis of the beard and rare folliculitis et perifolliculitis suffodiens et abscedens of the scalp. In all three, buried dead hairs are an incitement to inflammation and, in our patient in particular, to keloidal scar formation.

Treatment, ideally, is surgery. The total instant removal of an area which has plagued the patient for over a decade is highly gratifying. With direct excision down to the fascia and primary closure, the cosmetic result is good, because significantly incisional keloids do not often develop. In the unusually large lesions, grafting may be necessary. Although surgery offers the greatest chance of cure, recurrence may occur just above the scar or graft site, since the genetic predisposition persists.

However, in this patient with juvenile diabetes, extensive surgery poses an unacceptable risk. He is even a poor candidate for the popular helpful intralesional triamcinolone hexacetonide injections. After ascertaining that his diabetes is well controlled, we restrict ourselves to two primary goals—topical sterilization and epilation. To achieve the first, Vleminckx's solution (Vlem-Dome, one packet to a pint of very warm water) is used as a local compress for 15 minutes daily. It is not pleasant, has the odor of rotten eggs, tarnishes silver and must be used in a well-ventilated room and applied carefully by someone wearing rubber gloves. But it is remarkably effective in combating the infection. Our patient is also cautioned to keep from touching, squeezing and manipulating the area. Reaching the second goal is equally arduous. It calls for regular once-a-week manual epilation of all hairs, grown or ingrown, in the lesion and in its penumbra. This is best done with professional hair tweezers used under 3 to 5 powered magnification. Understandably, when confronted with this regimen over a period of months, any but the most dedicated patient-physician team will falter.

This is a disease that deserves more research. Why is the primary lesion a perfect perifollicular keloid? Should we not be looking for an intrafollicular organism which stimulates the surrounding fibrocyte system to produce collagen in excessive amounts?

Cosman, B., and Wolff, M.: Acne Keloidalis. Plast. Reconstr. Surg., *50*:25-30, 1972.
  Review of 14 cases of this folliculitis keloidalis: little understood idiopathic chronic inflammation around scalp hair follicles of posterior upper neck.

Bayles, M. A. H.: Coiffure Keloids. Brit. J. Derm., *86*:415-416, 1972.
  Patterned keloid in a Zulu woman, related to tension on hair from braided coiffure.

Pinkus, H., and Mehregan, A. H.: *A Guide to Dermatohistopathology.* Appleton-Century-Crofts, New York, 1969, pp. 203-204.
  Buried dead hairs, infection and keloid formation produce folliculitis keloidalis.

Varadi, D. P., and Saqueton, A. C.: Perifollicular Elastolysis. Brit. J. Derm., *83*:143-150, 1970.
  An instructive analogue: ballooning follicular papules from destruction of elastic tissue by elastase of intrafollicular staphylococci.

Cohen, J. O.: *The Staphylococci.* John Wiley and Sons, Inc., New York, 1972, 548 pp.
  Anatomy, chemistry, genetics, enzymology of *S. aureus* and *S. epidermidis,* as well as clinical, epidemiologic, immunologic and therapeutic aspects of staphylococcal disease.

Kenney, J. A.: Management of Dermatoses Peculiar to Negroes. Arch. Derm., *91*:126-129, 1965.
  Initial treatment of folliculitis keloidalis: manual epilation of hairs, intralesional triamcinolone, topical antibiotic and steroid creams.

Malherbe, W. D. F.: Sycosis Nuchae and Its Surgical Treatment. Plast. Reconst. Surg., 47:269-271, 1971.
  Excellent results with total excision — primary closure in 7 patients. Initial retraction of head so marked, patient asked for good book on astronomy !

18

For the past five months this woman has had **multiple abscesses, ulcers and deep draining sinuses of her soles** *as well as a large purulent ulcerative area on the right heel. Relatively painless and noninflammatory, these failed to heal despite hospitalization and intensive systemic treatment with penicillin, erythromycin and tetracycline.*

The patient has had deforming rheumatoid arthritis for five years, requiring corticosteroid therapy to the point of Cushingoid changes during the past two years.

No evidence of osteomyelitis was seen on roentgenograms. Cultures repeatedly showed vast numbers of **Pseudomonas aeruginosa** *sensitive to carbenicillin, gentamicin and colistin.*

Pseudomonas Infection

The diagnosis here is a triumph for the microbiologist. Often his reports are the sterile exercises of a bacterial accountant, but this time he has the answer loud and clear. This is the infection that doesn't respond to any of the oral antibiotics. This is the infection that finds its home in the tissues of the debilitated and of the steroid consumer. This is the infection that has replaced staphylococcal infection as the most important one in hospitals today. And this is a disease which requires the microbiology laboratory for its identification.

True, the clinician may suspect that infection is responsible for this five-month disabling sequence of abscesses, ulcers and draining sinuses. He knows, however, that the skin of the rheumatoid arthritis patient, and especially one who has taken steroids for years, is susceptible to a strange assortment of ulcers. Some of these are vasculitic and can only be detected by means of a biopsy specimen, which he hesitates to take from this area. Others are neuropathic, reflecting trauma to a poorly innervated, insensitive area, being a form of malum perforans as seen in tabes, diabetes or poliomyelitis, and a few are the picture of pyoderma gangrenosum. In addition, he wonders about the possibility of osteomyelitis, deep fungal infection or even a factitial origin. His vision is limited, since in a way ulcers are not lesions but rather an absence of

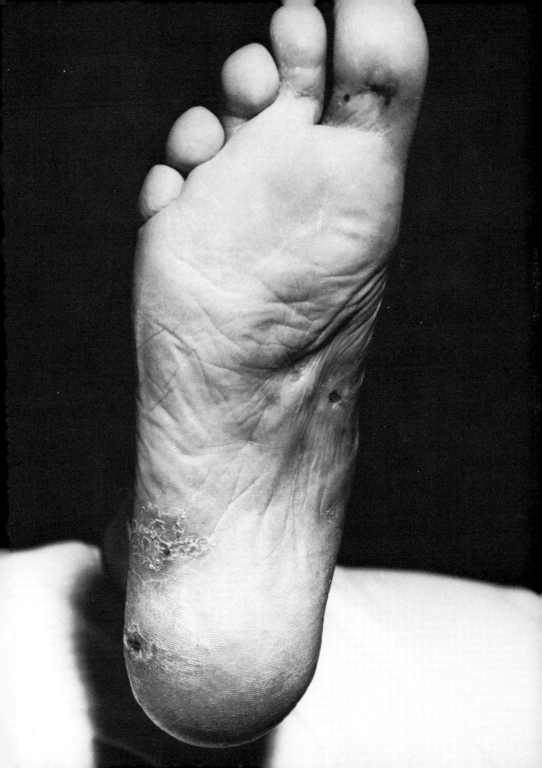

lesions. He needs laboratory help, and this time the assistance comes from the culture plates of microbiology. It is on these plates that the causative Pseudomonas is first sighted.

Pseudomonas aeruginosa is a remarkable pathogen. A gram-negative, aerobic bacillus, it is indifferent to a variety of antiseptics, disinfectants and antimicrobials. pHisoHex, Vioform and quaternary ammonium compounds only favor its growth by eliminating the competitive gram-positive bacteria. Likewise, systemic oral antibiotics induce a similar ecologic shift. Equally remarkable is the fact that Pseudomonas organisms can meet their nutritional needs on little more than distilled water. Thus, they can live and be winged about hospitals in the microdroplets of water from a humidifier. Moisture is their milieu, so that anything from mop-pails to Hubbard tanks may contain them. Not surprisingly, in our otherwise sterile modern antiseptic and antibiotic world, the Pseudomonads have slipped through our defense to become suddenly the most important cause of nosocomial infections today.

Pseudomonas aeruginosa and a few pathogen cospecies produce an amazing array of clinical findings. When it grows in the skin it may evoke the distinctive blue-green pus which results from its elaboration of the blue-green pigments, pyocyanin and pyoverdin. The latter pigment is fluorescent and can be detected by Wood's light illumination, a procedure especially helpful in rapid screening of burns for this organism. Neither sign is present at this time in our well-compressed patient. Pseudomonas has keratinases, lecithinases and lipases to give clout for direct invasion of the skin of defense-deficient individuals. It can induce cellulitis as well as these ulcers you see here.

When Pseudomonas grows in the paronychium, a dramatic green-colored nail is the result. When it grows between the toes, the web becomes hyperkeratotic, thick and white, with the pyoverdin showing greenish fluorescence under Wood's light. In the ear canal, it can be responsible for otitis externa. And here, if ignored, it can be malignant, leading to mastoiditis and death in elderly diabetics. In the eye, Pseudomonas can produce corneal ulcers and subsequent loss of vision. In the bone, it manifests itself as osteomyelitis.

But it is in the blood that Pseudomonas is most lethal and frightening. And it is here that the clinician can be most helpful, because there is an early cutaneous sign pathognomonic of Pseudomonas septicemia. This sign is *ecthyma gangrenosum*. It is neither ecthyma nor pyoderma gangrenosum but rather a hemorrhagic bullous lesion which rapidly becomes necrotic and ulcerative. One or more of these are often located in the axillary, anogenital and inframammary areas. They are the signs of a Pseudomonas septicemia and result from actual bacterial invasion of the vessel walls. At times they are so destructive that they lead to ulcers requiring skin grafting. A smear of the lesion shows myriad gram-negative bacteria, and biopsy reveals this phenomenal invasion of the vessel walls by Pseudomonas. Although petechial, purpuric and cellulitic eruptions are also seen, ecthyma gangrenosum is the truly diagnostic sign, permitting recognition and treatment of the septicemia long before blood cultures can be helpful. Know and look for this life-saving sign in any debilitated, leukemic, severely burned or multiantibiotic-treated patient.

The Pseudomonad appears invincible, untreatable, and ineradicable. And it virtually was until a few years ago. True, it could be killed by desiccation, but how could one dry the toe webs, let alone an ulcerative lesion? True, it could be killed with 5 per cent acetic acid, but how can this be introduced into other than the toe web? True, surgical debridement and irrigation were helpful, but usually only temporarily. But today we have three specific antibiotics tailored for the Pseudomonads. The first is polymyxin B, a surface-active compound which attacks the vital phospholipids which are in especial abundance in the Pseudomonas cell membrane. When used in a variety of topical creams and ointments, it is helpful, as is its newer analogue, colistin (polymyxin E), but strain resistance occurs and its toxicity limits systemic use. The second weapon is gentamicin, available as a 0.1 per cent cream and ointment (Garamycin). Again, ototoxicity and nephrotoxicity have reduced its value for systemic use. The third and newest antibiotic is carbenicillin (Geopen, Pyopen), a semisynthetic penicillin which acts against Pseudomonas as well as against other gram-negative and gram-positive organisms. It is truly the life-saving drug in Pseudomonas septicemia and is indicated in our patient. Marvelously nontoxic, it can be given in the tremendous dosage necessary—as much as 40 grams a day. Even though the entire amount must be administered intravenously, Pseudomonas is no longer invincible, and our hospital infectious disease teams can glow with pride.

It is evident that not only the diagnosis but also the treatment of this patient is a triumph for the microbiologist. The clinician is his grateful handmaiden.

Dyck, P. J., Conn, D. L., and Okazaki, H.: Necrotizing Angiopathic Neuropathy. Mayo Clin. Proc., *47*:461-475, 1972.
Setting the stage: peripheral neuropathy common in rheumatoid arthritis. Fiber degeneration due to ischemia produced by necrotizing angiopathy in epineurial arterioles.

Hall, J. H., Callaway, J. L., Tindall, J. P., and Smith, J. G., Jr.: *Pseudomonas aeruginosa* in Dermatology. Arch. Derm., *97*:312-324, 1968.
A reference to be treasured.

Savin, J. A.: *Pseudomonas aeruginosa* Infections in a Skin Ward. Trans. St. Johns Hosp. Derm. Soc., *53*:75-79, 1967.
Pseudomonas infected ulcers of soles followed hemorrhagic blisters when steroid creams were applied under occlusion.

Givler, R. L.: Necrotizing Anorectal Lesions Associated with Pseudomonas Infections in Leukemia. Dis. Colon Rectum, *12*:438-440, 1969.
Five terminal patients presenting noninflammatory necrotic ulcers, with myriad gram-negative rods within walls of surrounding blood vessels.

Dorff, G. J., Geimer, N. F., Rosenthal, D. R., and Rytel, M. W.: Pseudomonas Septicemia. Illustrated Evolution of Its Skin Lesion. Arch. Intern. Med., *128*:591-595, 1971.
Learn to recognize ecthyma gangrenosum, the hemorrhagic bullous pathognomonic sign of Pseudomonas septicemia. Color photos.

Taplin, D., Bassett, D. C. J., and Mertz, P. M.: Foot Lesions Associated with Pseudomonas Cepacia. Lancet, *2*:568-571, 1971.
Sodden, white, hyperkeratotic lesions in toe webs, typical for Pseudomonas infection.

Shellow, W. V. R., and Koplon, B. S.: Green Striped Nails: Chromonychia Due to *Pseudomonas aeruginosa*. Arch. Derm., *97*:149-153, 1968.
Each band marked an episode of pseudomonal paronychia.

Dinapoli, R. P., and Thomas, J. E.: Neurologic Aspects of Malignant External Otitis: Report of Three Cases. Mayo Clin. Proc., *46*:339-344, 1971.
Persistent external otitis in elderly diabetic can lead to mastoiditis, osteomyelitis, cranial nerve palsies, meningitis, deaths. Cause: *Pseudomonas aeruginosa.*

Golden, B., Fingerman, L. H., and Allen, H. F.: Pseudomonas Corneal Ulcers in Contact Lens Wearers. Arch. Ophthal., *85*:543-547, 1971.
Identification demands immediate culture.

Minnefor, A. B., Olson, M. I., and Carver, D. H.: Pseudomonas Osteomyelitis Following Puncture Wounds of Foot. Pediatrics, *47*:598-601, 1971.
Barefoot boys' disease; detect with x-ray and culture.

Tong, M. J.: Septic Complications of War Wounds. J.A.M.A., *219*:1044-1047, 1972.
Pseudomonas aeruginosa **is most common organism found in extremity wounds after five days in hospital.**

Foley, F. D.: Pathology of Cutaneous Burns. Surg. Clin. N. Amer., *50*:1201-1210, 1970.
Suspect Pseudomonas infection when hemorrhagic purpuric discoloration occurs in or near burn wound.

Polk, H. C., Ward, G., Clarkson, J. G., and Taplin, D.: Early Detection of Pseudomonas Burn Infection. Clinical Experience with Wood's Light Fluorescence. Arch. Surg., *98*:292-295, 1969.
Pseudomonads elaborate a fluorescent material seen under 360 nm. illumination.

Libit, S. A., Ulstrom, P. A., and Doeden, D.: Fecal *Pseudomonas aeruginosa* as a Cause of the Blue Diaper Syndrome. J. Pediat., *81*:546-547, 1972.
Pseudomonads also produce pyocyanin, which is blue-green under ordinary light.

Forkner, C. E.: Pseudomonas aeruginosa *Infections*. Grune & Stratton, Inc., New York, 1960.
Basic reference text on the number one nosocomial infection of today. 465 references.

Gilardi, G. L.: Characterization of Pseudomonas Species Isolated from Clinical Specimens. Appl. Microbiol., *21*:414-419, 1971.
Isolated 227 strains of Pseudomonads; 90 morphologic and physiologic characteristics.

Teplitz, C.: Pathogenesis of Pseudomonas Vasculitis and Septic Lesions. Arch. Path., *80*:297-307, 1965.
Bacterial invasion of vessel walls; reproducible in animals.

Baehner, R. L.: Disorders of Leukocytes Leading to Recurrent Infection. Pediat. Clin. N. Amer., *19*:935-956, 1972.
Newborn's susceptibility to gram-negative infections due to lack of IgM necessary for phagocytosis. Modern review of host defenses. 188 references.

White, P. M.: *Pseudomonas aeruginosa* in a Skin Hospital. Brit. J. Derm., *85*:412-417, 1971.
Indifferent to many sterilizing agents, it abounds in the moisture of air humidifiers, sinks, tanks, distilled water, food and feces.

Phillips, I., Lobo, A. Z., Fernandes, R., and Gundara, N. S.: Acetic Acid in the Treatment of Superficial Wounds Infected by *Pseudomonas aeruginosa*. Lancet, *1*:11-12, 1968.
Five per cent acetic acid effective against Pseudomonas but ineffective against *Staphylococcus aureus* **and Proteus.**

Goldschmidt, M. C., Kuhn, C. R., Perry, K., and Johnson, D. E.: EDTA and Lysozyme Lavage in the Treatment of Pseudomonas and Coliform Bladder Infections. J. Urol., *107*:969-972, 1972.
Chelating agent uncovers mucopolypeptide layer of Pseudomonas, permitting lysis by lysozyme.

Alexander, J. W., Fisher, M. W., and MacMillan, B. G.: Immunological Control of Pseudomonas Infection in Burn Patients. A Clinical Evaluation. Arch. Surg., *102*:31-35, 1971.
Vaccine reduced Pseudomonas septicemia mortality from 14 to 3 per cent.

Hoeprich, P. D.: The Polymyxins. Med. Clin. N. Amer., *54*:1257-1265, 1970.
Polymyxin B and Colistin (Polymyxin E) are cationic decapeptides and act as surfactant antibiotics, attacking phospholipid wall of Pseudomonas.

Finland, M., and Hewitt, W. L.: Second International Symposium on Gentamicin. An Aminoglycoside Antibiotic. J. Infect. Dis., *124*:S1-300, 1971.
A great advance in the therapy of Pseudomonas infection but ototoxic and nephrotoxic.

Solberg, C. O., Kjellstrand, K. M., and Matsen, J. M.: Carbenicillin Therapy of Severe *Pseudomonas aeruginosa* Infections. J. Chron. Dis., *24*:19-28, 1971.
Given like sugar (30 to 40 grams a day, I. V.) costing like gold (75 to 100 dollars a day), acting like magic, carbenicillin can be life-saving in Pseudomonas septicemia.

19

Known to be a family trait for eight generations, these **dappled nonpigmented areas** *appeared* **on the right knee** *and stomach of this youngster three weeks after birth. Although more evident by contrast in the summer months, they have persisted unchanged despite psoralen-ultraviolet light therapy. The vellus hairs of the area have never normally pigmented, remaining white.*

This girl's hearing, intellectual development, and neurologic studies, including sensory studies of the piebald spots, are all normal. An only sister was born with a white forelock and similar achromic areas, as were their father and his sister.

Biopsy — absence of melanin in epidermis.

Dopa stain — occasional large dopa-positive melanocytes.

Piebaldism

Only one thing is missing in this clinical picture — melanin pigment. And it makes for a fascinating story etymologically and genetically. Through the centuries, the white forelock of this disorder has been a strange and singular predictable familial mark. Generation after generation carried it, some families memorializing it in their names! Thus came the Whitlocks, the Horlicks and the Blaylocks, the white, the gray and the blanched eponyms of skin color. Interestingly, the medical term piebaldism may in turn be construed as an ornithological eponym, if you will. "Pie," as in pied piper, refers to the magpie, an English bird of black and white plumage, and "bald" may be related to the bald eagle, famed for its white-feathered head.

Genetically, the story of the inheritance of this white forelock and patches of white skin had been written since the early days of Egyptian history. It was known to affect each generation (a mendelian dominant), to affect both sons and daughters (an autosomal trait) and to persist a lifetime (a genetic defect). But what mechanism was defective?

From a curiosity, a source of superstition, piebaldism has gradually evolved into a neurocutaneous disease. We recognize that the essential skin color source is the melanocyte, which produces the pigment melanin. It is a nerve cell which arises in the neural crest and makes the

120

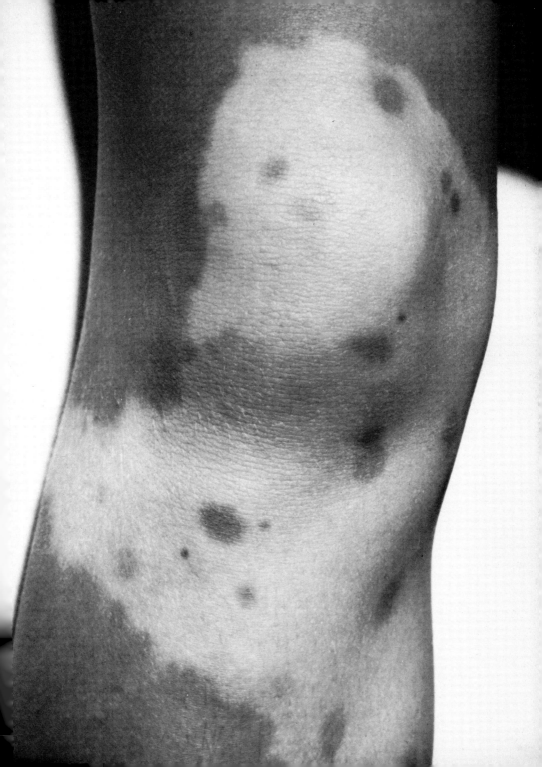

long embryonic voyage to the epidermis. In our patient it somehow failed to make the trip, hence, these restricted areas that lack color. Therefore, there is no machinery for the normal manufacture of melanin and its contact transfer to the adjacent keratinocytes. Significantly, melanin is a very insoluble pigment, so that any anticipated coloring by diffusion does not take place. The borders of the lesion outline precisely the sites devoid of melanocytes, and the dappling represents clones of melanocytes which are present as islands in an achromic sea.

We have come to learn that occasionally the piebald patient may have a sensorineural hearing loss (Waardenburg's), motor coordination defects, ataxia or even mental retardation. A defect in the gene controlling development and migration of the melanoblast apparently can have pleiotropic neural effects. The white forelock thus signals a special neurologic alert during the early developmental years of infancy when these genetic problems of unpredictably variable penetrance can appear.

How do we separate piebaldism from other white spotting disease? Piebaldism lacks the universality and eye involvement of albinism even though some scholars label it partial albinism. And it lacks the melanocytes that the albino does have, nonfunctional and empty but still visible under the electron microscope. Piebaldism is present at birth, becoming evident after the few weeks necessary for the normal melanocytes to respond to their removal from intrauterine darkness. It is thus not vitiligo or any of the acquired depigmentations or losses of color of later life. It does not blend in with the surrounding skin on diascopy as does the nevus anemicus, which shows a remarkable congenital area of color lack due to vasoconstriction. It does not present the ash leaf hypomelanotic macules with its perifollicular pigmentation seen in another congenital problem, tuberous sclerosis. All in all, piebaldism is a gloriously unique and easy diagnosis usually made by the patient's family.

Treatment is limited to protection of the affected areas from sunburn by the use of the classic topical sun screens, e.g., para-aminobenzoic acid preparations. Cosmetic camouflage may be needed when the sites of involvement are facial or otherwise disturbing. Many modern commercially available make-up preparations are effective and gratifying. The parents of infants must be made aware of the need for audiologic and, at times, neurologic review. Early audiologic investigation of every infant born into this family is especially important, since in the home congenital hearing loss can escape detection for a long time and thereby delay the early institution of remedial measures so critical for the development of language in a deaf child.

The virtual absence of melanocytes from the achromic area does not suggest that local or systemic remedies could be helpful. Epidermal grafting is still in an experimental developmental stage. Thus, although this disease may be the geneticist's delight, it remains the therapist's fright.

Witkop, C. J.: Albinism. *In* Harris, H., and Hirschhorn, K. (Eds.): *Advances in Human Genetics*, Vol. 2, Plenum Press, New York, 1971, pp. 61-142.
Surpassingly fine survey of genetic amelaninism, both universal (oculocutaneous albinism) and circumscribed (piebaldism). 309 references.

Telfer, M. A., Sugar, M., Jaeger, E. A., and Mulcahy, J.: Dominant Piebald Trait (White Forelock and Leukoderma) with Neurological Impairment. Amer. J. Hum. Genet., 23:383-389, 1971.
Neurosensory hearing loss, cerebellar ataxia and mental retardation occasional components of piebaldism.

Reed, W. B., Stone, V. M., Boder, E., and Ziprkowski, L.: Pigmentary Disorders in Association with Congenital Deafness. Arch. Derm., 95:176-186, 1967.
With loss of pigment, look for loss of hearing.

Hurwitz, S., and Braverman, I. M.: White Spots in Tuberous Sclerosis. J. Pediat., 77:587-594, 1970.
Café au lait spots — neurofibromatosis; "au lait" spots — tuberous sclerosis.

Greaves, M. W., Birkett, D., and Johnson, C.: Nevus Anemicus: A Unique Catecholamine-Dependent Nevus. Arch. Derm., 102:172-176, 1970.
Pale skin areas due to continuous local adrenergic vasoconstriction.

Fitzpatrick, T. B., and Mihm, M. C.: Abnormalities of the Melanin Pigmentary System. *In* Fitzpatrick, T. B., et al. (Eds.): *Dermatology in General Medicine.* McGraw-Hill Book Co., New York, 1971, pp. 1591-1637.
Vitiligo and 25 other diagnoses to consider when you see a white spot!

Breathnach, A. S., Fitzpatrick, T. B., and Wyllie, L. M. A.: Electron Microscopy of Melanocytes in Human Piebaldism. J. Invest. Derm., 45:28-37, 1965.
Absent or reduced in number.

Grupper, C., Prunieras, M., Hincky, M., and Garelly, E.: Albinism Partial Familial (Piebaldism): Etude ultrastructurale. Ann. Derm. Syph., 97:267-286, 1970.
Melanocytes replaced by Langerhans' cells.

Schaible, R. H.: Identification of Variegated and Piebald-Spotted Effects in Dominant Autosomal Mutants. *In* McGovern, V. J., and Russell, P. (Eds.): *Mechanisms in Pigmentation,* Vol. 1, S. Karger, New York, 1973, pp. 14-19.
Genetic jiujitsu to explain why nonpigmented areas of piebaldism may on occasion have amelanotic melanocytes.

Fitzpatrick, T. B., and Quevedo, W. C., Jr.: Biological Processes Underlying Melanin Pigmentation and Pigmentary Disorders. *In* Borrie, P. (Ed.): *Modern Trends in Dermatology,* Vol. 4, Appleton-Century-Crofts, New York, 1971, pp. 122-149.
Suggests that piebaldism is due to neural crest defect or unfavorable local milieu.

Maciejasz, A.: Long-Lasting Mydriasis After Atropine in Congenital Albinism. Klin. Oczna, *41*:431-433, 1971.
In normal, atropine effect lasts 10 days; in eye without melanin to bind drug and produce depot, effect lasts less than 2 days.

Falabella, R.: Epidermal Grafting. An Original Technique and Its Application to Achromic and Granulating Areas. Arch. Derm., *104*:592-600, 1971.
Epidermis removed by suction used as grafts on recipient site denuded by liquid nitrogen. Promising.

Allende, M. F.: The Enigmas of Pigmentation. J.A.M.A., *220*:1443-1447, 1972.
Sympathy, reassurance, good camouflaging advice will not perform miracles but will help.

20

Necrotizing Vasculitis

20

For the past seven years this middle-aged woman has had repeated attacks of **painful, necrotizing lesions of the shins.** *Results of extensive medical hospital studies were normal on two occasions. Previous attacks cleared following systemic steroid therapy.*

Biopsy — crusted ulcer, necrotic vessels with nuclear debris.

Necrotizing Vasculitis

You are looking at a cutaneous infarct. This is focal gangrene of the skin due to specific obliterative inflammation of the underlying small vessels. The excruciating pain, the deep necrosis, the archipelagic patterning all point to a destructive vasculitis. But it is the biopsy which provides the conclusive evidence.

And indeed it is the biopsy which has established the vital concept of cutaneous vasculitis. Although we are still in the nascent period of nosologic confusion, we do realize that any number of clinical reaction patterns in the skin may result from specific vascular damage to vessels of varying size and location. Thus, a vasculitic process in the dermal papillae, if occlusive, may destroy the epidermis (toxic epidermal necrolysis) or, if hemorrhagic, may lead to petechiae and purpura (pigmented purpuric eruptions, Henoch-Schönlein). Another form may account for capillary leakage (chronic urticaria, erythema perstans). A more severe occlusive change in the larger vessels is necrotizing, i.e., it induces the gangrene (ulceration, scarring) we see in this patient. When deeper or even larger vessels are involved, inflammatory nodular lesions occur (erythema nodosum, nodular vasculitis). And in a more chronic form, we may see strange rare painful plaques (erythema elevatum diutinum).

It is not surprising that the concept has been long aborning, since the pathologist has but fleeting, peripheral glances at the vasculitis itself. He sees but a sample of the total clinical lesion, often of inadequate size and depth, and taken at an indeterminate time during the varying dynamic sequence of this process. Add to this the fact that all inflammatory diseases in the skin produce nonspecific vascular changes. But despite all

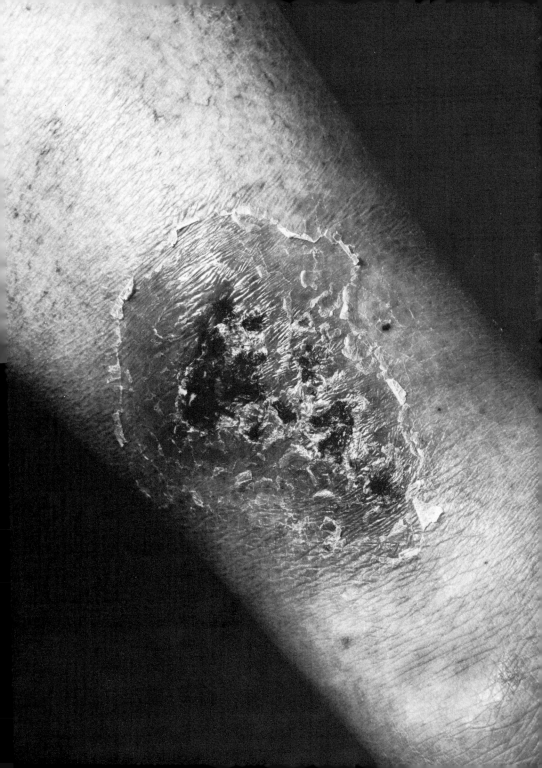

this, the pathologist does clearly discern primary microangiopathy in the skin, and this patient's problem exemplifies one of its few well-defined classes, namely, necrotizing vasculitis.

This type of angiitis is leukocytoclastic, that is, the vessel-wall changes of necrosis are associated with marked infiltration of polymorphonuclear leukocytes which in turn are rapidly destroyed. This remarkable leukocytoclasia leaves only nuclear remnants, at times only nuclear dust. Although the necrotic vessels usually defy precise anatomic identification, the primary site of the leukocyte involvement appears to be in the capillaries and veins, not the arterioles. The leukocytoclastic aspect is evident on routine slides; to learn more, immunofluorescent techniques must be employed.

It is with these new techniques that necrotizing vasculitis was found to be allergic. It is now generally assumed that vasculitis is an immune antigen-antibody complex disease, since immunoglobulins, at times complement and on rare occasions even antigen can be demonstrated in the involved sites. Presumably, in these patients, circulating antigen-antibody complex is deposited in vessels at sites of injury — thermal, mechanical or chemical. This in turn sets off a train of events reminiscent of the Shwartzman reaction, with leukocyte invasion and local necrosis. Certainly the localization of our patient's lesions is at the site of repeated physical injury — over the shins.

But what is the antigen? We don't know, since necrotizing vasculitis is but a reaction pattern. We do know that streptococcal as well as candidal antigens have been tagged in this type of vasculitis reaction. And we know that skin tests to bacterial antigens can clinically reproduce the disease, but generally such tests are not helpful unless histologically monitored for the presence of a primary vasculitis. One can suspect streptococci from the pharynx or Candida from the gut entering the blood stream to induce antibodies and form vasculitis-inducing complexes. All of this still remains tentative and shadowy. The globulins and the bacterial antigens observed in the vascular lesions may have been deposited fortuitously, and their only guilt is that by association. Yet we do know that bacterial infections elsewhere in the body can initiate necrotizing vasculitis at sites of cutaneous trauma. Drugs are another potential antigen. Penicillin, thiazides and even aspirin must be under suspicion as a cause. The heterogeneity of antigen sources is remarkable and underscores the need for hospitalization again for thorough search for malignant disease, autoimmune disease, dysproteinemias and focal infections. Necrotizing vasculitis can be another of the tantalizing cutaneous signs of internal disease.

But what to do for this patient in whom we find no underlying cause? First and foremost is bed rest. The legs must be elevated to aid the blood flow and prevent further sludging and immune-complex deposition. Secondly, the black hemorrhagic crusts must be compressed round the clock with open compresses containing Burow's solution until they can be gently debrided or soaked away. They are no ordinary crusts but rather a tenacious eschar with necrobiotic strands of collagen mooring them down. But they must be removed, since they can harbor bacterial flora capable of triggering even more leukocytoclasia and necrosis.

Another primary need is for a good general systemic antibiotic. Empirically, this is of value even though it may have to be chosen blindly. We favor erythromycin, ampicillin or Avlosulfon, provided that there is no evidence of drug sensitivity. And for just this latter reason we would avoid analgesics, sedatives, tranquilizers, mouthwashes, lozenges and the dozens of casual antigen contacts patients make every day. Systemic steroids are helpful and may be used if our patient's problem worsens. Immunosuppressive drugs are also of value but are generally reserved for the widespread intractable examples of vasculitis.

It is evident that cutaneous infarcts, like myocardial ones, can be serious and require bed rest as well as hospitalization.

Winkelmann R. K., and Ditto, W. B.: Cutaneous and Visceral Syndromes of Necrotizing or "Allergic" Angiitis: A Study of 38 Cases. Medicine, *43*:59-89, 1964.
Splendid introduction to recondite area: destructive immune reactions within walls of blood vessels.

Copeman, P. W. M., and Ryan, T. J.: The Problems of Classification of Cutaneous Angiitis with Reference to Histopathology and Pathogenesis. Brit. J. Derm., *82(Suppl. 5)*:2-14, 1970.
A confusion of classifications.

Moschella, S. L.: The Clinical Significance of Necrosis of the Skin. Med. Clin. N. Amer., *53*:259-274, 1969.
Fifty-six causes for your differential.

Groth, O., Lindemark, C. O., and Sjöberg, S. G.: Necrotizing Angiitis with Multiple Widespread Hemorrhagic Infarctive Lesions of the Skin. Acta Med. Scand., *180*:565-570, 1966.
Drug induced.

Desser, K. B., Santiano, G. P., and Cooper, J. L.: Lupus Livedo and Cutaneous Infarction. Angiology, *20*:261-261, 1969.
Cold induced.

Pevny, I., and Metz, J.: Positiver Intracutantest, Fern- und Aufflammphanomen mit Streptokokken—Antigen bei Vasculitis Allergica. Hautarzt, 23:350-353, 1972.
Bacteria induced.

Cox, A. J.: Pathologic Changes in Hypersensitivity Angiitis. *In* Helwig, E. B., and Mostofi, F. K.: *The Skin.* Williams & Wilkins Co., Baltimore, 1971, pp. 279- 292.
Not simply perivascular lymphocytic infiltrate or endothelial cell proliferation; must see fibrinoid deposits, necrosis and polymorphonuclear leukocytes within walls.

Copeman, P. W. M.: Investigations Into the Pathogenesis of Acute Cutaneous Angiitis. Brit. J. Derm., 82(Suppl. 5):51-65, 1970.
Localization by injury; caused by sludging out of immune complexes in capillaries and veins.

Copeman, P. W. M., and Ryan, T. J.: Cutaneous Angiitis Patterns of Rashes Explained by (1) Flow Properties of Blood, (2) Anatomical Disposition of Vessels. Brit. J. Derm., 85:205-214, 1971.
Inflammatory processes occur in slower flowing, relatively ischemic venous end of circulation.

Schroeter, A. L., Copeman, P. W. M., Jordon, R. E., Sams, W. M., Jr., and Winkelmann, R. K.: Immunofluorescence of Cutaneous Vasculitis Associated with Systemic Disease. Arch. Derm., 104:254-259, 1971.
May see immunoglobulin G and complement in vessel wall.

Parish, W. E.: Studies on Vasculitis. Clin. Allerg., 1:97-121, 1971.
And now the intralesional demonstration of antigens (streptococcal, candidal) which may form vasculitis-inducing antigen-antibody complexes.

Cunliffe, W. J., and Menon, I. S.: The Association Between Cutaneous Vasculitis and Decreased Blood Fibrinolytic Activity. Brit. J. Derm., 84:99-105, 1971.
Drugs which enhance fibrinolysis helpful, e.g., phenformin.

Borrie, P., and Stansfeld, A.: Cutaneous Vasculitis. *In* MacKenna, R. M. B. (Ed.): *Modern Trends in Dermatology*, Vol. 3, Butterworths, London, 1966, pp. 167-195.
Rx: corticosteroids, skin grafting, even amputation.

Skinner, M. D., and Schwartz, R. S.: Immunosuppressive Therapy. New Eng. J. Med., 287:221-227, 281-286; 1972.
Detailed review on an area of therapeutic promise for vasculitis.

Kauppinen, K.: Cutaneous Reactions to Drugs with Special Reference to Severe Bullous Mucocutaneous Eruptions and Sulfonamides. Acta Dermatovener., 52:Suppl. 68:1-89, 1972.
Cautious oral challenge as a way of identifying drug sensitivity. A classic.

21

Poikiloderma Atrophicans Vasculare

21

*For the past few years, this 69-year-old woman has had **large plaques of mottled, atrophic skin over her upper arms, chest and neck.** In some areas telangiectasia is present, in others a mild scaly lichenification, but all are pruritic. Two hospitalizations for complete review failed to reveal systemic disease.*

Multiple skin biopsies — nonspecific inflammatory changes.

Poikiloderma Atrophicans Vasculare

This is the dermatitis of aliases. It has been named, renamed, and re-renamed, only to be named over again.

The simplest label for this woman's problem is an old descriptive one — poikiloderma atrophicans vasculare. Poikiloderma, from the Greek for mottled skin, certainly describes the pattern of pigmentation seen. The atrophic element is evidenced by the fine wrinkling and the vascular change is one of telangiectasis, best appreciated by close inspection of the patient's skin itself.

Like opera, the diagnosis sounds better in a foreign language, but what does it mean? Actually, poikiloderma atrophicans vasculare is a rare reaction pattern we may see in a variety of settings. It is the hallmark of chronic radiodermatitis. It can be a component of systemic lupus erythematosus and is commonly an element of dermatomyositis. Most importantly, it can be the clinical portrait of the cutaneous lymphoma, mycosis fungoides. All these have been ruled out by careful study of this patient. There is no history of radiation exposure, the tests for systemic lupus are negative, and the patient denies any muscle weakness or pain. Repeated skin biopsies failed to show any evidence of lymphoma. And yet, our patient's problem is closely related to this latter problem, for we have come to recognize that these mottled atrophic vascular lesions are prelymphomatous.

Our patient, thus, has a premalignant, prereticulotic, premycotic dermatosis. And the swirl of synonymy continues, this change being known also as parapsoriasis. But it is a special poikilodermatous type.

The parapsoriasis family has had a long and complex etymologic history. But today there are only two surviving members, a benign form and this premalignant one. The benign type, parapsoriasis en plaques, looks somewhat like pityriasis rosea, but persists for years, even decades, despite attention or even inattention. No doubt it was parapsoriasis en plaques that inspired the bon mot, "They never get well, and they never die."

Our patient has the other form, the premalignant form. The lesions are also plaques but here they are large, in sharp contrast to the multiple small discrete lesions in the benign type. It has thus been called

large plaque type of parapsoriasis,
atrophic parapsoriasis.
poikiloderma vasculare atrophicans,
prereticulotic poikiloderma,

or, as we like to straddle-term it, poikilodermic parapsoriasis. Somehow, the distinction between this prelymphomatous type and the benign type must be maintained if we are to avoid a Tower of Babel.

The premalignant form usually involves the major flexures, the buttocks and, in women, the breasts. Exquisitely chronic, the process may remain unchanged for 20 or even 30 years. On occasion the patches may extend to virtually encompass the trunk and extremities with mottled erythematous skin, showing slight wrinkling. Scaling is minimal and pruritus variable. The histologic features are not dramatic, some round cells invading the epidermis from a mild subepidermal infiltrate of lymphocytes and reticular cells.

We have stressed that this poikiloderma atrophicans vasculare or poikilodermic parapsoriasis is prelymphomatous, but usually the patient dies with this disease rather than because of it. Its potential to become frankly malignant is small, 1 chance in 20. It can behave like the actinic keratosis that never becomes a squamous cell epithelioma. Our patient's allotted life span may allow her to see only this mottled, slightly atrophic reddened skin, never its ultimate conversion to malignant lymphoma. This suggests to us that her immune defenses achieve a lifelong homeostasis with a latent lymphoma.

Nothing should be done to shift the balance of power in favor of the invader. Rather, provide reassurance and whatever mild emollient creams, general guidance and annual reviews that seem indicated. Sunlight, ultraviolet light or grenz-ray therapy may be of significant help. If the pruritus increases, or there is any infiltrative clinical change, biopsy should be repeated for evidence of the malignant infiltrate of a

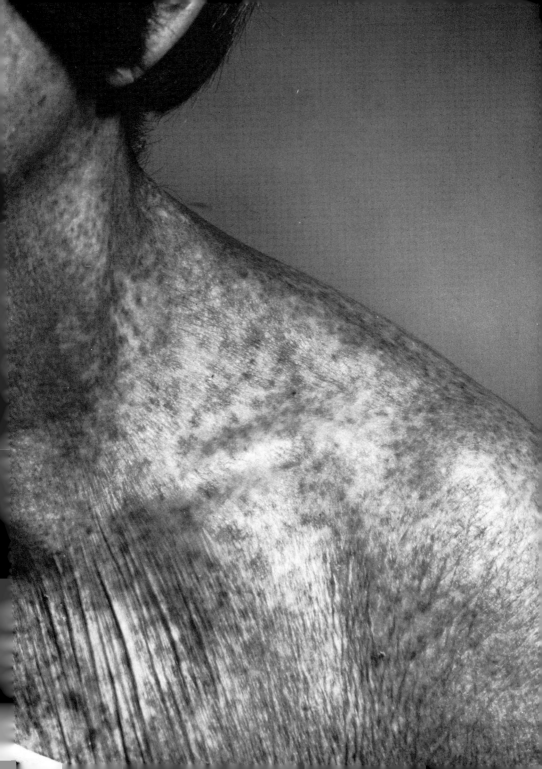

lymphoma. If such evidence is present, intensive treatment with topical nitrogen mustard can be most beneficial.

And remember that poikiloderma atrophicans vasculare by any other name deserves the same careful lifelong attention.

Samman, P. D.: The Natural History of Parapsoriasis en Plaques (Chronic Superficial Dermatitis) and Prereticulotic Poikiloderma. Brit. J. Derm., *87*:405-411, 1972.
Poikiloderma atrophicans vasculare (prereticulotic poikiloderma, large plaque type of parapsoriasis en plaques, atrophic parapsoriasis or lichenoid parapsoriasis) may rarely evolve into malignant cutaneous lymphoma (mycosis fungoides) or leukemia.

Dowling, G. B., and Freudenthal, W.: Dermatomyositis and Poikiloderma Atrophicans Vascularis: A Clinical and Histological Comparison. Brit. J. Derm., *50*:519-539, 1938.
Poikiloderma atrophicans vasculare: mottled hypo- and hyperpigmentation, with atrophy, telangiectasia and preceding scaly lichenoid papules.

Keil, H.: Parapsoriasis en Plaques Disséminées and Incipient Mycosis Fungoides. Arch. Derm., *37*:465-494, 1938.
Parapsoriasis en plaques: patches of dermatitis on trunk and extremities, showing an indifference to treatment and lasting for decades.

Pinkus, H., and Mehregan, A. H.: *A Guide to Dermatohistopathology.* Appleton-Century-Crofts, New York, 1969, pp. 180-181.
Poikiloderma atrophicans vasculare patterning appears in parapsoriasis (plaque, lichenoid or retiform), mycosis fungoides, dermatomyositis, lupus erythematosus, sunlight damage (Civatte's disease), congenital disorders (Thomson's syndrome) and x-ray dermatitis.

Mishima, Y., and Rudner, E.: Erythromelanosis follicularis faciei et colli. Dermatologica, *132*:269-287, 1966.
Has poikilodermatous features.

Nekam, L.: *Corpus Iconum Morborum Cutaneorum.* Barth Verlag, Leipzig, 1938, 3 vols.
Invaluable rogues' gallery of 4566 photographs. Poikiloderma section on pp. 563-571.

Woolfson, H., and McQueen, A.: Poikiloderma Atrophicans Vasculare Associated with Muscular Dystrophy. Arch. Derm., *107*:115-117, 1973.
Facioscapulohumeral syndrome, Marfan's syndrome and poikiloderma atrophicans vasculare all in one boy.

Good, R. A.: Relations Between Immunity and Malignancy. Proc. Nat. Acad. Sci., *69*:1026-1032, 1972.
Surveys the immunologic barrier to malignancy. 95 references.

Van Scott, E. J., and Winters, P. L.: Responses of Mycosis Fungoides to Intensive External Treatment with Nitrogen Mustard. Arch. Derm., *102*:507-514, 1970.
Complete clinical and histologic remission of plaque stage in majority of instances.

Wolf, D. J., and Selmanowitz, V. J.: Poikiloderma Vasculare Atrophicans. Cancer, *25*:682-686, 1970.
Poikiloderma vasculare atrophicans of 30 years' duration in a 74-year-old patient: exquisitely detailed study revealed no evidence of reticulosis, lymphoma or connective tissue disorder.

22

This young girl has shown keratotic growths since infancy. Manifested in the first few weeks of life as **subungual thickening,** *this hyperkeratosis later became evident as discrete acuminate horny excrescences on the knees and elbows. After she began to walk, sharply circumscribed thick* **calluses and corns with underlying deep bullae** *appeared and have persisted precisely at the pressure points on her soles. At present the buttocks, posterior thighs and palms show numerous* **follicular hyperkeratoses and cutaneous horns.** *Leukokeratotic changes are present on the palate and lower lip. She also exhibits hyperhidrosis of the palms and soles.*

She is an only child and there is no history of consanguinity nor any nail or skin problems in the past three generations.

Pachyonychia Congenita

This child was born with the gene for claws and horns! An extremely rare event, it has been recorded in the world's medical annals less than a hundred times. This is pachyonychia congenita, a genodermatosis. It is one in which the inheritance pathway can be singularly well studied, since the gene marker of thickened nails is fully apparent to all. And the pathway has proved to be an autosomal dominant one, traced in some instances for over six generations. In our patient, however, the syndrome has sprung full blown, de novo, and we assume a mysterious mutation has occurred.

What can we make of this hoof, nail and follicle disorder? The unifying theme is hyperkeratinization in response to physical stress. This is a pressure keratoderma, named for the first site to be affected, the nail bed. This is a disease of the keratinocyte, the major cell of the epidermis, responsible for the elaboration of the protective and insoluble surface protein, keratin. It is one of controlled yet superabundant production of stratum corneum. Clinically, it is initiated in the crib with simple acts such as scratching. The nail plate pull serves as a stimulus to the hyponychium to overproduce keratin. The result is a nail plate lifted high by subungual keratin. As might be expected, all of 20 nails are involved. Secondarily, the nail plate becomes deformed, warped, twisted

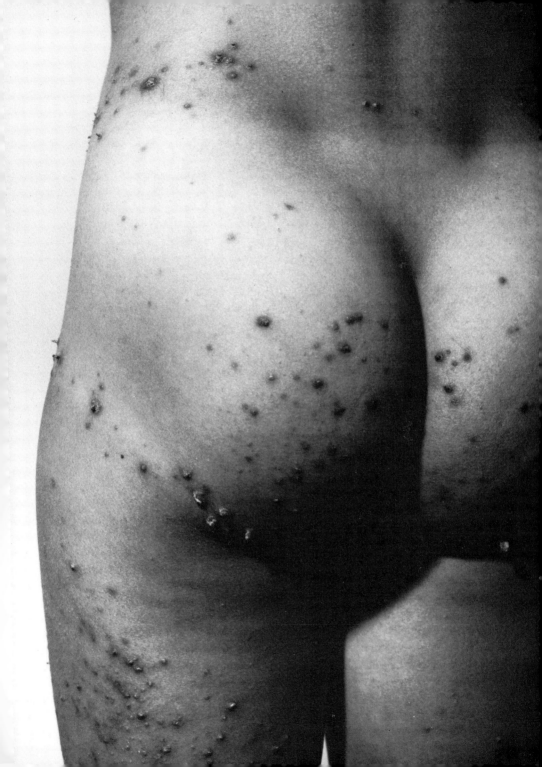

or abnormal as the keratin mass exerts an effect on the nail matrix. This is the thickened nail of pachyonychia—a very precise change, not just a thick nail.

As our infant grows, new points of trauma behave in an identical fashion, producing minarets of keratin at focal sites of follicular trauma. These are the giant magnified versions of keratosis pilaris, i.e., cutaneous horns. Even the leukokeratoses of the mucosa record the tendency to keratinize excessively. In early infancy these may be confused with thrush until the total picture is realized, and the scrapings for mycelia are repeatedly unsuccessful. We should be aware, incidentally, that pachyonychia congenita is a mucocutaneous genodermatosis inasmuch as the nasal, laryngeal, corneal, vaginal and rectal mucosa may be similarly involved. Probably the fact that some of these affected infants are born with a few fully erupted teeth is also relevant to an altered keratinizing potential.

The most dramatic change, however, comes with walking. The consequent pressure on relatively few plantar sites induces enormous calluses of keratin on the soles. Understandably, these can literally shear away the epidermal attachments to the dermis when she runs. It is this that is responsible for the sublesional bullae of the soles. These are not the lesions of epidermolysis bullosa despite a superficial resemblance. The calluses and corns of her feet reflect the intermittent pressures exerted there and not a local defect, since skin from elsewhere grafted to the sole has been shown to produce the same massive keratin growths. Her entire epidermis has, as it were, the capabilities of producing "keloids" of keratin.

A great deal can be done to help this child, although we can do nothing to reverse the mutant gene or to prevent its transmission to any children she might have. We can help because we know that her problem is triggered by pressure and physical trauma. It cannot be overemphasized that the keratin growths serve as a vicious self-perpetuating mechanism. The rubbing of any keratotic excrescence or simply sitting on a cutaneous horn provides a selective stimulus for even greater keratinocyte activity. The little become big, and the big grow larger. This self-amplification of lesions is nowhere better shown than on the feet, once localized thickenings occur at the normal pressure points, the entire body weight is virtually transferred to these alone, with progressive keratodermic growth and inevitable consequence. Her feet need our initial attention to break this vicious cycle. Moreover, the bullae which have followed are a source of painful disability and, because of her hyperhidrosis, can easily become infected. Special shoes should be made for her which have a latex molded sole to reduce pressure on the callused areas and to distribute the weight more evenly. Regular shaving of excess keratin as a part of good podiatric care is essential.

The keratinous horns elsewhere can be suppressed by topical retinoic acid (Retin-A) applied daily. Salicylic acid, if used in restricted areas, is also valuable for removal of the horny growths. We find that a liquid preparation 15 parts salicylic acid, 80 parts ethyl alcohol and 5 parts propylene glycol is also well tolerated and effective, especially if applied under Saran Wrap. The feet may be safely treated each night with 60 per cent propylene glycol in water, likewise applied under Saran Wrap. This aids in debridement of the excess keratin. The thickened nails can be treated similarly but are less responsive. Regular cutting of the nails after prolonged soaking is best done with large professional nail clippers. We are reminded by this that Jadassohn, who first described this syndrome at the turn of the century, had to use a hammer and chisel on the hardened nails of his patient.

A few patients may require plastic surgical excision of the entire matrix and nail bed to achieve permanent total removal of the nail. This is certainly preferable to yielding to the patient who pleads for amputation of his finger tips as a way to be rid of his grotesque, misshapen, painful and at times infected nails. Others who develop massive chronic ulcers at the sites of bullae on their feet may require grafting.

Be aware of the fact that, although this is a birth defect, it is not a neurocutaneous one. It does not involve the melanocyte and hence is not associated with neurologic problems or mental retardation. Also, it should be recognized that the lesions are not premalignant, not even the leukokeratotic ones. Confusion has arisen in this regard, since the diffuse keratodermas of the palms and soles may be associated with mucosal carcinoma, particularly in the esophagus. Pachyonychia congenita is a focal punctate keratoderma and is not premalignant.

Pachyonychia congenita is a remarkable experiment of nature from which we should learn much more about the keratinocyte and how it responds to physical forces. For this is truly a piezo-keratoderma.

Moldenhauer, E., and Ernst, K.: Das Jadassohn-Lewandowsky Syndrom. Hautarzt, *10*:441-447, 1968.
World literature describes only 93 cases of pachyonychia congenita: pachyonychia in

90 of these; keratoderma of sole, 67, and of palm, 44: oral leukokeratosis, 50; bullae, 35; hyperhidrosis, 22; sparse thin hair, 11; premature dentition, 11; granulosis rubra nasi, 4.

Akesson, H. O.: Pachyonychia Congenita in Six Generations. Hereditas, *58*:103-110, 1967.
Dominant autosomal transmission revealed in detailed survey of 18 cases in 6 generations.

Velasquez, J. P., and Bustamante, J.: Sebocystomatosis with Congenital Pachyonychia. Int. J. Derm., *11*:77-81, 1972.
A complication not really evident until puberty.

McKusick, V. A.: *Mendelian Inheritance in Man. Catalogs of Autosomal Dominant, Autosomal Recessive and X-linked Phenotypes.* 3rd ed. Johns Hopkins Press, Baltimore, 1971.
Invaluable for keeping up to date on cutaneous genetic syndromes.

Videbaek, A.: Hereditary Onychogryphosis. Ann. Eugenics, *14*:139-141, 1948.
Not to be confused with pachyonychia congenita; develops late in childhood, involves only a few digits, skin and hair normal.

Dubowitz, V., Cooke, P., Colver, D., and Harris, F.: Mental Retardation, Unusual Facies and Abnormal Nails Associated with a Group-G Ring Chromosome. J. Med. Genet., *8*:195-201, 1971.
Nail changes limited to pachyonychia and shedding of great toe nails.

Lucas, G. L., and Opitz, J. M.: The Nail-Patella Syndrome. J. Pediat., *68*:273-288, 1966.
These dystrophic nails suggest presence of potentially fatal renal disease!

Baden, H. P.: The Physical Properties of Nail. J. Invest. Derm., *55*:115-122, 1970.
In human nail, γ type keratin aligned perpendicularly to growth axis; in claw, orientation is parallel.

Robson, J. R. K., and El-Tahawi, H. D.: Hardness of Human Nail as an Index of Nutritional Status: A Preliminary Communication. Brit. J. Nutr., *26*:233-236, 1971.
Nails from malnourished children much harder than normal as shown by Knoop test with diamond indentor.

Hashimoto, K.: Ultrastructure of the Human Toe Nail Cell Migration, Keratinization and Formation of the Intercellular Cement. Arch. Derm. Forsch., *240*:1-22, 1970.
Shows how substances may pass through nail by way of a maze of ultra-microintercellular channels.

Logan, W. S.: Vitamin A and Keratinization. Arch. Derm., *105*:748-753, 1972.
Lack of vitamin A produces generalized hyperkeratosis with follicular keratinous plugging: phrynoderma. 68 references.

Kuokkanen, K.: Replica Reflection of Normal Skin and of Skin with Disturbed Keratinization. Acta Dermatovener., *52*:205-210, 1972.
Magnificently detailed silicone rubber replicas, useful for objective evaluation of therapy.

Garb, J.: Pachyonychia Congenita Regression of Plantar Lesions on Patients Wearing Specially Made Rubber Base Foot Molds and Shoes. Arch. Derm., *62*:117-124, 1950.
Res ipsa loquitur.

Gunther, S.: Vitamin A Acid in the Treatment of Palmoplantar Keratoderma. Clinical Investigations and Experimental Results with 13 Patients. Arch. Derm., *106*:854-857, 1972.
All improved when using 0.1 per cent retinoic acid in petroleum jelly.

Rosten, M.: The Treatment of Ichthyosis and Hyperkeratotic Conditions with Urea. Aust. J. Derm., *11*:142-144, 1970.
Ten cases of hyperkeratosis of hands and feet: good results with 10 per cent urea cream.

Goldsmith, L. A., and Baden, H. P.: Propylene Glycol with Occlusion for Treatment of Ichthyosis. J.A.M.A., *220*:579-580, 1972.
Four cases of keratosis palmaris et plantaris responding to 60 per cent propylene glycol in water, under Saran Wrap occlusion.

Chowdhury, S. R. D., and Banerjee, A. K.: Sodium Laevothyroxine in Pachyonychia Congenita. J. Indian Med. Assoc., *51*:246-248, 1968.
Thyroid therapy associated with temporary alleviation.

Hadida, M. E., Sayag, J., Marill, F. G., and Timsit, E.: Pachyonychia congenitale avec keratodermie et keratoses disseminée de la peau et des muqueuses. Bull. Soc. Franc. Derm. Syph., *76*:411-412, 1969.
Vitamin A in large dosage helpful.

Cosman, B., Symonds, F. C., Jr., and Crikelair, G. F.: Plastic Surgery in Pachyonychia Congenita and Other Dyskeratoses. Case Report and Review of Literature. Plast. Reconstr. Surg., *33*:226-236, 1964.
May have to totally remove nail bed and matrix; graft plantar ulcers.

Austin, R. T.: A Method of Excision of the Germinal Matrix. Proc. Roy. Soc. Med., *63*:757-758, 1970.
How to remove a nail — permanently.

23

*This 17 year old has had **oval brown atrophic plaques of his lower back** and abdomen for the past year. Gradually increasing in number, they are asymptomatic, noninflammatory and without induration.*

Biopsy—epidermis shows an increase in melanin; dermis is atrophic with normal elastic tissue.

Atrophoderma (Pasini-Pierini)

Here is a disease for the aficionados of dermatologic curiosa. Rare and mysterious, it is a slow, insidious disappearance of the dermis in localized patches. The skin sinks down into plateaus, with but the mark of melaninism to dramatize this atrophy.

We can describe this atrophoderma but only in a hollow way that gives no insight into its mystery. We know it begins usually in the late teens or early twenties, nearly always on the back, at times in a seemingly metameric patterning. It is asymptomatic, but it continues to extend with the appearance of new areas of pigment and a deepening of the earlier depressions, even to the point of unveiling the deep large blue venous channels. Years later, it stops as quietly as it began. But the atrophic imprint remains, essentially for life. It will not respond to treatment. It has no medical antecedents, counterparts or markers, and gives no augury of other disease.

Many observers have tried to dismiss it all as an atrophic form of morphea. But it is not such circumscribed scleroderma despite the fleeting pigmentary and atrophic resemblance. It is not indurated at any time, and histologically it is purely an atrophy of the dermis, exhibiting none of the hyalinization of the collagen typical of scleroderma. The diagnostic lilac ring of morphea is also absent. Nor is our patient's problem one of the macular atrophies, also known as anetodermas. All these lack both pigmentation and elastic tissue, the latter accounting for the wrinkling and herniation of such lesions, never seen in the atrophoderma of Pasini and Pierini. Furthermore, it is not a nevoid atrophoderma, diffuse, nonprogressive and appearing at birth. It stands alone as

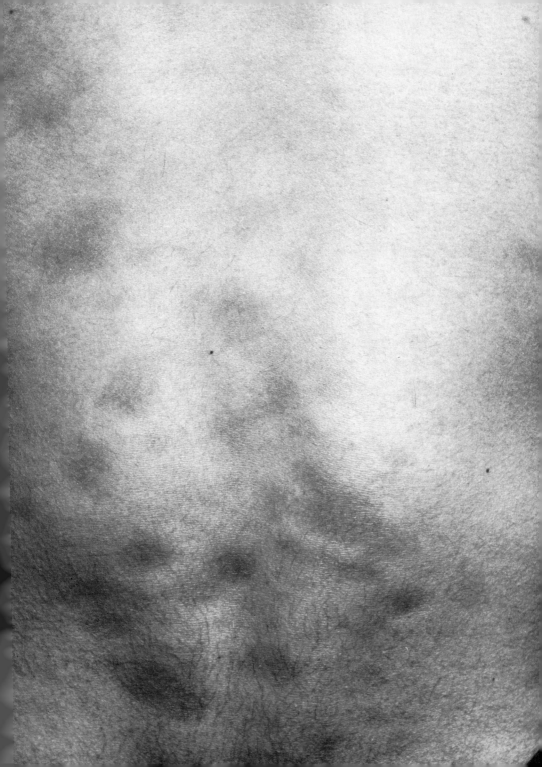

a true entity, described and recognizable, although largely in a negative atrophic sort of way.

Few problems are as baffling and as poorly defined. We cannot say what has happened. We still lack knowledge of the forces that maintain the dimensions of the dermis, since collagen turnover is so extremely slow. We can suspect a relationship to morphea and lichen sclerosus atrophicus and to neural influences, since isolated cases reports provide possible linkages. But the answer remains with tomorrow.

It should be explained to this patient that his chronic ailment will persist indefinitely, but that it is benign, nonhereditable and noncontagious. It is not premalignant, and not a sign of internal disease. Accordingly, he should treat it with the indifference accorded a cosmetic defect.

But for us, it still remains a hallmark of ignorance.

Pierini, L. E., Abulafia, J., and Mosto, S. J.: Atrophodermie Idiopathique Progressive et Etats Voisins. Ann. Derm. Syph., 97:391-416, 1970.
  Circular oval brown to bluish asymptomatic depressions on thorax, beginning ages 13 to 28, progressive, self-limited, permanent, idiopathic, rare; distinguish from nevoid atrophoderma and atrophic scleroderma.

Jablonska, S., and Szczepanski, A.: Atrophoderma Pasini-Pierini: Is It An Entity? Dermatologica, 125:226-242, 1962.
  Yes.

Canizares, O., Sacks, P. M., Jaimovich, L., and Torres, V. M.: Idiopathic Atrophoderma of Pasini and Pierini. Arch. Derm., 77:42-60, 1958.
  First American report clearly separates process from morphea. Details 5 cases.

Miller, R. F.: Idiopathic Atrophoderma. Report of a Case and Nosologic Study. Arch. Derm., 92:653-660, 1965.
  Feels it is abortive atypical form of morphea.

Szczepanski, A.: Atrophoderma Pasini-Pierini Coexisting with Circumscribed Scleroderma in the Light of Clinical Observations and Skin Function Tests. Przegl. Derm., 57:631-636, 1970.
  Describes morphea occurring in association with Pasini-Pierini atrophoderma, both at the same and different sites.

Stevanovic, D. V.: Primary Atrophoderma Associated with Hemiatrophy, Essential Telangiectasie Lichen Sclerosus and Tumor of the Skull. Arch. Derm. Forsch., 243: 255-264, 1972.
  Relates tumor of skull, hemiatrophy, Pasini-Pierini atrophoderma, and lichen sclerosus et atrophicus all in one patient.

Pinkus, H., and Mehregan, A. H.: *A Guide to Dermatohistopathology.* Appleton-Century-Crofts, New York, 1969, p. 281.
  Biopsy specimen must include adjacent normal skin, since atrophy of dermis only finding.

Grant, M. E., and Prockop, D. J.: The Biosynthesis of Collagen. New Eng. J. Med., *286*:194-199, 242-249, 291-299; 1972.
The best modern review on how the collagen of the dermis is put together...

Nordwig, A.: Collagenolytic Enzymes. *In* Nord, F. F. (Ed.): *Advances in Enzymology,* Vol. 34, Interscience Publishers, New York, 1971, pp. 155-205.
...and a review on how it can be taken apart.

24

For ten years this man has had a chronic eczematous dermatitis of the face, neck and dorsa of his hands. General medical and dermatologic studies, including patch-testing, scrapings and porphyrin surveys of blood and urine, have been normal. Biopsies showed nonspecific dermatitis.

Two years ago, photo-patch-testing revealed a marked eczematous reaction at the ultraviolet light-irradiated test sites for bithionol and trichlorocarbanilide, as well as for a variety of antiseptic soaps and shampoos he had been using. The nonirradiated patch-test sites showed no change.

Avoidance of all antiseptic-containing materials, use of a para-aminobenzoic acid sun screen, and administration of systemic steroids were followed by improvement, but **plaques of infiltrated eczematous skin remain on the cheeks and hands.**

Photosensitivity

Most people are afraid of the dark. Here is a man who has to be afraid of the light! He is allergic to it. Specifically he has become sensitized to the invisible part of light, the ultraviolet rays. The sun at high noon can cripple and disable him. Even ordinary fluorescent lighting has the terror of poison ivy for him. Only complete and total darkness protects him.

His problem is not an error in metabolism, such as in one of the porphyrias. Nor is his skin photosensitive as a result of a genetic incapability in repairing sunlight damage, as in xeroderma pigmentosum. Nor does he have a skin disease such as lupus erythematosus which shows sensitivity to sunlight. On the contrary, he has acquired a photosensitivity as a result of using soaps, shampoos and creams containing a phenolic germicide, bithionol. He has an immune delayed hypersensitivity, an ordinary contact dermatitis to bithionol, but with the striking exception that it can be triggered only by ultraviolet light. It is thus a *photo-contact dermatitis*, occurring in all the areas exposed to both bithionol and sun. It is completely reproducible in unexposed areas by patch-testing with bithionol and irradiating the site. Bithionol alone or ultraviolet light alone is without effect.

146

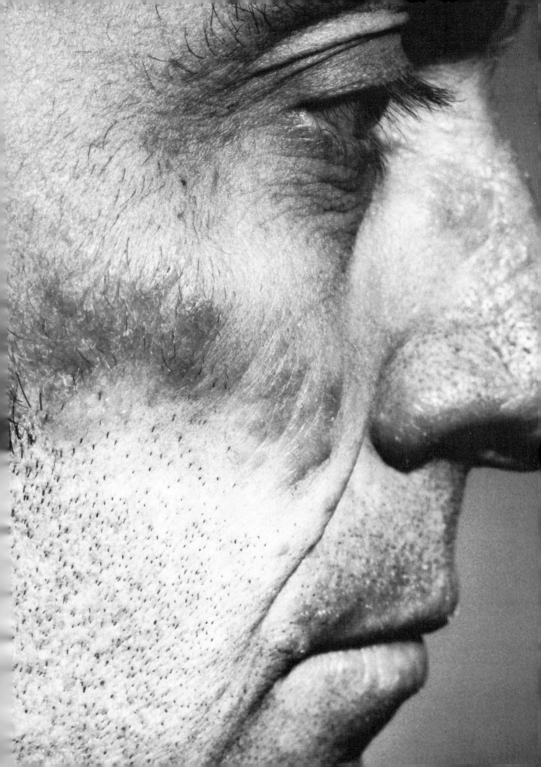

His problem becomes less simplistic when it is realized that congeners of bithionol such as trichlorocarbanilides are also photo-contact allergens for him. But this is the analogue of cross sensitivity so commonly observed in classic contact dermatitis, and chemically unrelated compounds are totally without this photosensitizing effect.

More surprising is the fact that our patient still has his photodermatitis despite the fact that he has had no known contact with bithionol or related germicides for a full two years. He has thus become a *persistent light reactor*. Ordinarily, removal of a contact allergen is followed by cure, but avoidance of the photo-contact allergen, to the best of this patient's ability, has strangely not been curative. There are several explanations to be considered. Despite no external contact with bithionol, traces may remain in the skin. He may have become cross sensitized to other photoallergens such as ragweed, oils in the skins of citrus fruits, furocoumarins in perfumes, tars in our polluted air or even sun screens. He may even be exposed unknowingly to photosensitizers such as phenothiazines which appear in insecticides and have served as an antioxidant in oils. The world abounds in hidden hazards for this man. Moreover, we have not been able to remove him from the sea of light which bathes us all. Sun screens are still screens, not doors of oak, and we know that the long ultraviolet rays follow us indoors through the windows, even though the rays of the sunburn spectrum cannot. Even more disturbing, inadvertent exposures to fluorescent lights are a daily event.

But there is a third level of complexity, for not only has our patient a proved photo-contact dermatitis and a persistent light reactivity, despite avoidance of bithionol and related phenylphenols, he now also has the clinical patterning of *polymorphous light eruption*. In other words, only certain plaques of skin are reactive, not the entire sun-exposed area. These may be the sites of maximal ultraviolet light challenge or areas of residual photo-allergen. In any event, as you see at this time he no longer has an eruption over the total area of exposure, as seen in simple photo-contact dermatitis.

Although photo-testing is the *sine-qua-non* diagnostic maneuver, there must first be a clinical awareness of photosensitivity. The clinical appearance is deceptive, simply that of an eczematous contact dermatitis and the biopsy repeats this with its epidermal vesiculation, spongiosis and nonspecific inflammatory infiltrate in the dermis. The clue comes from observing that the areas of involvement are those that are exposed to light—his face and neck and the dorsa of the hands. Areas "in the shade," e.g., the upper eyelids and the subnasal and submental zones, are spared. Significant involvement of heavily clothed sites would have shed doubt on the diagnosis.

Yet despite all our insight, this patient's problem remains. Its management requires not only insight but an infinite meticulous attention to detail. First, the avoidance of photo-contact allergens must be absolute. Injunctions against bithionol or salicylanilide are largely academic, since these have disappeared from the cosmetic market. It was the salicylanilide germicidal soaps that launched 10,000 cases of photo-contact allergy in England alone, but now they have come and gone to a large degree. Even hexachlorophene, one of the contact photosensitizers, and cyclamate, a systemic photosensitizer, are under the wraps of prescription use only. But in their stead are still more of the related phenylphenol derivates. Our patient must thus avoid all antibacterial, germicidal medicated shampoos, soaps, shaving creams and sprays. He must not use dispenser soaps at work, in rest rooms or on trips. Everything is suspect. His cosmetic life must be ascetic. He cannot use pre-shave or after-shave lotions, colognes, hair tonics, perfumed deodorants or antiperspirants.

He must not handle limes, figs, citrus fruits or dyes such as eosin, neutral red or fluorescein. Any fluorescent chemicals can be his undoing, since it is the chemicals that absorb radiation that cause photo-allergy. He should avoid contact with buckwheat, ragweed and celery (pink rot). He should be alert to other hidden hazards as in insecticides, fungicides and antioxidants and should avoid these.

Inasmuch as photosensitivity can reflect internal as well as external photo-allergens, our patient must be instructed to avoid drugs in general. In particular, he should not take thiazides, phenothiazines, dimethylchlorotetracycline, nalidixic acid and griseofulvin, since all these are known to be potentially dangerous in terms of photosensitivity. Alcohol should be avoided, since it is a hepatotoxin and could be associated with the formation of metabolic photosensitizers.

The other side of the therapeutic coin is the avoidance of that invisible band of ultraviolet light of from 300 to 400 nm. He cannot see or sense it so he must simply avoid light. Going outdoors only in the early and late hours of the day, walking on the shady side of the street and being fully clothed, wearing hat and gloves, are his rules. He must never work in a room illuminated with fluorescent light. Any compromise is a ticket to years of chronicity for his photodermatitis. However, only one of our patients achieved the true ideal, by becoming a coal miner.

An inert blocking sun screen is the best that can be prescribed for the unclothed sites. We recommend RVPlus, containing red petrolatum, titanium dioxide and mica. His photodermatitic skin of ten years should be protected from the potential sensitizing agents (e.g., cinnamates) of the more complex sun screens.

Topical and systemic steroids are helpful, but only in a temporary way, and their use must be judiciously geared to specific need for suppression of the immune reaction.

One can see in photo-contact dermatitis the methodology for reproducing a disease with a doublet of causes. In what disorder will we find the algorithm for analyzing a triplet of causes?

Epstein, J. H.: Adverse Cutaneous Reactions to the Sun. *In* Malkinson, F. D., and Pearson, R. W. (Eds.): Yearbook of Dermatology 1971. Year Book Medical Publishers, Chicago, 1971, pp. 5-43.
Cutaneous photobiological reactions produced largely by mid-ultraviolet spectrum, 290 to 320 nm.; photosensitivity reactions, by long ultraviolet, 320 to 400 nm. Introductory survey, 192 references.

Pathak, M. A., and Epstein, J. H.: Normal and Abnormal Reactions of Man to Light. *In* Fitzpatrick, T. B., et al. (Eds.): Dermatology in General Medicine. McGraw-Hill Book Co., New York, 1971, pp. 977-1036.
Biophysics and biochemistry of reactions due to light alone or light in conjunction with exogenous chemical, metabolite or skin disease. Monographic, 506 references.

Epstein, J. H.: Photoallergy—A Review. Arch. Derm., *106*:741-748, 1972.
Most important contact photosensitizing agents are halogenated salicylanilides and related antibacterial and antifungal compounds.

Jillson, O. F., and Baughman, R. D.: Contact Photodermatitis from Bithionol. Arch. Derm., *88*:409-418, 1963.
The phenolic germicide of soaps and shampoos, bithionol, can induce eczema precisely limited to areas exposed to ultraviolet light; reproducible by photo-patch-testing; may persist for years.

Adams, R. M.: Photoallergic Contact Dermatitis to Chloro-2-phenylphenol. Arch. Derm., *106*:711-714, 1972.
Bithionol, halogenated salicylanilides, hexachlorophene, dichlorophene and this new germicide are only known photo-allergens in phenol class.

Herman, P. S., and Sams, W. M., Jr.: Soap Photodermatitis: Photosensitivity to Halogenated Salicylanilides. Charles C Thomas, Springfield, Illinois, 1972.
A monograph on the strange story of skin sensitivity due to soap and sun.

Epstein, J., Wuepper, K., and Maibach, H. L.: Photocontact Dermatitis to Halogenated Salicylanilides and Related Compounds. A Clinical and Histological Review of 26 Patients. Arch. Derm., *97*:236-244, 1968.
Twenty patients: 11 were photosensitive to bithionol; 6 became persistent light reactors in absence of further exposure to photo-allergen; 3 developed polymorphous light eruption.

Willis, I., and Kligman, A. M.: The Mechanism of the Persistent Light Reactor. J. Invest. Derm., *51*:385-394, 1968.
Persistence can be due to inability of body to destroy and eliminate photoallergen.

Magnus, I. A.: Photobiology in Relation to Dermatology. *In* Borrie, P. (Ed.): *Modern Trends in Dermatology,* Vol. 4, Appleton-Century-Crofts, New York, 1971.
Persistence can be due to irradiation from fluorescent lights.

Frain-Bell, W., Mackenzie, L. A., and Witham, E.: Chronic Polymorphic Light Eruption (A Study of 25 Cases). Brit. J. Derm., *81*:885-896, 1969.
Shows spotty response unlike uniform involvement of exposed skin in photo-contact dermatitis.

Epstein, S., Enta, T., and Mehregan, A. H.: Photoallergic Contact Dermatitis from Antiseptic Soaps. A Histologic Study. Dermatologica, *136*:457-476, 1968.
Nonspecific eczematous patterning, identical to that in contact dermatitis.

Castrow, F., II, and Owens, D. W.: Office Screening for Photosensitivity. Texas Med., *68*:112-114, 1972.
Practical details on equipment, procedures, interpretation of photo-setting.

Gardiner, J. S., Dickson, A., Macleod, T. M., and Frain-Bell, W.: The Investigation of Photocontact Dermatitis in a Dye Manufacturing Process. Brit. J. Derm., *86*:264-271, 1972.
Phototoxic contact sensitivity to anthraquinone dye not reproduced until testing was done with visible light.

Willis, I., and Kligman, A. M.: Diagnosis of Photosensitization Reactions by the Scotch Tape Provocative Patch Test. J. Invest. Derm., *51*:116-119, 1968.
Stripping stratum corneum greatly enhances the sensitivity of photo-patch-testing by increasing the penetration of both light and drug into the living portions of the skin.

Harber, L. C., and Baer, R. L.: Pathogenic Mechanisms of Drug Induced Photosensitivity. J. Invest. Derm., *58*:327-342, 1972.
Contact photo-allergy is a form of cell-mediated hypersensitivity identical to ordinary contact allergy except for the requirement of light.

Alani, M. D.: Studies on the Induction of Allergic Photodermatitis in Newborn Guinea Pigs. Acta Allerg., *27*:50-54, 1972.
Newborns, unlike adults, cannot be photo-contact sensitized.

Herman, P. S., and Sams, W. M., Jr.: Requirement for Carrier Protein in Salicylanilide Sensitivity: The Migration-Inhibition Test in Contact Photoallergy. J. Lab. Clin. Med., *77*:572-579, 1971.
Salicylanilide acts as photo-allergen, inhibiting migration of sensitized cells only if chemically bound to albumin as result of irradiation.

Horkay, I., and Meszaros, C.: A Study on Lymphocyte Transformation in Light Dermatoses. Acta Dermatovener., *51*:268-270, 1971.
Positive photolymphocyte transformation test characteristic of polymorphous light eruption.

Bickers, D. R., and Harber, L. C.: Diagnosis and Treatment of Selected Photodermatoses. Postgrad. Med., *52*:Nov., 65-71, 1972.

Sun screens include absorbing agents (para-aminobenzoic acid and esters, cinnamates, salicylates, benzophenones) and blocking agents (red petrolatum, titanium dioxide). Systemics include aminoquinolines (antimalarials) and psoralens.

Torosian, G., and Lemberger, M. A.: O-T-C Sunscreen and Suntan Products. J. Amer. Pharm. Assoc., *12*:571-575, 1972.

Details on 52 choices facing consumer.

Fusaro, R. M., Runge, W. J., and Johnson, J. A.: Protection Against Light Sensitivity with Dihydroxyacetone/Naphthoquinone. Int. J. Derm., *11*:64-70, 1972.

Helpful in 51 of 77 patients, polymorphic light eruption.

Herd, J., Sturrock, I., and Frain-Bell, W.: The Use of Plastic Material for the Protection of Patients with Severe Photodermatoses. Brit. J. Derm., *88*:283-285, 1973.

Yellow plastic shades for windows to screen out ultraviolet rays but not visible light.

Swanbeck, G., and Wennersten, G.: Treatment of Polymorphous Light Eruptions with Beta-Carotene. Acta Dermatovener., *52*:462-466, 1972.

The latest: an oral dose of 100 mg. daily increases light tolerance by factor of five.

25

Varicella

25

For four days this 62-year-old man has had a generalized vesicular eruption. **Residual hemorrhagic crusted lesions of varying size remain on the trunk** *and extremities, as well as on the face and scalp. He has been receiving melphalan daily for four years for the treatment of multiple myeloma. For the past two months, hospitalized for severe back pain, he has been receiving cyclophosphamide, prednisone, procarbazine and blood transfusions, as well as radiotherapy to the spine.*

A Tzanck smear of the base of a fresh vesicular lesion showed numerous multinucleated giant cells.

Varicella

You are looking at a medical oddity—chickenpox in an adult. Normally the immunity acquired during everyone's childhood attack of chickenpox is sufficient to give a lifetime of absolute protection against a second attack. Even when that immunity falters with aging, the varicella virus can induce disease only from the privileged protected environ of the neuron. It is there that this same virus can reappear to cause herpes zoster.

But this man is different. His immune resistance has been ravaged by his malignant disease, by the steroid and immunosuppressant drugs and possibly by the radiotherapy. Hence, at this point the virus has re-emerged from its latent state or has been introduced again by inadvertent exposure, e.g., to a zoster patient in his hospital setting. He now has not zoster but chickenpox for a second time. It is so unusual that some observers call it an atypical generalized zoster, but it is simply chickenpox. It is the disease of the debilitated. It is the sign of the compromised immune system.

We recognize it by its vesicular element, its distribution and the clinical scene. We confirm it by the Tzanck smear of the base of a fresh lesion. It is here we see on Giemsa stain the characteristic giant multinucleate cells of the herpes virus group (simplex, varicella and zoster). A biopsy offers little more than the sight of these same DNA viruses

154

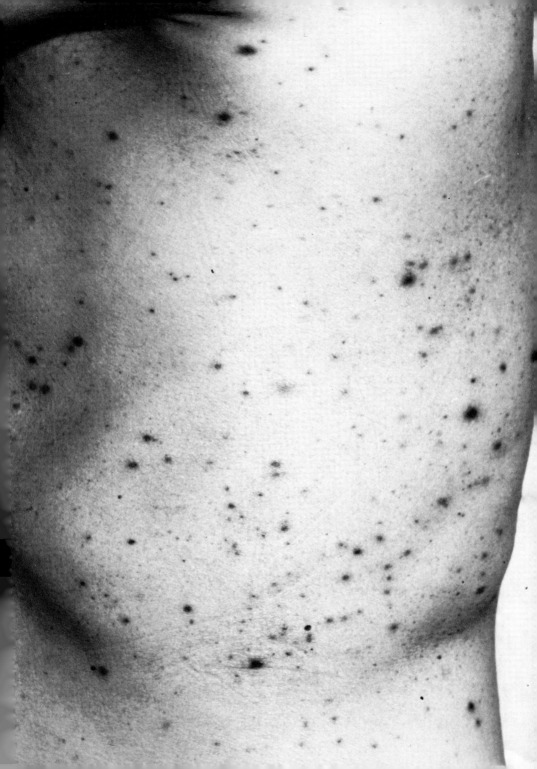

growing as intranuclear viral inclusion bodies. Had we access to electron microscopy we could see the distinctive 100 nm. icosahedral viral particles themselves in the vesicle fluid or crust. Had we used gel precipitin techniques we could specifically identify the virus as varicella. And should we go to tissue culture, confirmatory evidence could be forthcoming by showing the destructive effects of growth of the virus in human embryonic fibroblasts. Finally, serum complement-fixation antibody studies should show a low titer consistent with his depressed immune status. In this regard skin-testing these patients with dinitrochlorobenzene (DNCB) fails to elicit the normal sensitization as seen in patients with zoster.

This patient should be watched closely for complications, the mild eruption itself not posing a major problem, either diagnostically or therapeutically. Pneumonia is perhaps the most frequent of these, occurring 15 to 25 per cent of the time. Cough, dyspnea and cyanosis alert one to the need for roentgen screening for pulmonary infiltrates. In these instances, the sputa may also reveal telltale inclusion bodies. Much less common are inflammatory changes clinically referable to the heart, liver and kidney, but these may become evident as well as thrombocytopenia and rare thromboembolic phenomena.

Treatment of the skin lesions should be low key. A drying lotion or just tincture of time should suffice. This varicella is but a rock in the foothills of this patient's medical problems with myeloma. If pneumonia or systemic signs of varicella supervene — and this is a virus which can infect any organ or system — one can consider the popular yet unproved cytosine arabinoside therapy. This is given in a surge intravenous daily dose of 100 to 150 mg. per square meter of body surface, for just three or four days. Delayed effects of hematopoietic suppression, e.g., thrombocytopenia, may be seen, so that the procedure is not innocuous.

Hyperimmune serum is of no help at this stage but it should be remembered that in any case of known exposure of a high-risk patient, a single injection of zoster immune globulin (ZIG) is valuable prophylactically. This ZIG is prepared from the blood of donors who have had zoster within the past five weeks and is available from the U.S.P.H.S. Center for Disease Control, Atlanta, Georgia.

Varicella is just one of the growing number of cutaneous viral diseases of childhood which reappear in the patients whose immune barriers are being knocked down by disease and immunosuppressants. We will see them more often in the years to come.

Schimpff, S., Serpick, A., Stoler, B., Rumack, B., Mellin, H., Joseph, J. M., and Block, J.: Varicella-Zoster Infection in Patients with Cancer. Ann. Intern. Med., 76:241-254, 1972.

Six adult cases: no antecedent zoster, widespread lesions, no crops, cutaneous anergy to DNCB, often Hodgkin's disease in background.

Triebwasser, J. H., Harris, R. E., Bryant, R. E., and Rhoades, E. R.: Varicella Pneumonia in Adults. Report of Seven Cases and a Review of the Literature. Medicine, 46:409-423, 1967.

Most frequent and most severe of complications of varicella in adult.

Brunton, F. J., and Moore, M. E.: A Survey of Pulmonary Calcification Following Adult Chicken-pox. Brit. J. Radiol., 42:256-259, 1969.

Think varicella, not T.b. — 16,191 people surveyed: 463 had had adult chickenpox, 8 had residual pulmonary calcific deposits.

Taylor-Robertson, D., and Caunt, A. E.: *Varicella Virus.* Springer-Verlag, New York, 1972, 88 pp.

An exhaustive source of virologic, clinical, experimental and therapeutic data.

Juel-Jensen, B. E., and MacCallum, F. O.: Herpes Simplex Varicella and Zoster. J. B. Lippincott Co., Philadelphia, 1972, 194 pp.

Another splendid new monographic source book.

Park, R. K., Goltz, R. W., and Carey, T. B.: Unusual Cutaneous Infections Associated with Immunosuppressive Therapy. Arch. Derm., 95:345-350, 1967.

Chronic recurrent isolated varicella lesions in one patient.

Merigan, T. C., Waddell, D., Grossman, M., Ritchie, J. H., and Mo, G.: Modified Skin Lesions During Concurrent Varicella and Measles Infections. J.A.M.A., 204:333-335, 1968.

Halo around each varicella lesion, spared by rubeola rash.

Naveh, Y., and Friedman, A.: Transient Circumscribed Hypertrichosis Following Chickenpox. Pediatrics, 50:487-488, 1972.

Patches of temporary hair growth around residual scars in 6-month-old patient.

Charkes, N. D.: Purpuric Chickenpox: Report of a Case, Review of the Literature, and Classification by Clinical Features. Ann. Intern. Med., 54:745-759, 1961.

Due to vascular damage; even arterial thrombosis can occur.

Glick, N., Levin, S., and Nelson, K.: Recurrent Pulmonary Infarction in Adult Chickenpox Pneumonia. J.A.M.A., 222:173-177, 1972.

Result of thrombi in vessels showing endothelial damage by varicella virus.

Geeves, R. B., Lindsay, D. A., and Robertson, T. I.: Varicella Pneumonia in Pregnancy with Varicella Neonatorum: Report of a Case Followed by Severe Digital Clubbing. Aust. N. Z. J. Med., 1:63-68, 1971.

Pneumonia-induced circulatory change responsible for clubbing of all fingers and toes of mother. 55 references.

Griffith, J. F., Salam, M. V., and Adams, R. D.: The Nervous System Diseases Associated with Varicella. Acta Neurol. Scand., 46:279-300, 1970.

Strangely not due to direct viral invasion.

Thomas, M., and Robertson, W. J.: Dermal Transmission of Virus as a Cause of Shingles. Lancet, 2:1349-1350, 1971.

Zoster not invariably due to reactivation of latent virus; can follow dermal exposure to virus.

Stevenson, J., Hambling, M. H., and Bradshaw, D. B.: Collecting Vesicle Fluid. Brit. Med. J., *1*:181-182, 1972.
Use 30 needle and disposable tuberculin syringe, cap, tape and ship to lab.

Macrae, A. D., Field, A. M., McDonald, J. R., Meurisse, E. V., and Porter, A. A.: Laboratory Differential Diagnosis of Vesicular Skin Rashes. Lancet, *2*:313-316, 1969.
Electron microscopy best: disclosed herpes virus varicella in 31 of 32 instances of suspect chickenpox; precipitin antibody test positive in only 10 of 30; and culture in only 11 of 16.

Uduman, S. A., Gershon, A. A., and Brunell, P. A.: Rapid Diagnosis of Varicella-Zoster Infections by Agar-Gel Diffusion. J. Infect. Dis., *126*:193-195, 1972.
Specific; can use vesicular fluid or crusts.

Gold, E.: Serologic and Virus Isolation Studies of Patients with Varicella or Herpes-Zoster Infection. New Eng. J. Med., *274*:181-185, 1966.
Virus no longer present after third day.

Armstrong, R. W., Gurwith, M. J., Waddell, D., and Merigan, T. C.: Cutaneous Interferon Production in Patients with Hodgkin's Disease and Other Cancers Infected with Varicella or Vaccinia. New Eng. J. Med., *283*:1182-1187, 1970.
Greatly reduced.

Wallis, K., Gross, M., and Henczeg, E.: Varicella as the Cause of Death in an Infant Affected by Lymphopenic Thymic Dysplasia with Dysgammaglobulinemia. Acta Pediat. Scand., *61*:98-104, 1972.
Ordinarily benign, chickenpox is lethal in person without lymphocytes and gamma globulin.

Savage, M. O., Moosa, A., and Gordon, R. R.: Maternal Varicella Infection as a Cause of Fetal Malformations. Lancet, *1*:352-354, 1973.
Chickenpox joins German measles in posing serious teratogenic threat in first trimester of pregnancy!

Brunell, P. A., Gershon, A. A., Hughes, W. T., Riley, H. D., and Smith, J.: Prevention of Varicella in High Risk Children: A Collaborative Study. Pediatrics, *50*:718-722, 1972.
Zoster immune globulin (ZIG) given (5 ml. I. V.) within 48 hours of exposure will prevent or attenuate varicella.

Stevens, D. A., and Merigan, T. C.: Uncertain Role of Cytosine Arabinoside in Varicella Infection of Compromised Hosts. J. Pediat., *81*:562-565, 1972.
Cytosine arabinoside is used to treat varicella, but unless double-blind studies are done, efficacy remains in doubt.

Davis, C. M., Van Dersarl, J. V., and Coltman, C. A.: Failure of Cytarabine in Varicella-Zoster Infections. J.A.M.A., *224*:122-123, 1973.
Cytosine arabinoside used under double-blind protocol failed to prevent dissemination of herpes zoster.

Davis, C. M.: Modern Management of Cutaneous Viral Infections. Postgrad. Med., *52*(Nov.):109-114, 1972.
Treatment of chickenpox is symptomatic: drying lotions, flexible collodion, cool oatmeal baths, sedation with antihistamines.

26

Lichen Sclerosus et Atrophicus

26

Twenty-one years ago this 56-year-old woman developed a pruritic white band at the site of an episiotomy. This extended to involve the vulvar and perianal areas. Gradually through the years pruritic white atrophic areas have appeared on her trunk, as well as at points of obvious trauma on her hips, buttocks and shins. Here, on her thigh, a typical **shiny white plaque** *is seen, with atrophy evident in the crinkly surface. Its irregular border is* **fringed by a purplish inflammatory zone.** *Oral chloroquine and topical fluorinated steroid creams under occlusion have provided the greatest help.*

Biopsy — epidermal atrophy, subepidermal edema, hyalinized collagen.

Lichen Sclerosus et Atrophicus

Few dermatoses have a more distinctive appearance and distribution than lichen sclerosus et atrophicus. And few are more mysterious from an etiologic standpoint. Here is a dermatosis almost invariably white and nearly always involving the genital area. But why?

The white is not merely the white of a loss of pigment, but the ivory or porcelain white of an atrophic translucent epithelium stretched over an edematous hyalinized corium. This is the white spot disease of primitive nosology. Basically, it begins as flat-topped papules, later melding into plaques with an inflammatory halo of erythema. Grossly, there is a hyperkeratotic surface, but more importantly there are focal follicular, poral and delled areas of keratin accumulation. Microscopically, edema in the dermis is so prominent at times as to virtually lift the epidermis away, initially producing pruritus from the stretch of the fine nerves subserving the epidermal itch organ. Later erosions may evolve in areas of friction. In other instances the vessels may be sheared, producing purpura and dramatic subepidermal hemorrhage. In the later atrophic period, telangiectasia may become evident in the white matrix of scarred collagen.

The genital localization is as remarkable as the white scarring. This is a disease of the vulva, the labia and the clitoris in over 95 per cent of all

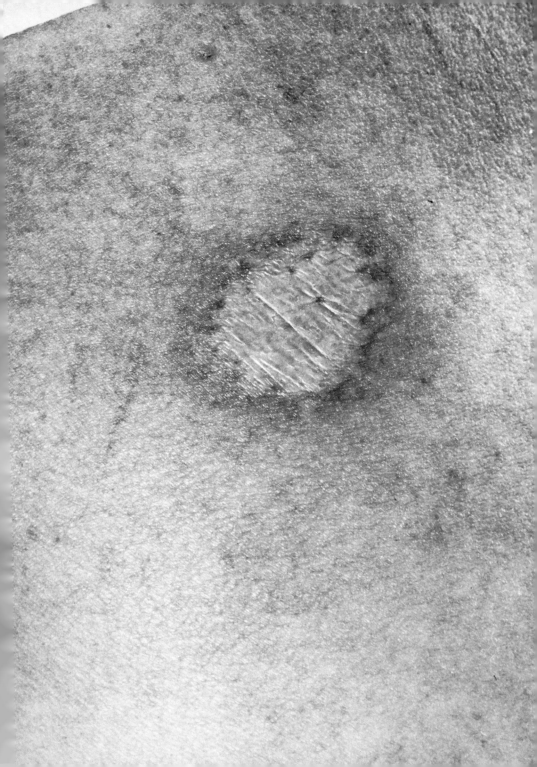

women affected. In at least half there is involvement of anal area as well, with the resultant double encirclement forming a dramatic topographic figure eight. Although lichen sclerosus et atrophicus is characteristically an atrophic disease of middle-aged women, it can occur at any age and in a small percentage of instances is seen in men and children as well. In the men, the same genital predilection is manifest in a localization of the lesions on the prepuce or glans penis. All this is reflected in an earlier name, balanitis xerotica obliterans, now simply a synonym for the male version of lichen sclerosus et atrophicus.

It is important to recognize that all the atrophic diseases of the vulva are not lichen sclerosus et atrophicus. There is a primary atrophy as well as an atrophy of aging, and at times lichen planus induces a dramatic atrophy in this area. Equally significant, recall that all that develops in the vulvar area of a lichen sclerosus et atrophicus patient is not the disease itself. These individuals are not immune to intertrigo, bacterial infections, candidiasis, trichomoniasis or the pruritus of diabetes. Indeed, these overlying problems can make the immediate diagnosis of any underlying lichen sclerosus virtually impossible. Although features of this disease remind one of morphea, vitiligo and lichen planus, lichen sclerosus et atrophicus is morphologically distinct. Indeed, we recognize that occasionally any one of these three may coexist with lichen sclerosus et atrophicus, a remarkable association of possibly more than chance significance.

We are singularly lacking in clues as to the nature of this rare disorder which in its scarred atrophic state remains for a lifetime. We know that lichen sclerosus et atrophicus does not herald any internal disease or disorder. We learn that histochemical stains, even electron microscopy, tell us nothing specific about the structureless acellular collagen gel of this atrophic skin. We are taunted by discouragingly few "genetic" glimpses — no family trees, only a few twigs of sibling incidence and one striking branch of a mother with the vulvar form and her son with penile lichen sclerosus et atrophicus. We are intrigued that mechanical injury can localize lesions as in this patient. We recognize a role for female hormones, in that lesions may disappear at puberty or first appear at menopause. Nonetheless, long decades of study of the natural history, the epidemiology and the gross and microscopic characteristics of lichen sclerosus et atrophicus gives us the comfort of recognition but not of understanding.

What is its natural history? What can be anticipated? Our patient's

21-year course attests to the benignity of the process. Yet, in the vulvar area it proves to be premalignant in about 1 in 20 patients. It is this area which must be repeatedly and regularly watched for the early signs of premalignant leukoplakia. Small foci of hyperkeratoses evolve and over the years can convert to squamous cell epithelioma. Such is the unusual but important avenue of change. The average woman shows simply a band of atrophic scar tissue which may be accompanied by a shriveling of the labia and clitoris as well as a contracture of the introitus. This latter may in part account for the dyspareunia experienced by some. Fusion of the labia minora may also occur. In the men, the same obliterative constricting change is to be expected, with a resultant phimosis or meatal stricture, depending on the site of involvement. In both women and men there is local atrophy and disappearance of sebum, sweat and mucous glands, accounting for the special adjectival terms in *kraurosis* vulvae and balanitis *xerotica* obliterans. Nearly all these changes are lifelong and unremitting, since, once the acute phase has passed, permanent scarring persists. But there is an exception. Lichen sclerosus et atrophicus of the vulva in young girls can be expected to involute or markedly improve at the menarche, suggesting an ameliorative hormonal change. Conversely, many women develop the disease at menopause, possibly owing to the loss of a critical protective estrogen. Thus, it is evident that prognosis is tempered by the sex and the age of the patient, as well as by the location of the lesions. What can be viewed with equanimity on this patient's thigh is watched with concern on her vulva.

Fluorinated topical steroids afford the patient the greatest symptomatic relief. In the genital area, however, they may lead to further atrophy and erosions if used indefinitely, and their use should therefore be carefully supervised. In some areas intralesional steriods are well worthwhile. Liquid nitrogen cryotherapy is another adjuvant of benefit.

Surgery is undertaken occasionally for plastic correction of a constricted vaginal or meatal orifice, or circumcision in the cases of phimosis. It is also the treatment of choice for any sequential leukoplakia or squamous cell epithelioma. But conservative removal of specific sites is always to be preferred to total radical vulvectomy, with its adverse psychologic and sexual effects. Every one of these patients needs not only annual review but a full awareness that changes or sores that remain for more than three weeks demand review forthwith. But in all instances, an unreasoning fear of cancer on the part of the patient or the physician is as much to be avoided as an ostrich-like indifference.

Wallace, H. J.: Lichen Sclerosus et Atrophicus. Trans. St. Johns Hosp. Derm. Soc., *57*:9-30, 1971.
Simply the best article ever written on the subject: a 20-year personal study of 395 patients.

Ridley, C. M.: A Review of the Recent Literature on Diseases of the Vulva. Brit. J. Derm., *86*:641-647, *87*:58-69; *87*:163-170, 1972.
Differential dermatologic diagnosis in the area most commonly affected by lichen sclerosus et atrophicus.

Klosterman, G. F., and Ipsen, V.: Vulva—Beteiligung bei Lichen Sclerosus. Hautarzt, *18*:529-532, 1967.
A closer look at this lesion in its home base where it can prelude dyspareunia, leukoplakia, and squamous cell carcinoma.

Stevanovic, D. V.: Annular, En Bande, and Plaque Lichen Sclerosus. Arch. Derm., *103*:226-228, 1971.
Variants.

Purres, J., and Krull, E. A.: Lichen Sclerosus et Atrophicus Involving the Palms. Arch. Derm., *104*:68-69, 1971.
Prefers anogenital area. May appear anywhere on skin or mucous membrane.

Apisarnthanarax, P., Osment, L. S., and Montes, L. F.: Extensive Lichen Sclerosus et Atrophicus in a 7-Year-Old Boy. Arch. Derm., *106*:94-96, 1972.
Rare; primarily a disease of women.

Gordon, W., Kahn, L. B., and Dove, J.: Lichen Sclerosus et Atrophicus and Scleroderma. S. A. Med. J., *46*:160-163, 1972.
May coexist with localized scleroderma.

Montgomery, H.: *Dermatopathology*. Harper & Row, New York, 1967, pp. 753-759.
L S & A means spotty hyperkeratosis, epidermal atrophy, subepidermal edema, and homogenized collagen.

Tagami, H.: Eosinophilic Infiltration in Lichen Sclerosus et Atrophicus. Arch. Derm., *105*:606-607, 1972.
Rare; associated with severe pruritus.

Whimster, I. W.: The Natural History of Skin Malignancy. Brit. J. Derm., *77*:534-535, 1965.
Lichen sclerosus skin excised from vulva, transplanted to thigh, became normal, and normal skin from thigh, grafted on vulvectomy wound, developed lichen sclerosus!

Pillsbury, D. M., and Shelley, W. B.: Intradermal Steroid Therapy: Hemorrhagic Lichen Sclerosus et Atrophicus. Arch. Derm., *87*:338-341, 1963.
Most effective therapy is corticosteroid, topical or intralesional.

Zderkiewicz, B.: Lichen Sclerosus et Atrophicus Hemorrhagicus Treated by a New Method. Przegl. Derm., *59*:55-59, 1972.
Freezing with ethyl chloride.

27

Henoch-Schönlein Purpura

27

For two weeks this 16-year-old girl has had ankle edema, as well as a **purpuric eruption of her legs**, *buttocks and arms. Her ankles and elbows have been very painful and she has had episodic emesis and epigastric pain. Yesterday she noted her urine was reddish-brown in color. One month ago she had a streptococcal pharyngitis.*

Urinalysis—proteinuria, red cell casts.

Roentgenogram—filling defects in terminal ileum.

Negative studies include coagulogram, blood cultures, L. E. preparations, antinuclear antibodies, protein electrophoresis.

Henoch-Schönlein Purpura

A delightfully easy diagnosis is made in this patient who has bleeding into her skin, arthralgia, visceral crises and gross hematuria. We readily recognize this as a sharply defined clinical constellation of signs and symptoms, described in part by Schönlein and later more fully by Henoch over a century ago. It remains a clinical disease for which there is no diagnostic laboratory test. But our delight in the ease of diagnosis is quickly replaced by dismay over our inability to determine its cause or to modify its course.

Interestingly, this disease is sighted on the two great radar nets of the body, the skin and the kidney. The skin with its vast surface area monitored continuously for sensory input, and inspected diurnally for defects, gives evidence of bleeding. And the same signal comes from the kidney, which provides a continuous product for frequent noninvasive laboratory sampling and analysis. Red cells are escaping from the fine capillaries, the sign of a coagulation or vascular defect. Once the normal coagulogram is obtained, it is evidence that the defect resides in the vessel. This is not a thrombocytopenic purpura, but one of vasculitis. A biopsy of the skin would show a leukocytoclastic type of inflammatory change in the small vessels. In the kidney, an inflammatory, at times destructive, process in the glomerular capillary produces a proliferative glomerulonephritis.

Such vascular wall damage is responsible for the edema as well as

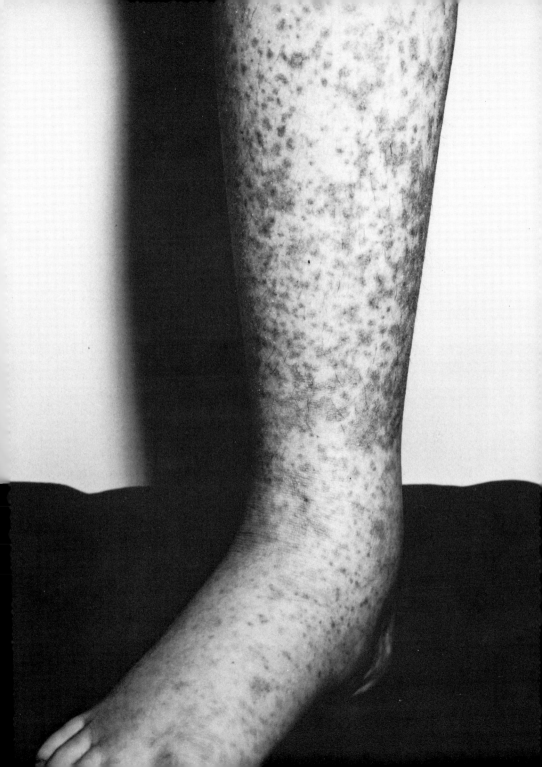

the proteinuria. Many of these patients have marked urticaria in addition to the purpura. As would be expected, the purpura and edema are most obvious in the dependent areas, the extremities and the buttocks, where the intraluminal pressures become greatest and leakage is most marked. Thus, in crib-bound infants, urticaria is often most pronounced over the scalp and may swell the eyelids to complete closure. Even the patterning of the purpuric areas on the leg reflects to a degree the uneven reticular patterning of the blood flow. Central nonpurpuric light areas correspond to the sites of rapid low venous pressure flow, whereas the slower sluggish high venous pressure flow results in extravasation of red cells which remain in the dermis for long periods. Not only dependency but cold and trauma are also critical determinants of the localization of purpura. Chilling slows the blood flow, and trauma damages vessel walls; both at times initiate urticarial and petechial episodes.

The vascular signs are not limited to the skin and kidney. Although probably widespread, they are regularly displayed in the joints and in the gastrointestinal tract. The joints ache, no doubt the result of the same inflammatory change in the synovium. Although the roentgenogram detects no change and there is no residual deformity, we suspect that inflammatory exudate and red cells are present within the joint cavity during the attacks. In the gastrointestinal tract the signs are more evident. The episodic colicky pain is associated with purpura on the inside and the outside of the bowel. Edematous swelling may be so marked as to reverse peristalsis and produce vomiting. It is also clearly visible on her roentgenogram. Extravasation of blood from the gut mucosa explains the positive tests for occult blood, hematochezia and melena. In youngsters hematomas within the bowel may lead to intussusception, and more severe vasculitis with thrombosis and necrosis results in a second reason for immediate surgical intervention, intestinal perforation.

The diagnosis is not always as simple as in this patient. At times the noncutaneous signs appear first and are thus confusing. In others, meningococcemia, lupus erythematosus, dysproteinemias, bacterial endocarditis, leukemias and hemorrhagic diseases may pose complex diagnostic problems which require careful laboratory and clinical study.

As to the cause, Henoch-Schönlein purpura has suffered more than its share of *post hoc ergo propter hoc* reasoning. Article after article up to the present day anecdotally names an antecedent drug, a food or an illness as a cause. Understandably, only a few patients have been challenged with these suspects, and to our knowledge none of the challenges has unequivocally reproduced the full syndrome. Rather, they have induced cutaneous purpura or urticaria, as with thiazides, milk or the yellow dye tartrazine. Similarly, there is no evidence that the streptococci of the commonly cited antecedent pharyngeal infection play any causal role. At this point, all we can say is that the picture is reminiscent of experimental circulating immune complex disease. Much more must be learned of the nature of vasculitis before the mystery is removed. Henoch-Schönlein is but one distinctive line in a spectrum of vasculitic disease. It is a spectrum which extends from the benign capillaritis of the peculiar progressive pigmentary disease of Schamberg to the necrotizing of larger vessels previously reviewed.

Treatment is based on the scout motto, "Be prepared." Know your patient and be prepared for the complications. Ordinarily this is a disease of kindergarteners and is as short lived as most of their infectious diseases. After several weeks of episodic petechiae, joint pain, colic and gross or microscopic hematuria, the syndrome vanishes as inexplicably as it came. During this period, systemic corticosteroids will relieve the pain and reduce the edema and urticaria, but there is no evidence that they do more. In some patients, dapsone appeared helpful. The purpura requires no attention, being a diagnostic sign, not a therapeutic problem. Be prepared for abdominal crises, recalling that in this patient intussusception and perforation are very unlikely, but thrombotic accidents do occur. The patient needs good general medical monitoring and close attention paid to new signs or symptoms.

But it is the kidney that requires the closest attention because of the serious functional effect of the focal necrotizing glomerulonephritis. It is the kidney which largely accounts for the 3 per cent mortality rate in this disease. The course can be assessed by urinalysis, blood studies, and even renal biopsy. But it cannot be altered by treatment, whether it be systemic corticosteroids or immunosuppressants. Even prolonged bed rest is of no help and poses the known harm of deep vein thrombosis and atrophy of muscle and bone, to say nothing of the stress of being removed from the normal social environment. Should there be months and years of renal crippling, supportive aid must be provided by the internist most experienced in this area.

Thus the acute changes of this patient's skin may portend chronic changes in her kidneys. Watch for them.

Silber, D. L.: Henoch-Schönlein Syndrome. Pediat. Clin. N. Amer., *19*:1061-1070, 1972.
Critical overview of a mysterious vasculitis involving skin, joints, G.I. tract and kidneys.

Cream, J. J., Gumpel, J. M., and Peachey, R. D. G.: Schönlein-Henoch Purpura in the Adult. A Study of 77 Adults with Anaphylactoid or Schönlein-Henoch Purpura. Quart. J. Med., *39*:461-484, 1970.
Superb clinical research on the purpura, arthralgia, diarrhea, hematuria syndrome in adults.

Meadow, S. R., Glasgow, E. F., White, R. H. R., Moncrieff, M. W., Cameron, J. S., and Ogg, C. S.: Schönlein-Henoch Nephritis. Quart. J. Med., *163*:241-258, 1972.
Definitive report. Renal biopsies from 88 patients: proliferative glomerulonephritis. Numerous crescents of glomerular sclerosis: poor prognosis.

Wolfert, R., and Beck, A. R.: Intussusception in Henoch-Schönlein's Purpura. Mt. Sinai J. Med., *39*:397-403, 1972.
Subserosal and submucosal purpura, common. Intussusception and perforation are rare.

Rodríguez-Erdmann, F., and Levitan, R.: Gastrointestinal and Roentgenological Manifestations of Henoch-Schönlein Purpura. Gastroenterology, *54*:260-264, 1968.
Edema of mucosa produces reversible "thumbprint" and pseudo-tumor filling defects, also seen in other hemorrhagic conditions.

Sahn, D. J., and Schwartz, A. D.: Schönlein-Henoch Syndrome: Observations on Some Atypical Clinical Presentations. Pediatrics, *49*:614-616, 1972.
Thirty-eight per cent incidence of testicular involvement in males.

Efstratopoulas, A. D., and Sdougou, J.: Ascites Due to Allergic Purpura. Lancet, *2*:168-169, 1971.
Preceded Henoch-Schönlein syndrome by 2 weeks.

Danemann, H. A., and Texter, E. C.: Adult Celiac Disease and Henoch-Schönlein Syndrome. Amer. J. Dig. Dis., *12*:939-946, 1967.
Henoch-Schönlein followed by gluten enteropathy!

Beard, M. E. J., and Taylor, D. J. E.: Renal Vein Thrombosis in Cases of Polyarteritis Nodosa and of the Henoch-Schönlein Syndrome. J. Clin. Path., *22*:395-400, 1969.
Induced by vasculitis of venous vasa vasorum.

Lewis, I. C., and Philpott, M. G.: Neurological Complications in the Schönlein-Henoch Syndrome. Arch. Dis. Child., *31*:369-371, 1956.
Subarachnoid hemorrhage in two cases.

Rogers, P. W., Bunn, S. M., Jr., Kurtzman, N. A., and White, M. G.: Schönlein-Henoch Syndrome Associated with Exposure to Cold. Arch. Intern Med., *128*:782-786, 1971.
Chilling seemed to provoke attacks in one case.

Copeman, P. W. M., and Ryan, T. J.: Cutaneous Angiitis Pattern of Rashes Explained by (1) Flow Properties of Blood (2) Anatomical Disposition of Vessels. Brit. J. Derm., *85*:205-214, 1971.
Cooling and dependency critical factors in localizing lesions by slowing blood flow.

Cream, J. J.: Cryoglobulins in Vasculitis. Clin. Exp. Immunol., *10*:117-126, 1972.
Are present, suggesting circulating immune globulins as cause.

Trygstad, C. W., and Stiehm, E. R.: Elevated Serum IgA Globulin in Anaphylactoid Purpura. Pediatrics, *47*:1023-1028, 1971.
In half of patients studied. Other immunoglobulins normal.

Ayoub, E. M., and Hoyer, J.: Anaphylactoid Purpura: Streptococcal Antibody Titers and β_{1C} Globulin Levels. J. Pediat., *75*:193-201, 1969.
No evidence for causal relation between group A streptococcal infection and Henoch-Schönlein syndrome.

Criep, L. H.: Allergic Vascular Purpura. J. Allerg. Clin. Immunol., *48*:7-12, 1971.
Purpura but not Henoch-Schönlein syndrome reproduced by challenge with tartrazine, a common yellow dye.

Lindenauer, S. M., and Tank, E. S.: Surgical Aspects of Henoch-Schönlein Purpura. Surgery, *59*:982-987, 1966.
Rare indications: intussusception and perforation.

Goldbloom, R. B., and Drummond, K. N.: Anaphylactoid Purpura with Massive Gastrointestinal Hemorrhage and Glomerulonephritis. An Unusual Case Treated Successfully with Azathioprine and Corticosteroids. Amer. J. Dis. Child., *116*:97-102, 1968.
Required 22 liters of blood!

Stremple, J. F., Polacek, M. A., and Ellison, E. H.: The Acute Non-Surgical Abdomen of Henoch-Schönlein syndrome in the Elderly Patient. Amer. J. Surg., *115*:870-873, 1968.
As in zoster, abdominal symptoms may precede cutaneous sign: treat conservatively.

Ashton, H., Frenk, E., and Stevenson, C. J.: The Management of Henoch-Schönlein Purpura. Brit. J. Derm., *85*:199-203, 1971.
Symptomatic.

28

*This 24-year-old man has sharply **circumscribed coin-shaped lesions** on his anterior thighs. Remarkably, they have reappeared each springtime in five of the last eight years, invariably clearing in the summer. He also gives a history of having had psoriasis and presents typical psoriatic pitting of all his finger nails.*

KOH examination of scales negative for hyphae.

Trichophytin skin test — no eczematous response.

Nummular Eczema

This is a "not" diagnosis.

— It is not tinea corporis, although clinically identical.

— It is not a pyoderma, although it may be heavily colonized by staphylococci.

— It is not atopic dermatitis, although atopic patches may be round.

— It is not psoriasis, although it has the same nummary plaques which can show central involution.

— It is not dry skin dermatitis, although it has a predilection for the same asteatotic extremities.

— It is not contact dermatitis, although in a nickel-sensitive patient contact with a nickel-containing coin could reproduce its appearance.

— It is not an id reaction, although stasis, fungal and seborrheic dermatitis each can induce distant lesions like this.

— It is not a dermatitis that fits into any nosologic niche other than its own, viz., nummular (coin-shaped) eczema (dermatitis).

Actually, nummular eczema is a familiar clinical picture, an authentic old portrait but of uncertain provenance. Known since 1857, it has a modest biography. We do know that it is a malady of adults, one that preferentially affects the low sweat, low sebum extensor surfaces of the legs and arms. It appears as round, or later, ring-shaped erythematous patches of a vesicular and papulovesicular nature. Crusting and scaling are common, and new lesions appear almost fully formed. The degree of involvement may vary from coin-shaped patches of depigmentation to exudative crusted lesions simulating the squamous cell epithelioma in

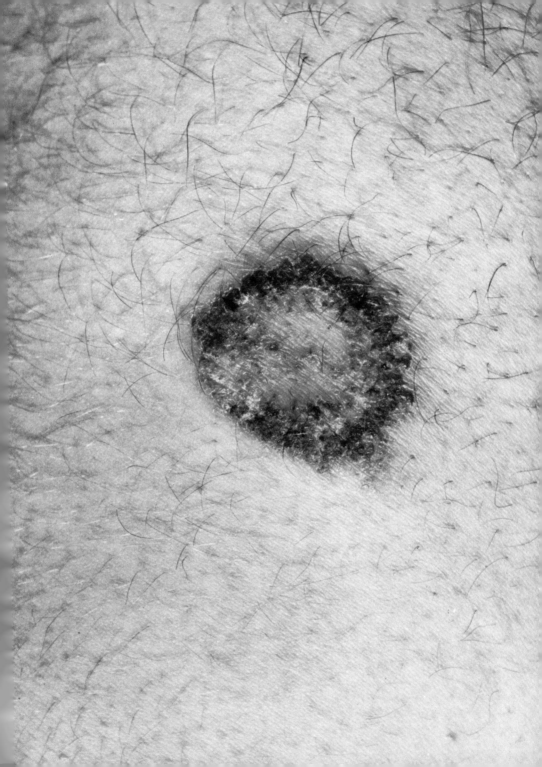

situ (Bowen's disease). It commonly comes in the winter, only to fade in the warmth of summer. Strangely, recurrences at precisely the same spot do occur. Pruritus is a variable finding, and the whole picture is commonly blurred by primary irritants, soaps and overtreatment. This is particularly true of the hands of housewives, in which case the process may present as a patchy eczematoid dermatitis.

Nummular eczema is a microvesicular eczematous process. Some observers feel that the epidermal change is secondary to a vasculitis seen histologically. Others view the microscopic picture as a blend of an eczema and psoriasis patterning.

Once the process is recognized, we are likely to pursue the practical therapeutic goals more vigorously than the investigative pathogenetic ones. We should, however, be able to rule out atopic dermatitis by the absence of a family or personal history of eczema in infancy, asthma or hay fever, as well as by the absence of flexural involvement. Drugs should be discontinued and foci of infection eliminated when possible. Should there be a history of heavy alcohol intake or stress, appropriate moderation is advisable. We have eliminated the likelihood of any fungus infection by multiple KOH examinations of scrapings. A trichophytid is equally unlikely in the presence of a negative eczematoid trichophytin test, but on occasion systemic griseofulvin is still indicated on a trial basis.

Crude coal tar and steroids are the indispensable topical aids in the care of this type of eczema. We have found an extemporaneous 3 per cent crude coal tar in Valisone cream helpful. In resistant cases, a few applications of tar paint (acetone 4, flexible collodion 4, crude coal tar q.s. ad 30) are often very effective. Vioform-hydrocortisone cream is a remedy of long-standing merit, and Cortisporin cream is equally effective for others. In extensive instances, generalized ultraviolet light serves a useful purpose, but it is not to be used in conjunction with the powerful photosensitizing tar paint. Generally, one should be certain that at least the patient's bedroom is humidified. The restricted use of soap and water is highly advisable to avoid overdrying of the skin. Caution the patient not to try to remove by scrubbing what he considers the "infection." A bland soap such as Neutrogena and a dispersible bath oil are welcome adjuvants. Finally, rough or woolen clothing should be interdicted.

We can search for a cause, but as detectives on this case we frankly admit that it is much more likely that we will restore the stolen goods than ever identify the thief.

Hellgren, L., and Mobacken, H.: Nummular Eczema—Clinical and Statistical Data. Acta Dermatovener., *49*:189-196, 1969.
A monumental study of 755 patients with coin- or ring-shaped dermatitis; most common on the legs of laborers in the winter.

Calnan, C. D.: Eczema for Me. Trans. St. Johns Hosp. Derm. Soc., *54*:54-64, 1968.
General background for understanding nummular eczema which may appear in the less tidy forms of large scallop-bordered plaques and scattered papulovesicles.

Rollins, T. G.: From Xerosis to Nummular Dermatitis. J.A.M.A., *206*:637-637, 1968.
Dry skin, an important etiologic factor in some instances.

Krueger, G. G., Kahn, G., Weston, W. L., and Mandel M. J.: IgE Levels in Nummular Eczema and Ichthyosis. Arch. Derm., *107*:56-58, 1973.
Nummular eczema patients do not have elevated IgE levels seen in atopic eczema.

Krogh, H. K.: Nummular Eczema. Its Relationship to Internal Foci of Infection. A Survey of 84 Case Records. Acta Dermatovener., *40*:114-126, 1960.
No clear relationship.

Graham, J. H., Marques, A. S., Johnson, W. C., and Gray, H. R.: Stasis Dermatitis. *In* Graham, J. H., et al. (Eds.): *Dermal Pathology.* Harper & Row, New York, 1972, pp. 333-361.
Nummular eczema shows primary vasculitis with secondary epidermal changes.

Pinkus, H., and Mehregan, A. H.: *A Guide to Dermatohistopathology.* Appleton-Century-Crofts, New York, 1969, pp. 118-119.
Nummular eczema combines eczematous and psoriasiform features.

Braun-Falco, O., and Petry, G.: Zur Feinstructur der Epidermis bei chronischem nummularen Ekzem. Arch. Klin. Exp. Derm., *222*:219-241, 1965.
Electron micrography reminiscent of psoriasis.

Fowle, L. P., and Rice, J. W.: Etiology of Nummular Eczema. Arch. Derm., *68*:69-79, 1953.
Nummular lesions heavily colonized by staphylococci.

Cowan, M. A.: Nummular Eczema. A Review, Follow-up and Analysis of a Series of 325 Cases. Acta Dermatovener., *41*:453-460, 1961.
Favors topical tar, steroids and x-ray for therapy.

29

*The right **axilla** and antecubital fossa of this 6-year-old boy have shown **yellowish, irregular, verrucous growths** since birth.*

Biopsy — vacuolization and hyperplasia of the epidermis as well as hyperkeratosis.

Epidermal Nevus

This is the lifelong mark of a tiny flaw in the genetic flow of information in this patient's embryonic ectoderm. What we see is the resultant malfeasant overgrowth of the epidermis. This rugose warty surface is not that of an epithelioma, but rather the result of an orderly programmed growth of an excessive number of fully differentiated and functional epidermal cells.

Warty, papillomatous, fimbriated, even cerebriform growths are always the outward sign of these epidermal nevi. Often linear, they may occur on an extremity or the neck, stretched out, as it were, from the initial ball of protoplasm (nevus unius lateris, systematized nevus). They may also involve the mucosa as well as the epidermis and on occasion are darkly pigmented owing to a related overgrowth of melanocytes.

All these are keratinocyte nevi, analogues of the common mole, the melanocytic nevus. There are many other siblings in this large family. Accordingly, one may see nevoid growths of any of the epidermal appendages, the vessels, the nerves, the connective tissue, and even the fat. Undoubtedly, such a spectrum of nevoid dysplasia occurs in many organs of the body, but only on the broad canvas of the skin is it so vivid and distinct.

The fimbriae of this boy's growths hauntingly suggest a grotesque exaggeration of epidermal ridging, hence, an epithelial process. But we must turn to the microscope for real understanding. And it is here that a most illuminating revelation occurs. This boy's lesion is not the ordinary epidermal nevus with just acanthosis, papillomatosis and elongated rete ridges. It has a unique hallmark of balloon cells — vacuolated keratinocytes in the mid and granular zones of the epidermis.

It is this histologic aberration which links this epidermal nevus with

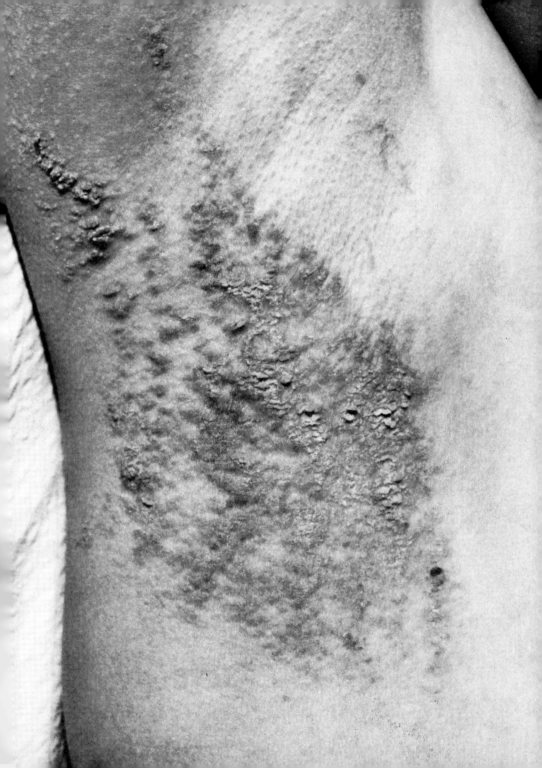

a rare congenital ichthyosiform process covering the entire body. In both there is an identical microscopic picture of vacuolated keratinocytes, i.e., epidermolysis. Even more dramatic is the fact that in both there are serried rows of fimbriate epidermal overgrowth grossly evident in the flexural areas. Thus, our patient has a circumscribed version of this very same process, both grossly and microscopically. Both can be labelled epidermolytic hyperkeratosis. What we see in our patient's axilla and antecubital fossa is but a fragment of a genetic defect that can be monstrously deforming and universal. It is the histologic finding of vacuolated keratinocytes which is the common bond and leads to our realization that patients with this generalized epidermolytic hyperkeratosis (bullous congenital ichthyosiform erythroderma) are actually covered with a giant universal epidermal nevus. Conversely, the relationship is highlighted by the fact that our patient's localized epidermal nevus has long been also known as ichthyosis hystrix, an etymologic allusion to the scales of fish and the wavy excrescences of the porcupine. Our perception of this remarkable clinical, histologic and nomenclatural interrelationship is complete as we become aware that patients with epidermal nevi of this type may have children with generalized epidermolytic hyperkeratosis. Often, as might be expected, the genetic chain breaks at this point with no further progeny.

The clinical picture is not always tidy, since associated organoid or appendageal growths of the sebaceous gland or hair follicles, or sweat glands, are relatively common in patients with localized epidermal nevi. This adds complexity to both the clinical and histologic pictures, begetting terms such as organoid nevus, nevus sebaceus, nevus comedonicus, and nevus syringocystadenomatosus papilliferus. Furthermore, vascular and neural elements may abound. Not only are there these localized associations of hamartomas, but distant ones occur as well. A close and careful inspection of this patient thus could reveal skeletal, vascular or central nervous system anomalies, therefore making his diagnosis the epidermal nevus syndrome.

It is unlikely that a routine family history will uncover any genetic background, but possibly one of his parents has an occult locus of epidermolytic hyperkeratosis, be it no more than a localized patch of palmar thickening. Although ichthyosis hystrix is an autosomal dominant trait, the genetic trail of these minor examples is blurred and obscure. Accordingly, genetic counseling is difficult.

Our patient's nevus is one for a lifetime, with no reasonable prospect of involution. On the contrary, it must be watched with particular care at puberty, when new apocrine gland elements may appear as a result of hormonal induction. It is also noteworthy that epitheliomatous change can occur within epidermal nevi, but this is extremely rare and thus is a late threat, so minimal that it generates little concern.

Removal of this epithelial nevus appears disarmingly simple. It would seem that electrodesiccation with curettage, dermabrasion or superficial tangential excision with a dermatome should be curative. Actually all these procedures are followed by a phoenix return of the nevus to its former dimensions. The only successful removal is one in which the underlying dermis is totally excised, thus eliminating the inductive forces within the collagen actually responsible for the epidermal proliferation. In our patient, this would require plastic surgery with skin grafting, a major approach not in keeping with the minor significance of his problem.

Finally, we can all take comfort in the good fortune that this little boy was but grazed by a genetic bullet that could well have maimed his entire skin for life.

Leider, M., and Rosenblum, M.: *A Dictionary of Dermatological Words, Terms and Phrases.* McGraw-Hill Book Co., New York, 1968, p. 297.
Nevus: anything odd, abnormal or faulty, that is related to conception, gestation and postnatal development and stems from a hereditable or embryogenic fault, abnormality, or oddity — a birthmark.

Solomon, L. M., and Esterly, N. B.: *Neonatal Dermatology.* W. B. Saunders Co., Philadelphia, 1973, pp. 60-64.
Epidermal nevi present as warty papillomatous growths, unilateral verrucous streaks, scaly whorls of hyperkeratosis, velvety acanthosis nigricans-like lesions. Nice introduction to taxonomy.

Adam, J. E., and Richards, R. N.: Ichthyosis Hystrix vs. Linear Verrucous Epidermal Nevus. Cutis, 5:1253-1260, 1969.
Distinguish these two epidermal nevi genetically (autosomal dominant = ichthyosis hystrix) and histologically (vacuolization of cells = ichthyosis hystrix).

Adam, J. E., and Richards, R. N.: Ichthyosis Hystrix. Epidermolytic Hyperkeratosis; Discordant in Monozygotic Twins. Arch. Derm., 107:278-282, 1973.
Why did only one twin have this autosomal dominant nevus? Bispermatic fertilization of binucleate egg?

Barker, L. P., and Sachs, W.: Bullous Congenital Ichthyosiform Erythroderma. Arch. Derm., 67:443-455, 1953.
Father was born with linear epidermal nevus (ichthyosis hystrix); his daughter was born with ichthyosiform erythroderma (epidermolytic hyperkeratosis).

Reed, R. J., Galvanek, E., and Lubritz, R. R.: Bullous Congenital Ichthyosiform Hyperkeratosis. Arch. Derm., 89:665-674, 1964.

Historical review of how we came to realize that localized variants of bullous congenital ichthyosiform erythroderma are epithelial nevi.

Shelley, W. B.: *Consultations in Dermatology*. W. B. Saunders Co., Philadelphia, 1972, pp. 140-145.
Review of epidermolytic hyperkeratosis (bullous congenital ichthyosiform erythroderma), a universal epithelial birthmark.

Ackerman, A. B., and Reed, R. J.: Epidermolytic Variant of Solar Keratosis. Arch. Derm., *107*:104-106, 1973.
Epidermolytic hyperkeratosis is seen in congenital ichthyosiform erythroderma, ichthyosis hystrix, keratodermas, neoplastic processes and keratoses.

Altman, J., and Mehregan, A. H.: Inflammatory Linear Verrucose Epidermal Nevus. Arch. Derm., *104*:385-389, 1971.
Twenty-five patients with epidermal nevi which were psoriasiform, both grossly and microscopically.

Solomon, L. M., Fretzin, D. F., and Dewald, R. L.: The Epidermal Nevus Syndrome. Arch. Derm., *97*:273-285, 1968.
Twelve patients with epidermal nevi (nevi unius lateris, ichthyosis hystrix) revealed on careful study associated congenital skeletal disorders and central nervous system disease. Literature review.

Swint, R. B., and Klaus, S. N.: Malignant Degeneration of an Epithelial Nevus. Arch. Derm., *101*:56-58, 1970.
May develop squamous cell epithelioma in situ.

Pack, G. T., and Sunderland, D. A.: Naevus Unius Lateris. Arch. Surg., *43*:341-375, 1941.
Monographic review of literature and 160 epidermal nevi: superficial removal or destruction invariably followed by reappearance.

Schorr, W. F., and Papa, C. M.: Epidermolytic Hyperkeratosis Effect of Tretinoin Therapy on the Clinical Course and the Basic Defects in the Stratum Corneum. Arch. Derm., *107*:556-562, 1973.
Therapy with 0.1 per cent vitamin A acid cream reduces hyperkeratosis.

30

Mycosis Fungoides

30

For 16 years this 39-year-old man has had a slowly enlarging **plaque over his left hip. It is scaling, erythematous and atrophic**, *resembling a radiodermatitis. A clinical and histologic diagnosis of poikiloderma vasculare atrophicans had been made 12 years ago. The lesion becomes painfully tender and bright red eight hours after ingestion of chocolate. General medical studies were negative.*

Biopsy — mycosis fungoides.

Mycosis Fungoides

Here is a disease that takes life away — slowly. Its pace is one of years, its course one of decades, and its termination inexorably fatal. Through the window of the skin we see the entire internecine struggle, from its early nonspecific pruritus, erythema or eczematous change, through its geographic plaques over the entire body, to the final years or months of malignant ulcerative tumors capable of invading any organ in the body. We see death come finally, often in the form of a blessed infection. This is the story of the primary malignant lymphoma of the skin, mycosis fungoides.

Named for its mushroom-like tumors over a century ago by the master French dermatologist, Alibert, mycosis fungoides has come to be recognized as the most diversified and chronic of all skin diseases. It may make its entrance as an inexplicable severe pruritus, strange ephemeral erythema, patchy eczema or, as in this man, a poikilodermic plaque that looked like radiodermatitis. It may come imitating psoriasis, seborrheic dermatitis, pemphigus or a fungous infection. It may come as urticaria, dyshidrosis, alopecia or a trivial scaling area.

In this first stage the biopsy findings are as uninformative as the outward clinical signs. The patient is well and there are no laboratory signals of disease. Spontaneous temporary remissions may occur. But as the days pass into months and the months into years, and as the fleeting erythemas become eczema and the pruritus becomes lichenification, the suspicion of mycosis fungoides must grow. But still the diagnosis cannot

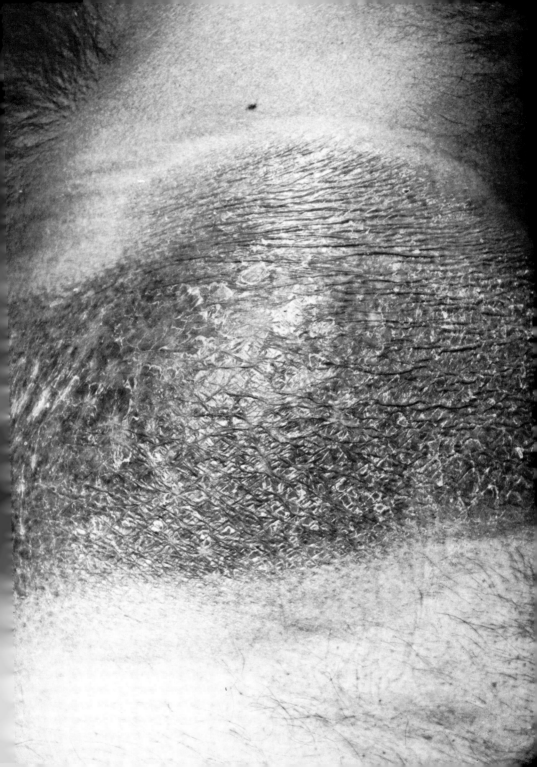

be made in this *premycotic* stage, clinically or histologically. It is made only retrospectively.

The diagnosis first comes with assurance from either the clinician or the pathologist. The clinician can identify mycosis fungoides in its classic second stage of widespread, sharply circumscribed, infiltrated plaques. These figurate, annular, circinate, polycyclic and geographic red scaling areas make for a "doorway" diagnosis. Again, laboratory support is only in the cutaneous histopathology, although some patients may have a concurrent eosinophilia and an elevated uric acid. The blood picture and bone marrow are normal. Lymphadenopathy may be present but usually the biopsy specimen shows the nonspecific changes of dermatopathic lymphadenopathy.

In the other instances, including the present one, the diagnosis comes from the pathologist. With serial biopsy specimens, just as with repeated clinical visits, there comes a time when the diagnosis is finally apparent. The signal finding is the multiplicity of cell types seen in the dermal infiltrate. Thus, the cytology of mycosis fungoides is as pleomorphic as its clinical facies. All cell types seem to be represented, particularly the reticulum or histiocytic cells. The histiocyte with its serpentine convoluted nucleus, so clear on ultra-thin sectioning or electron microscopy, seems to be the distinctive yet not diagnostic cell of mycosis fungoides. The epidermis often shows striking round loci of monocytic cell infiltrates, the microabscesses discerned by Pautrier.

What is this puzzling chronic disease we identify more by gross or histologic configuration than by anything else? It is one that comes out of the shadows of the reticulum of the skin. Existing almost as an abstraction, the reticular cells are the primitive progenitors of hemal and lymphoid cells as well as stromal reticulum fibers. From these cells come lymphocytes, monocytes, histiocytes, plasma cells and tissue mast cells as well as erythrocytes and granulocytes. Thus, a stimulus to these cells can give rise to an amazingly pleomorphic array of descendents! The result is proliferative lymphopoietic tissue simulating and later turning into neoplastic tissue. Apparently, it is this unknown stimulus which accounts for the foci of infiltrating cells.

In the early stage, the stealthy infiltrate is announced only by the immune mechanisms it may call into play in the epidermis and dermis. It is this that underlies the pruritus, eczema and urticaria of mycosis fungoides. Later, the infiltrates, be they hyperplastic or neoplastic, become clinically obvious as the increasing number of pleomorphic cells gives the pathologist diagnostic certitude. In the final stages, a cell lineage may differentiate into the monomorphic reticulum cell sarcoma, or lymphosarcoma, with malignant terminal extension to the lymph nodes, the blood (Sézary's syndrome) or any organ. It is good modern medical care which has made this last scene possible. Even a generation ago, when death came earlier, it was felt that mycosis fungoides was a tumor of the skin and the skin only!

But mycosis fungoides is not always this neat. Many times the disease is foreshortened, stages are skipped, and bizarre signs appear. The entire course may be one of an erythroderma. The microscopic examination is subject to interpretative waffling and judgment error. There are no unequivocal patterns. Even in the tumor stage the climax cytology may direct one to a lymphoma, and the trail of mycosis fungoides may be lost. Yet in the majority of instances the clinical and histologic outlines of a chronic polymorphic eruption allow us to recognize most examples of this most remarkable disease.

There are no cures for mycosis fungoides—only delaying tactics. It is a disease of such chronicity that chance favors the disease outliving the patient! Everything is done to favor this end and treatment is given to match the stage and the lesions of the patient, heavier artillery being brought in as necessary. Initially, ultraviolet light and topical high concentration fluorinated steroid preparations under Saran Wrap may be adequate. Grenz-ray therapy is an additional weapon of merit.

In a patient such as this man, with plaques of proven mycosis fungoides, topical nitrogen mustard is the treatment of choice. Daily application of an aqueous dilution (10 mg. in 40 ml.) of nitrogen mustard, applied at the moment of preparation, is very helpful in controlling the plaque stage. One to three weeks of treatment is generally adequate. It contact-sensitizes some individuals, but this can be ameliorated by systemic steroids.

Actually, systemic steroids in high dosage are effective in many examples of mycosis fungoides, but these should be reserved for the later stages, since its effect on the immune defense system may militate against a long-term détente between the proliferating lymphoreticular tissue and the host. Radiation therapy is the most effective modality in suppressing advanced mycosis fungoides. The employment of x-rays, beta rays of ^{90}Sr or the electron beam depends largely on local facilities. Finally, chemotherapy is another alternative. Methotrexate and Cytoxan are currently in favor, but undoubtedly the development of new agents for the treatment of lymphomas will change this, since to date nothing has been found to be selectively destructive.

Judicious use of these therapies cannot yet effect a cure, but it does give hope, help and precious remissions.

Bluefarb, S. M.: Mycosis Fungoides. *In* Bluefarb, S. M. (Ed.) *Cutaneous Manifestations of the Malignant Lymphomas.* Charles C Thomas, Springfield, 1959, pp. 1-215.
Encyclopedic introduction to an exquisitely chronic yet fatal skin disease; progressing from premycotic eczematous change, through infiltrative plaques, to terminal tumor stage.

Saman, P.: The Natural History of Parapsoriasis en Plaques (Chronic Superficial Dermatitis) and Pre-reticulotic Poikiloderma. Brit. J. Derm., *87*:405-411, 1972.
Large, pigmented, atrophic, erythematous patches (poikiloderma atrophicans vasculare) are another prelude to mycosis fungoides.

Roenigk, H. H., and Castrovinci, A. J.: Mycosis Fungoides Bullosa. Arch. Derm., *104*:402-406, 1971.
An example of the incredible multiplicity of lesions seen in this disease.

Connor, B.: Mycosis Fungoides with Dermatomyositis. Proc. Roy. Soc. Med., *65*:251-252, 1972.
Dermatomyositis due to an *"overlying"* malignancy.

Rosai, J., and Spiro, J. M.: Central Nervous System Involvement by Mycosis Fungoides. Acta Dermatovener., *48*:482-488, 1968.
In late stages, any organ may be involved.

Moschella, S. L., and Mihm, M. C.: Gastrointestinal Hemorrhage in a Man with Mycosis Fungoides. New Eng. J. Med., *285*:1526-1532, 1971.
Due to an ulcerated tumor.

Caldwell, I., and Dayan, A. D.: Mycosis Fungoides and Progressive Multifocal Leukoencephalopathy. Brit. J. Derm., *82*:176-181, 1970.
Dementia due to opportunistic viral infection of brain due to impairment of immune defenses by disease and chemotherapy.

Brehmer-Andersson, E., and Brunk, U.: Tape-Stripping Method for Cytological Diagnosis of Mycosis Fungoides. Acta Dermatovener., *47*:177-180, 1967.
See atypical reticulum cells on tape.

Vesper, L. J., Winkelmann, R. K., and Hargraves, M. M.: The Mycosis Fungoides Cell: The Skin Window in Mycosis Fungoides. Brit. J. Derm., *84*:54-65, 1971.
Considers mycosis fungoides as a hyperplastic non-neoplastic disease of cutaneous reticuloendothelial system, since only large mononuclear cells appear at skin window.

Helwig, E. B.: Malignant Lymphomas and Reactive Lymphoid Hyperplasias. *In* Graham, J. H., et al. (Eds.): *Dermal Pathology.* Harper & Row, New York, 1972, pp. 683-713.
Diagnostic picture of mycosis fungoides: monocytic microabscesses in epidermis, polymorphic infiltrate of reticular cells (histiocytes), monocytes, lymphocytes in dermis.

Fisher, E. R., Horvat, B. L., and Wechsler, H. L.: Ultrastructural Features of Mycosis Fungoides. Amer. J. Clin. Path., *58*:99-110, 1972.
Diagnosis best made with ordinary, not electron, microscopy.

Flaxman, B. A., Zelazny, G., and Van Scott, E. J.: Non-specificity of Characteristic Cells in Mycosis Fungoides. Arch. Derm., *104*:141-147, 1971.
Allegedly unique abnormal cell is present, but not specific, being seen in wide variety of dermatoses.

Brownlee, T. R., and Murad, T. M.: Ultrastructure of Mycosis Fungoides. Cancer, *26*:686-698, 1970.
No method of treatment produced necrosis in the characteristic mycosis fungoides cell with the large infolded nucleus.

Kelly, D. F., Halliwell, R. E. W., and Schwartzman, R. M.: Generalized Cutaneous Eruption in a Dog, with Histological Similarity to Human Mycosis Fungoides. Brit. J. Derm., *86*:164-171, 1972.
First case.

Bierman, S. M.: The Role of Immunologic Aberrations in the Pathogenesis of Lymphoma with Particular Reference to Mycosis Fungoides and Exfoliative Erythroderma. Arch. Derm., *97*:699-711, 1968.
Possibility exists that patients may be harmed rather than benefited by chemotherapy.

Ratner, A. C., Waldorf, D. S., and Van Scott, E. J.: Alterations of Lesions of Mycosis Fungoides Lymphoma by Direct Imposition of Delayed Hypersensitivity Reactions. Cancer, *21*:83-88, 1968.
Plaques temporarily cleared when contact sensitivity to 2, 4 dinitrochlorobenzene was induced.

Farber, E. M., Zackheim, H. S., McClintock, R. P., and Cox, A., Jr.: Treatment of Mycosis Fungoides with Various Strengths of Fluocinolone Acetonide Cream. Arch. Derm., *97*:165-172, 1968.
Suppressive effect on early lesions if applied in high concentration under plastic film (Saran Wrap) occlusion.

Van Scott, E. J., and Winters, P. L.: Responses of Mycosis Fungoides to Intensive External Treatment with Nitrogen Mustard. Arch. Derm., *102*:507-514, 1970.
Complete clinical and histologic remission of plaque stages of mycosis fungoides achieved in majority of patients treated intensively with whole body applications of nitrogen mustard.

Stenram, U., and Liden, S.: Topical Fluorouracil Treatment of Senile Keratosis and Mycosis Fungoides. Arch. Geschwulstforsch., *39*:153-162, 1972.
Prolonged improvement followed experimental use on small lesions of mycosis fungoides.

Zackheim, H. S.: Treatment of Mycosis Fungoides with Topical Nitrosourea Compounds. Arch. Derm., *106*:177-182, 1972.
Experimental use of these potential carcinogens produced involution in plaque stage.

McDonald, C. J., and Calabresi, P.: Azaribine for Mycosis Fungoides. Arch. Derm., *103*:158-167, 1971.
An antimetabolite which resulted in complete clinical remission in 7 of 13 patients.

de Bast, C., Moriame, N., Wanet, J., Ledoux, M., Achten, G., and Kenis, Y.: Bleomycin in

Mycosis Fungoides and Reticulum Cell Lymphoma. Arch. Derm., *104*:508-512, 1971.
An antibiotic from streptomyces with antineoplastic effects: helpful in 4 cases of mycosis fungoides.

Macdonald, R. H., and Russell, A. R.: Mycosis Fungoides: Its Management with Superficial X-rays and Strontium 90 Therapy Compared. Brit. J. Derm., *85*:388-393, 1971.
Mycosis fungoides is usually sensitive to x-rays and beta rays.

Fuks, Z., and Bagshaw, M. A.: Total-Skin Electron Treatment of Mycosis Fungoides. Radiology, *100*:145-150, 1971.
Complete regression of disease in 56 of 107 patients following 3000 rads of 2.5 Mev. given in 6 weeks.

Barnes, P., and Rees, D.: *A Concise Textbook of Radiotherapy*. J. B. Lippincott Co., Philadelphia, 1972, 384 pp.
A penetrating account of the mysteries of x-rays, beta radiations and electron beams.

Epstein, E. H., Jr., Levin, D., Croft, J. D., and Lutzner, M. A.: Mycosis Fungoides Survival, Prognostic Features, Response to Therapy, and Autopsy Findings. Medicine, *51*:61-72, 1972.
Definitive review of 144 cases finds radiotherapy the best modality.

31

Aphthous Stomatitis

31

For the past two years this 26-year-old woman has had repeated attacks of **painful ulcers of the buccal mucosa, tongue and palatine arch.** *In the last two months she has lost 25 pounds because of her inability to eat solid food.*

Smear of fresh lesion showed no viral inclusions, balloon cells or hyphae. Alpha streptococci isolated from ulcers proved resistant to tetracycline but sensitive to cephalexin. Intradermal skin testing showed strongly positive reactions to a battery of streptococcal antigens. General medical studies were normal.

Aphthous Stomatitis

These small white erosions are making this woman's life miserable. The pain and tenderness take away her enjoyment of life. The simple delights of food and drink are changed to terrors, and the repetitive, recurrent nature of her lesions gives her the feeling of Job. Will it ever end? What are these canker sores?

Hippocrates had a word for them—aphthae, meaning spots. Twenty-four centuries later we are still calling them spots and in some ways we know little more about them than Hippocrates did. We do know that they are not contagious. Spouses do not acquire them. We do know that they are not patently congenital or hereditary. They usually appear in the 20 to 40 year age group, so commonly as to blur genetic analysis. We know that they are not precancerous. They heal slowly but spontaneously in a week or two, without scarring. But we still don't know their cause nor how to prevent them.

There is much to suggest that these aphthae might be viral. Recurrent herpes simplex produces similar lesions, although usually on mucosal surfaces bound down to periosteum as on the gums and hard palate. The viruses of varicella and zoster are equally capable of producing intraoral erosions as is the Coxsackie virus. Nevertheless, cytologic studies reveal no evidence of the presence of virus, and even the most sophisticated viral laboratories have failed to isolate any virus from such lesions.

There is mounting awareness that these erosions might reflect a defective white cell defense. We know that in cyclic neutropenia the periodic gaps in hematopoiesis are associated with mucosal ulceration. Func-

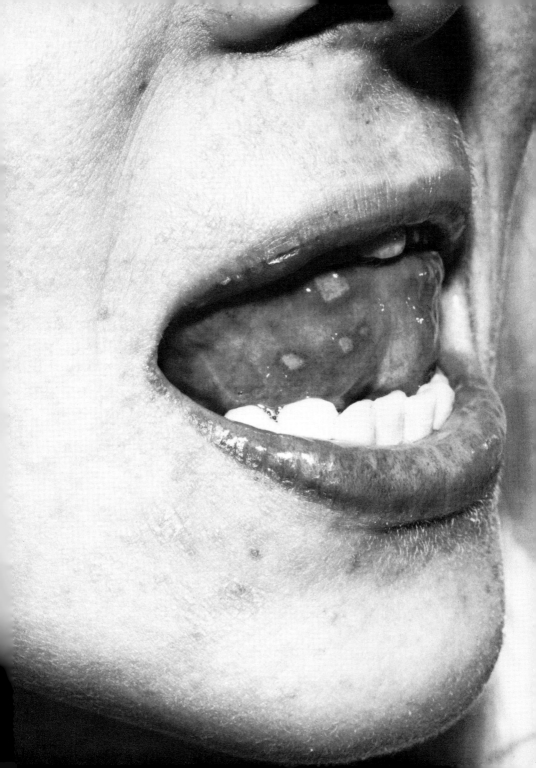

tional impairment of the neutrophil in its chemotactic, phagocytic or bactericidal activity could thus also be expected to show an association with mucosal ulceration. In this regard, immunosuppressants and leukemias are known determinants of serious mucosal ulceration. Yet, aphthous patients as a group show no essential hematologic abnormality.

There is a strong tendency of the laity to relate aphthous ulcers to a food intolerance. Many convincingly relate spices, cola drinks or milk to the onset of their attacks. Yet, rarely are there objective supportive data from blind challenges. Certainly the punctate nature of the initial lesions is far from the diffuse stomatitis we have seen from proven contact sensitivity to sage, for instance. Almost any antecedent, ranging from emotional tension to dyspepsia, may be causally related to an attack by the patient wishing to be removed from the unpleasantness of the unknown! And the experiences of one patient are rarely congruent with those of another.

There is currently the greatest scientific support for viewing aphthae as an immune phenomenon. The histopathologic finding of an early lymphocytic infiltrate is that seen in delayed hypersensitivity. The lymphocytes of patients with recurrent aphthae attack and destroy oral mucosal cells in tissue culture in an immune fashion. The majority of these patients show specific hemagglutinating antibodies to saline extracts of fetal oral mucosa. All this suggests that aphthae begin as an autoimmune response, possibly triggered by the minor mucosal trauma of eating. But there is more. Cultures of the erosions commonly show the presence of pleomorphic streptococci to which the patient may have exquisite hypersensitivity on intradermal skin testing. The same streptococcal antigens in vitro inhibit leukocyte migration, again suggesting a hypersensitive state. In contrast, the patient's lymphocytes fail to show an anticipated blast formation in the presence of the antigen. Undoubtedly, much more will be learned concerning the details of the immunologic conundrum of this common disease.

Any patient with recurrent or extensive aphthous or aphthoid lesions deserves careful study. Her skin should be examined minutely for the lesion she may want to hide or ignore. Are there the petechial vesicles of Coxsackie infection on the palms? Are there any target lesions of erythema multiforme on the extremities? Are there aphthae of the vulva? Any lichen planus? A scraping of a fresh erosion is next. Are there any viral inclusion bodies or giant multinucleated balloon cells? Are the spores of Candida present? A bacterial culture sensitivity test and a biopsy remain optional but should be considered if the history or course is aberrant. As a result of today's mores, the mucous patch of syphilis and oral ulcerations of gonorrhea are no longer a rarity. A blood count and serum protein electrophoresis should rule out leukemia, pernicious anemia and dysproteinemia as possible causes. A serologic test for syphilis and a serum folic acid determination round out the usual screen.

There is one and only one treatment for aphthous stomatitis which has real accreditation. Antihistamines, vitamins, gamma globulins, chemocauterants, topical steroids and lactobacillus tablets all yield in efficacy to tetracycline compresses. Almost routinely one can reduce the pain and accelerate the healing of even the most fibrinopurulent aphthae by applying a tetracycline compress for 20 minutes four to six times a day. The compress consists of wads of soft, finely woven white cotton soaked in a suspension of 250 mg. of tetracycline or a derivative in one ounce of water which are placed in apposition to the lesion. Within a day or two healing is achieved and the patient's gratitude is obvious. Simple use of the tetracycline as a mouthwash rinse or gargle is not adequate. The use of viscous Xylocaine for topical anesthesia is rarely necessary, since the tetracycline is so effective.

But our patient is the exception to prove the rule. The laboratory studies make it clear that she will not respond to tetracycline inasmuch as her oral streptococci have developed a resistance to this antibiotic. She must be instructed to use Keflex in compresses to obtain relief and promote healing.

Although prevention is far from an achievable goal, the avoidance of suspect food allergens, abrasive foods, spices, aspirin, lozenges, chewing gums, mouthwashes, toothpaste and menthol cigarettes is prudent. Our last two patients proved to have attacks triggered by milk and egg, respectively. An antihistaminic taken nightly for the two weeks before the menses can prevent or ameliorate premenstrual flares. Bacterial vaccines, staphylococcal or streptococcal, are worthy of trial, showing dramatic prophylactic effects on occasion. An attack may be aborted if prednisone is taken orally in a dose of 20 mg. once or twice during the prodromal symptomatic period. Finally, in some few patients, hospitalization with total environmental control may be necessary just as it is in chronic urticaria.

These patients need continuous observation in the hope of determining the correlates of recurrence. But their greatest help comes with the knowledge that they have tetracycline or an appropriate congener to treat any future attacks.

Zabrodsky, S., and Skach, M.: Recurrent Aphthae. Acta Univ. Carol. (Med.), *16*:599-673, 1970.
Monographic data on the nature and treatment of these common idiopathic, painful erosions of the mouth.

Collins, W. J., and Wells, R. F.: Aphthous Esophagitis. Gastrointest. Endosc., *17*:115-116, 1971.
Erosions occasionally extend into esophagus.

O'Brien, T. K., Saunders, D. R., and Templeton, F. E.: Chronic Gastric Erosions and Oral Aphthae. Amer. J. Dig. Dis., *17*:447-454, 1972.
May see gastric erosions in aphthous stomatitis, but rarely; association probably fortuitous.

Kansu, E., Ozer, F. L., Akalin, E., Guler, Y., Zileli, T., Tanman, E., Kaplaman, E., and Muftuoglu, E.: Behcet's Syndrome with Obstruction of the Venae Cavae. Quart. J. Med., *162*:151-168, 1972.
Recurrent aphthae of mouth and genitalia combined with relapsing iritis: Behçet's syndrome. A definitive review.

Schlappner, O. L. A., and Shelley, W. B.: Telangiectasia, Aphthous Stomatitis and Hypersplenism. Arch. Derm., *104*:668-670, 1971.
A strange concatenation.

Weathers, D. R., and Griffin, J. W.: Intraoral Ulcerations of Recurrent Herpes Simplex and Recurrent Aphthae: Two Distinct Clinical Entities. J.A.D.A., *81*:81-88, 1970.
Fifty-one cases of recurrent herpes simplex in mouth: distinguish by (1) presence of grouped erosions on gums or hard palate and (2) multinucleate giant cells on smear from early lesion.

Ship, I. I., and Galili, D. A.: Systemic Significance of Mouth Ulcers. Postgrad. Med., *49*:67-72, 1971.
Erosions may be sign of leukemia, pernicious anemia or immunosuppressant therapy.

Levy, E. J., and Schetman, D.: Cyclic Neutropenia. Arch. Derm., *84*:429-433, 1961.
Oral ulcerations recurring every 21 days, associated with sharp temporary drop in neutrophil count.

Rickles, N. H.: Allergy in Surface Lesions of the Oral Mucosa. Oral Surg., *33*:744-754, 1972.
Cinnamon oil induced aphthae: confirmatory positive skin patch-testing.

Sallay, K.: Le role du traumatisme dans la production des aphthes recidivants. Acta Stomat. Belg., *67*:273-280, 1970.
Mechanical trauma to mucosa can evoke aphthae.

Graykowski, E. A., Barile, M. F., Lee, W. B., and Stanley, H. R.: Recurrent Aphthous Stomatitis. Clinical, Therapeutic, Histopathologic and Hypersensitivity Aspects. J.A.M.A., *196*:637-644, 1966.
Incriminates pleomorphic streptococci as a cause of aphthae, stressing positive skin test results.

Dolby, A. E.: Mikulicz's Recurrent Oral Aphthae. Histopathological Comparison with Two Experimentally Induced Immunological Reactions. Brit. J. Derm., *83*:674-679, 1970.
Experimental delayed hypersensitivity reaction to dinitrochlorobenzene in guinea pig oral mucosa resembles aphthous stomatitis histologically. Favors idea of delayed hypersensitivity.

Wilgram, G. F.: A Possible Role of the Merkel Cell in Aphthous Stomatitis. Oral Surg., *34*:231-238, 1972.
Speculation: tension produces autonomic impulses, releasing catecholamine granules of Merkel cell, inducing focal vasoconstrictive necrosis of mucosa.

Lange, D. E., Meyer, M., and Hahn, W.: Oral Exfoliative Cytology in the Diagnosis of Viral and Bullous Lesions. J. Periodontol., *43*:433-437, 1972.
Absence of specific cell alteration confirms diagnosis of aphthae, rules out viral and neoplastic lesions. Photos.

Lehner, T.: Pathology of Recurrent Oral Ulceration and Oral Ulceration in Behçet's Syndrome: Light, Electron and Fluorescence Microscopy. J. Path., *97*:481-494, 1969.
Early lympho-monocytic infiltrate supports view that aphthae represent delayed hypersensitivity reaction.

Lehner, T.: Immunologic Aspects of Recurrent Oral Ulcers. Oral Surg., *33*:80-85, 1972.
Summation of the evidence that aphthae are a mucosal autoimmune phenomenon.

Wasastjerna, C., Kalliola, H., Rosanen, J. A., and Wager, O.: IgG Cryoglobulinaemia. Case Report and Immunological Studies of a Patient with Recurrent Ulcerative Stomatitis and High Content of Cold Precipitable Immunoglobulin in Serum. Scand. J. Haemat., *4*:473-484, 1967.
Aphthae as a rare immunopathy.

Dolby, A. E.: Mikulicz's Recurrent Oral Aphthae: The Effect of Anti-Lymphocyte Serum Upon the In Vitro Cytotoxicity of Lymphocytes from Patients for Oral Epithelial Cells. Clin. Exp. Immunol., *7*:681-686, 1970.
Lymphocytes from patients with aphthae are specifically cytotoxic for oral mucosal cells.

Nasz, I., Kulcsar, G., Dan, P., and Sallay, K.: A Possible Pathogenic Role for Virus-Carrier Lymphocytes. J. Infect. Dis., *124*:214-216, 1971.
Adenovirus and herpes simplex antigens more commonly found in lymphocytes of aphthous patients than in normals.

Donatsky, O., and Bendixen, G.: In Vitro Demonstration of Cellular Hypersensitivity to Strep 2 A in Recurrent Aphthous Stomatitis by Means of the Leucocyte Migration Test. Acta Allerg., *27*:137-144, 1972.
Eight of 17 aphthous patients showed streptococcal antigen induced inhibition of leukocyte migration, an in vitro parameter confirming positive skin tests.

Francis, T. C., and Oppenheim, J. J.: Impaired Lymphocyte Stimulation by Some Streptococcal Antigens in Patients with Recurrent Aphthous Stomatitis and Rheumatic Heart Disease. Clin. Exp. Immunol., *6*:573-586, 1970.
Although streptococcal antigen gives positive skin tests (and inhibits leukocyte migration), it fails to induce blast formation in lymphocytes of aphthous patients.

MacPhee, I. T., Sircus, W., Farmer, E. D., Harkness, R. A., and Cowley, G. C.: Use of Steroids in Treatment of Aphthous Ulceration. Brit. Med. J., *2*:147-149, 1968.
Controlled, statistically valid study failed to reveal any help from topical steroids.

Eggleston, D. J., and Nally, F. F.: Treatment of Aphthous Ulceration with Topical Azathioprine. Brit. J. Oral Surg., *9*:233-236, 1972.
A topical immunosuppressant is no help.

Guggenheimer, J., Brightman, V. J., and Ship, I. I.: Effect of Chlortetracycline Mouth Rinses on the Healing of Recurrent Aphthous Ulcers. A Double Blind Controlled Trial. J. Oral Ther. Pharm., *4*:406-408, 1968.
Reduced healing time by 50 per cent.

32

*This patient has soft, velvety, easily **stretchable skin.** Her **joints** are **hyperextensible,** and since childhood she has noted "black and blue" marks at sites of minor trauma. Her hair turned white when she was 12 years old. Massive varicose veins have been present since her first pregnancy. A venous ligation was accompanied by delayed healing and prominent scar formation. Both her father and her son exhibit hyperextensible skin and joints as well as easy bruisability.*

General medical studies, including a coagulogram, were normal except for the urogram, which showed a double collecting system on the right.

Skin biopsy — normal, with considerable elastic tissue.

Ehlers-Danlos Syndrome

This woman has ballet fingers. Her lissome joints result from her remarkable connective tissue. Thin and dramatically extensible, this defective tissue accounts not only for her double-joints but for her super-stretch skin. It is a defect genetically determined, one she shares with her father and son. This is the autosomal dominant syndrome described by Ehlers and Danlos.

These patients have a lineage of fragile tissue. They are often born prematurely as a result of the delicate fetal sheath. Their inadequate supportive tissues are responsible for their being characterized as floppy infants and for their possible dislocated hip, hematomas, hernias or rectal prolapse. Or, the thin dermis may give a charming china doll appearance, with blue sclerae and delicate vascular tracing in the skin. The defects may be more varied, such as a club foot, or subtle, such as we see in the ureteral reduplication in our patient.

As youngsters, they are the envy of their peers. It is no defect to virtually tie one's fingers in knots, to evert eyelids and to stick stretched ears into one's mouth. In ages past, such gymnastic stunts could have been the prelude to a distinguished career as a side show contortionist. But the dark lining of the cloud of cutis hyperelastica appears when body contact sports induce giant hematomas in these children. A fall from a

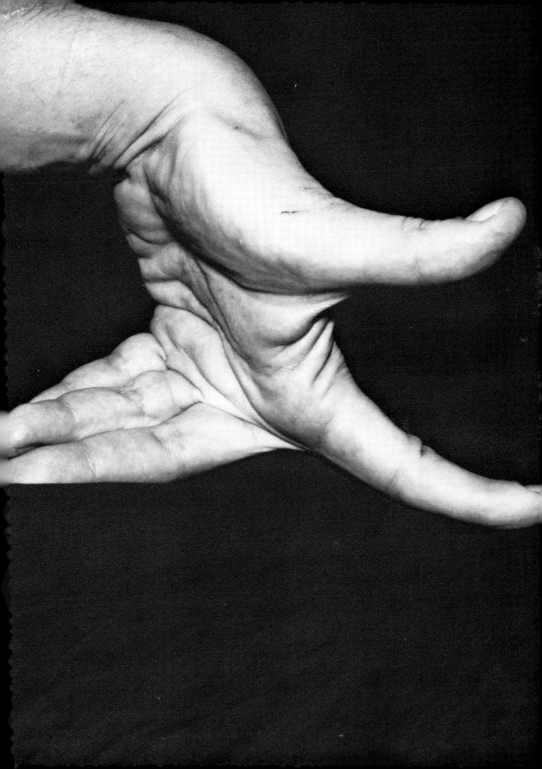

bike can be fatal for the Ehlers-Danlos child, whose vessel walls have no tough protective connective tissue sheath. This is the ecchymotic form, but nearly all patients suffer at least from easy bruisability. These are the fragile wall bleeders with normal coagulograms. Actual arterial rupture is a special risk in these patients, and varicose veins are very common in these vessels with so little resistance to stretch.

Much more lies beneath the surface, for the defect in these patients' connective tissue is universal. It extends throughout every tissue that contains any stroma of collagen. The bowel is subject to herniation through a weak abdominal wall, and to diverticula which may even perforate as a result of the stresses of obstipation. Pregnancy is a special threat, with tears, hematomas and poor healing to be anticipated. The eye is not exempt; there have been reports of lens dislocations and blindness following retinal detachment. Even the dentin of the teeth of these patients is defective.

Diagnosis has not been difficult; at times, a simple handshake is enough — the bag of bones feel is distinctive. In other instances, wide scars are a clue to the patient's weak skin. In all cases, the skin is abnormally stretchable but returns to a perfect fit. These changes are strikingly different from what we currently call cutis laxa, in which the skin hangs in great pendulous folds or dewlaps, as a result of the absence of elastic tissue.

The nature of the defect in Ehlers-Danlos syndrome has not been easy to discover. It is not found in any laboratory parameter or any medical study. It is not found in the histology under either micro- or ultramicroscopic visualization. Biophysical measurements do reveal a drop in tensile strength, and scanning electron microscopy of the skin shows fewer and smaller collagen bundles than normal, as well as defects in orientation. Yet, the ultimate answer is not in the gross wicker weave but in the molecular structure of collagen. The critical determinant of structural stability and normal resistance to stretch is in the side chains of collagen. These have been found to be reduced in number in Ehlers-Danlos syndrome, and it is this molecular change which explains the remarkable extensibility of this defective collagen.

Even more exciting is the latest discovery that a variant of Ehlers-Danlos syndrome results from a specific enzyme deficiency. In these individuals with joint laxity, recurrent dislocations, scoliosis, hyperextensible skin and thin scars, the skin collagen was specifically lacking in hydroxylysine. By means of fibroblast cultures from these patients it could be shown that this was associated with a marked reduction in lysyl-protocollagen hydroxylase. Although hydroxylysine numbers only 4 per 1000 amino acids in collagen, it serves as a critical cross linkage in the collagen molecule, and its lack results in the abnormal collagen responsible for the clinical findings. We are thus witnesses to the first biochemical elucidation of an inborn error of collagen synthesis.

Equally fascinating is the observation that the collagen from patients with classic Ehlers-Danlos syndrome fails to aggregate platelets in the normal protective fashion. It is apparent that this could account in part for the purpura and oozing which occur.

Our new insights into the pathogenesis of cutis hyperelastica grant us no therapeutic wand. We must still give genetic counsel. We must continue to alert our young patients to the perils of bumps and bruises. We must remain sensitive to the hazards of surgery for these individuals. We must always remember that anticoagulants and angiography are contraindicated. There can be no casual elective surgery, because their vessels may be torn by hemostats and sutures. For the present, Ehlers-Danlos patients must remain a surgically deprived group under all but life-threatening conditions.

Yet beyond all this, we can now see the dawn of an age when bioengineering will permit replacement of the genetically missing enzymes and erase their defect.

Beighton, P.: The Ehlers-Danlos Syndrome. Wm. Heineman Medical Books Ltd., London, 1970, 194 pp.
    The complete story of this cutis hyperelastica syndrome: familial super-stretch connective tissue.

Grahame, R., and Beighton, P.: Physical Properties of the Skin in the Ehlers-Danlos Syndrome. Ann. Rheum. Dis., 28:246-251, 1969.
    The exhibitionist's skin, thin with increased extensibility, allowing one patient to simultaneously hold six golf balls — in his mouth!

Goodman, R. M., Katznelson, M. B., and Frydman, M.: Evolution of Palmar Skin Creases in the Ehlers-Danlos Syndrome. Clin. Genet., 3:67-72, 1972.
    Dermatoglyphics normal but nongenetic secondary palmar creases appear as patient ages.

Beighton, P.: Articular Manifestations of the Ehlers-Danlos Syndrome. Semin. Arthritis Rheum., 1:246-261, 1972.
    Hyperextensible joints, dislocations, effusions and congenital spinal, thoracic and pedal abnormalities.

Barabas, A. P.: Vascular Complications in the Ehlers-Danlos Syndrome. With Special Reference to the "Arterial Type" or Sacks' Syndrome. J. Cardiovasc. Surg., 13:160-167, 1972.
    Easy bruisability, hematomas, varicose veins, fatal arterial rupture.

Beighton, P., Murdoch, J. L., and Votteler, T.: Gastro-intestinal Complications of the Ehlers-Danlos Syndrome. Gut, *10*:1004-1008, 1969.
Hernias, bleeding, rare bowel perforation.

Beighton, P.: Obstetric Aspects of the Ehlers-Danlos Syndrome. J. Obstet. Gynec. Brit. Commonw., *76*:97-101, 1969.
Premature delivery, tearing, hematomas, bleeding, uterine prolapse, delayed wound healing.

Beighton, P.: Serious Ophthalmological Complications in the Ehlers-Danlos Syndrome. Brit. J. Ophthal., *54*:263-268, 1970.
Major: retinal detachment, lens displacement. Minor: eyelid redundancy with easy eversion, blue sclerae, myopia.

Beighton, P., and Thomas, M. L.: The Radiology of the Ehlers-Danlos Syndrome. Clin. Radiol., *20*:354-361, 1969.
Subcutaneous calcified spheroids, postural deformities, scoliosis, kyphosis, subluxation of joints, diverticula of bowel. Avoid angiography — very dangerous.

Beighton, P., Price, A., Lord, J., and Dickson, E.: Variants of the Ehlers-Danlos Syndrome. Clinical, Biochemical, Haematological and Chromosomal Features of 100 Patients. Ann. Rheum. Dis., *28*:228-245, 1969.
Mitis, gravis, hypermobile, ecchymotic and X-linked variants of this autosomal dominant collagen disorder all have normal biochemical, hematologic and chromosomal findings.

Karaca, M., Cronberg, L., and Nilsson, I. M.: Abnormal Platelet-Collagen Reaction in Ehlers-Danlos Syndrome. Scand. J. Haemat., *9*:465-469, 1972.
Specific failure of Ehlers-Danlos connective tissue to induce platelet aggregation in part explains bleeding tendency.

Varadi, D. P., and Hall, D. A.: Cutaneous Elastin in Ehlers-Danlos Syndrome. Nature, *208*:1224-1225, 1965.
Ehlers-Danlos skin has only one fifth of tensile strength of normal skin. Elastin, chemically normal.

Barabas, G. M.: The Ehlers-Danlos Syndrome Abnormalities of the Enamel, Dentine Cementum and the Dental Pulp: An Histological Examination of 13 Teeth from 6 Patients. Brit. Dent. J., *126*:509-515, 1969.
Abnormalities were in dentin — consistent with collagenous nature of disease, since no elastic tissue present in dentine.

Julkunen, H., Rokkanen, P., and Inoue, H.: Scanning Electron Microscopic Study of the Collagen Bundles of the Skin in the Ehlers-Danlos Syndrome. Ann. Med. Exp. Biol. Fenn., *48*:201-204, 1970.
Collagen fibers decreased in number and irregular in orientation. Elastic fibers increased.

Hegreberg, G. A., Padgett, G. A., and Henson, J. B.: Connective Tissue Disease of Dogs and Mink Resembling Ehlers-Danlos Syndrome of Man. III. Histopathologic Changes of the Skin. Arch. Path., *90*:159-166, 1970.
Collagen fibers: irregularity in bundle size and orientation.

Goltz, R. W., and Hult, A. M.: Generalized Elastolysis (Cutis Laxa) and Ehlers-Danlos Syndrome (Cutis Hyperelastica): A Comparative Clinical and Laboratory Study. Southern Med. J., *58*:848-854, 1965.
Elastic fibers which snap skin back after it has been stretched: increased in Ehlers-Danlos; degenerate in cutis laxa, with resultant pendulous folds.

Steer, G., Jayson, M. I. V., Dixon, A. St. J., and Beighton, P.: Joint Capsule Collagen Analysis by the Study of Intra-articular Pressure During Joint Distention. Ann. Rheum. Dis., *30*:481-486, 1971.
Elasticity of collagen depends more on molecular cross linkages than on amount of collagen present. Reduction in cross linkages makes collagen easier to stretch.

Mechanic, G.: Cross-linking of Collagen in Heritable Disorder of Connective Tissue: Ehlers-Danlos Syndrome. Biochem. Biophys. Res. Commun., *47*:267-272, 1972.
He finds lack of reducible intermolecular cross links in dermal collagen in Ehlers-Danlos syndrome.

Krane, S. M., Pinnell, S. R., and Erbe, R. W.: Lysyl-Protocollagen Hydroxylase Deficiency in Fibroblasts from Siblings with Hydroxylysine-Deficient Collagen. Proc. Nat. Acad. Sci., *69*:2899-2903, 1972.
Variant of Ehlers-Danlos syndrome showing skin collagen specifically lacking in hydroxylysine, associated with hydroxylase enzyme deficiency. First inborn error of human collagen metabolism to be defined at biochemical level.

Beighton, P., and Horan, F. T.: Surgical Aspects of the Ehlers-Danlos Syndrome. A Survey of 100 Cases. Brit. J. Surg., *56*:255-259, 1969.
Skin cuts like cold porridge, tears easily; sutures pull out, vessels ooze, infections occur, scars widen. A surgeon's dread.

33

These **rimmed polycyclic plaques** *on the back of this girl's hands have been present for years. Beginning as small warty areas, they have gradually enlarged, always remaining asymptomatic, noninflammatory and treatment resistant.*

Porokeratosis of Mibelli

This is a dermatosis distingué. Once seen, such skin heraldry cannot easily be forgotten. It has the singular characteristic of a well-defined keratotic border. In contrast, the central zone of skin is rather unprepossessing in appearance. Only by study do we come to realize that not just the epidermis but also the epidermal appendages are atrophic. The area is anhidrotic and without lanugo hairs. Actually the central epidermis may be verrucous, scaly or hyperplastic, even pruritic and inflammatory, the one unmistakable diagnostic criterion for porokeratosis being the keratotic rim.

Under the microscope the keratotic rim is as striking and remarkable as in the patient. When properly oriented for cross section, the specimen shows an intrusive plug or band of thickened stratum corneum. This is the unique cornoid lamella of porokeratosis. Without it the diagnosis cannot be made. It is composed of keratin formed in excess and in haste, showing many retained keratinocyte nuclei (porokeratosis). Thus, the cornoid lamella which completely rings the lesion has been a puzzlement to all students of the disease since Mibelli first delineated porokeratosis in 1893.

Down through the years the search went on. The original view that this was a sweat pore disease was abandoned when it was found that, although the cornoid lamella might appear to arise in an acrosyringium on a single section, it actually was a ring coursing all around the lesion, involving sweat pores and hair follicles only when they fell in its narrow path. Furthermore, the lesions occur in the buccal mucosa, a stranger to sweat ducts. The conundrum persisted, as it was learned that the lesions could be familial; indeed, inheritance was considered to be autosomal dominant. Yet the process did not appear until childhood or later and

202

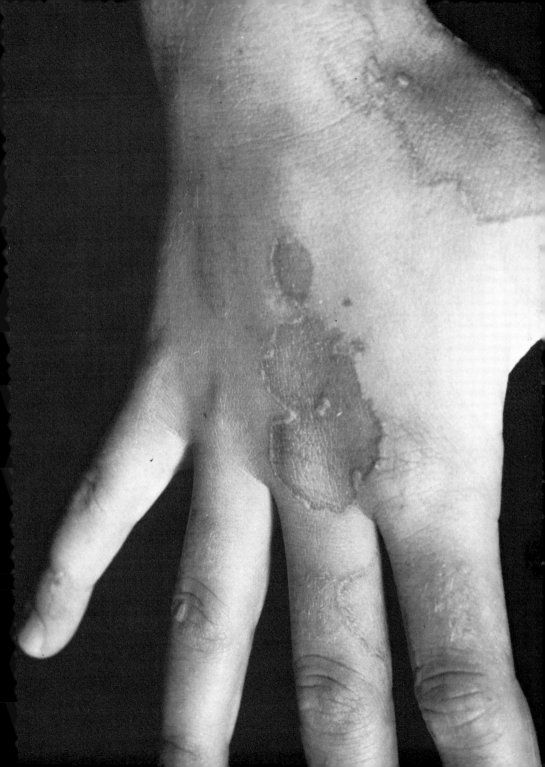

often there was no family history. It was not contagious nor could it be transferred to animals by inoculation. Observation of unilateral and linear forms gave no help, since they were only in dermatomes, not in nerve distribution per se. Extensive medical workups failed to disclose any clinical or metabolic concomitants. The slow insidious extension persisting for a lifetime, extending back into the biopsy scar, and rarely involuting, did not lessen the mystery. But two observations did have impact; first, the fact that sunlight could induce multiple diminutive porokeratoses, and second, the fact that some of these lesions did become squamous cell epitheliomas.

We have come to realize that in porokeratosis we are watching the quiet drama of a mutant cell and its progeny shoving aside and replacing the normal epidermis of this girl. Each lesion represents a clone of these new keratinocytes and the keratotic rim, the battle line between these invasive cells and the normal epidermal population. It is a quiet but mortal engagement. In some, the counter forces keep the lesions small, actually insignificant, and easily overlooked. Rarely, the invaders are pushed back, and the skin returns to normal. In others, as in our patient, the new cells show an evolutionary superiority. But note that the mutant strain fails to form new appendages, the old being destroyed as the wave of battle passes over. Moreover, the mutant epidermis is thin and sparsely colonized. It may be this atrophy which after decades of sunlight accounts for the further degeneration to squamous cell epithelioma in some of these patients.

We don't know what mutational forces are at work to initiate porokeratosis, but the predilection of the process for the sun-exposed areas suggests that such irradiation may be significant. It is interesting that the distinctive dike surrounding the lesions is reminiscent of the threadlike border we see encircling superficial basal cell epitheliomas. All this adds credence to the current view that porokeratosis is not as benign as its visage would suggest. True, it does not ulcerate or develop the gross dimensions of a tumor, yet its behavior is one of relentless low-key destruction, replacement and extension.

The diagnosis is apparent in our girl, but in the variants histologic study may be necessary to provide assistance to the clinician. At times the gross appearance may suggest

Actinic keratosis	Annular verrucae
Alopecia areata	Atrophic lichen planus
Annular lichen planus	Elastosis perforans serpiginosa

Epidermal nevi	Onychodystrophy
Granuloma annulare	Psoriasis
Ichthyosis hystrix	Superficial epitheliomatosis
Keratosis follicularis	Tinea corporis

But always alert the pathologist to orient the specimen for a cross-sectional view of the diagnostic cornoid lamella. Porokeratosis is a diagnosis which favors the prepared mind. Think of it.

Treatment is difficult. Partial removal by curettage and desiccation may be followed by recurrence. Topical fluorouracil has not proved as effective as in the treatment of actinic keratoses. Steroids, vitamin A, thyroid and keratolytics have all been tried with predictably poor results. Excision is the best approach but is limited to small areas. Liquid nitrogen cryotherapy is probably the best modality for a trial in this patient. In many instances the benignity of this new growth is such that it justifies simple long-term surveillance. In any event, the patient should be warned of the hazards of excessive sunlight and radiotherapy in these atrophic sites.

Porokeratosis provides us with a remarkable view of a Darwinian cellular struggle between normal and mutant keratinocytes. As a paradigm of clonal disease, it deserves further intensive study and observation.

Mikhail, G. R., and Wertheimer, G. W.: Clinical Variants of Porokeratosis (Mibelli). Arch. Derm., *98*:124-131, 1968.
Critical review of this strange rare genodermatosis which may be big or little, thick or thin, but is always surrounded by a distinctive dike!

Goldner, R.: Zosteriform Porokeratosis of Mibelli. Arch. Derm., *104*:425-426, 1971.
Looks like epidermal nevus, lichen striatus or keratosis follicularis.

Chernosky, M. E., and Freeman, R. G.: Disseminated Superficial Actinic Porokeratosis (DSAP). Arch. Derm., *96*:611-624, 1967.
Diminutive form and, like actinic keratosis, sunlight induced.

Guss, S. B., Osbourn, R. A., and Lutzner, M. A.: Porokeratosis Plantaris, Palmaris, et Disseminata. A Third Type of Porokeratosis. Arch. Derm., *104*:366-373, 1971.
Another variant of this autosomal dominant trait.

Welton, W. A.: Linear Porokeratosis in a Family with DSAP. Arch. Derm., *106*:263-263, 1972.
One man's family: one daughter developed porokeratosis of Mibelli; three daughters developed disseminated superficial actinic porokeratosis; another daughter, three sons, his wife and he himself had normal skin.

Cort, D. F., and Abdel-Aziz, A. M.: Epithelioma Arising in Porokeratosis of Mibelli. Brit. J. Plast. Surg., *25*:318-328, 1972.
Need for long-term surveillance; recounts 14 cases in which squamous cell epitheliomas developed within lesion.

Braun-Falco, O., and Balsa, R. E.: Zur Histochemie der cornoiden Lamelle. Ein Beitrag zur Pathogenese der Porokeratosis Mibelli. Hautarzt, *20*:543-550, 1969.
Diagnostic feature: marginal wedge of thickened porokeratotic stratum corneum. The so-called cornoid lamella at interface of atrophic and normal epidermis.

Reed, R. J., and Leone, P.: Porokeratosis — A Mutant Clonal Keratosis of the Epidermis. I. Histogenesis. Arch. Derm., *101*:340-347, 1970.
Best answer to the puzzle of porokeratosis: lesions are mutant clones of keratinocytes; keratotic ridge marks territorial edge.

Puck, T. T.: *The Mammalian Cell as a Microorganism.* Holden-Day, Inc., San Francisco, 1972, 219 pp.
Essential background for understanding how a mutant clone of keratinocytes can arise, invade and replace normal epidermis.

Chernosky, M. E., and Anderson, D. E.: Disseminated Superficial Actinic Porokeratosis. Clinical Studies and Experimental Production of Lesions. Arch. Derm., *99*:401-407, 1969.
Experimental induction of mutants with ultraviolet radiation.

Eyre, W. G., and Carson, W. E.: Linear Porokeratosis of Mibelli. Arch. Derm., *105*:426-429, 1972.
Small versions may be excised or destroyed with liquid nitrogen.

34

Generalized Vaccinia

34

This 17-year-old girl has a **generalized pustular eruption,** *temperature of 102° and malaise seven days after being vaccinated for smallpox. She had been successfully vaccinated before without incident. Her health has been excellent and she has had no skin disease.*

The vaccination site shows a large umbilicated pustule, but no necrosis. Elsewhere the pustules are variably sized, at times umbilicated and hemorrhagic. Note the highlighting of her physiologic adolescent **seborrhea.**

Most remarkable is a virtually confluent studding of miliary pustules over the right arm at the site of a concurrent typhoid-paratyphoid vaccine injection.

Generalized Vaccinia

This is a one in a hundred thousand chance event. This girl developed the usual viremia seen after vaccination but, for reasons not known to us, she failed to initiate promptly the appropriate humoral and cellular defense responses. As a result, the viremia became fulminant and at the points of capillary leakage, most notably in the area of the typhoid vaccine, the virus escaped to lodge in the epidermis. Here it produced the cell destruction responsible for the multilocular vesiculation and the pustules seen.

This is not the vaccinia of accidental *autoinoculation,* as found in infants. Nor is it the grave secondary infection of eczematous skin, *eczema vaccinatum,* as occurs in the atopic conditions. Neither is it the fearsome *progressive gangrenous vaccinia* that develops in someone whose immunity is compromised by immunosuppressants, steroids, or leukemia, or in someone with a congenital defect in immune response. It is simply generalized vaccinia, and as such it is an alarming yet benign cutaneous expression of her unchecked viremia.

With her history of a vaccination seven days ago, and these multiple replicas of her primary vaccination pustule, it seems almost superfluous to engage the laboratory in further study. Nonetheless, a Tzanck smear of the vesicle is appropriate to show on Giemsa stain the hematoxinophilic intracytoplasmic type B inclusion bodies (Guarnieri). Inciden-

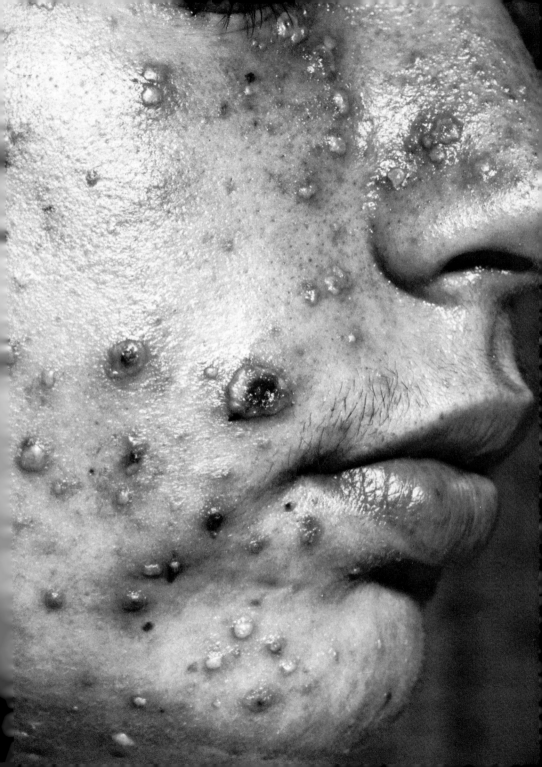

tally, such a smear should not be air-dried but should be fixed at once in 95 per cent ethyl alcohol to avoid artefacts. Further studies will probably reflect the interest and expertise of your laboratory. Electron microscopy is the most elegant and rapid approach, but immunofluorescent staining is equally valuable. The vaccinia virus may be grown and visualized as plaques on the fertilized chicken egg chorioallantoic membrane or in tissue culture. Serologic studies are of mainly retrospective interest, since they depend on a comparison of today's serum with convalescent sera. In this regard, complement fixing as well as neutralizing antibodies and hemagglutinin inhibition may be measured.

Vaccination is one of those anomalous situations in which a physician deliberately induces disease. It is this deliberate procedure of introducing live but minor virus into the skin, and hence into the lymphatics and blood stream, which has virtually eradicated smallpox and is one of medicine's proudest achievements. Nonetheless, it is not an entirely innocuous undertaking, as we see in this patient. Each time it is done, the antiviral immune defense system is fully tested, and should any major component be lacking, the results can be serious.

We recognize at least three protective components in the immune system: circulating antibodies, lymphocytes and interferon. It can be assumed that the circulating antibodies are capable of neutralizing the free virus in transit. Likewise, the lymphocyte may be involved in classic protective immune action against the virus as it attaches to the cell surface. Finally, interferon, a protein elaborated by infected cells, makes the keratinocyte resistant to the virus particles. The picture we have is still but a faint, misty sketch of what is actually occurring. However, it alerts us to the fact that experimental disease with a virus is potentially hazardous, since our pharmacologic cupboard is virtually bare of antiviral agents. Although the death rate in vaccination is one per million, it is dramatically higher in all those groups with inadequate defenses. Thus, vaccination must *not* be given to any patient with the humoral and cellular immunologic defects of dysgammaglobulinemia, leukemia or lymphoma. Furthermore, it should not be given to those whose cellular immunity has been depressed by steroids, immunosuppressants or radiotherapy. Pregnancy is an equally forceful contraindication in view of the potential threat of viremia to the fetus, with its primitive immune status.

Despite the threatening appearance of this patient's pox, it is basically benign and requires no heroic treatment. It does not have the frightening prognosis of progressive vaccinia despite its generalized nature. Hospitalization is advisable nonetheless for observation and assessment of the extent of her vaccinia as well as of any possible immune deficit. She must be kept strictly isolated, however, since she is a really lethal danger to the hospitalized patients who have severely reduced immunity.

Therapy consists of keeping the skin cleansed with gentle bathing and applications of 1 to 40 aluminum subacetate solution compresses. Super-infection with bacteria is best avoided by keeping the lesions dry and not covered with dressings. Systemic antibiotics are not necessary nor is thiosemicarbazone (Marboran) chemotherapy. Almost invariably, the natural defenses take hold at this time, aborting further extension. If any treatment is to be used it is the vaccinia immune globulin. A dose of 10 ml. given intramuscularly will aid in reducing the possibility of a prolonged viremia and the outcropping of further lesions. Within two weeks these lesions should all have involuted without scarring.

Experience with generalized vaccinia provides an instructive chapter in our understanding of the nature and pathogenesis of the viral poxes. It likewise gives us new respect for the considerable challenge vaccination thrusts upon our patient's immune system. It seems prudent to restrict the cutaneous inoculation of live vaccinia virus to individuals with zero defects in immunity.

Waddington, E.: Vaccination and Its Possible Complications. *In* Simons, R. D. G. P., and Marshall, J.: *Essays on Tropical Dermatology*. Excerpta Medica, Amsterdam, 1969, pp. 73-84.
(1) Viremic vaccinial lesions (generalized, fetal, gangrenous and eczema vaccinatum); (2) contact transfer vaccinia; (3) immune phenomena (erythema multiforme, purpura, urticaria); and (4) local necrotic ulcer.

Copeman, P. W. M., and Banatvala, J. E.: The Skin and Vaccination Against Smallpox. Brit. J. Derm., *84*:169-173, 1971.
Every successful vaccination associated with viremia. General review.

Lane, J. M., Ruben, F. L., Neff, J. M., and Millar, J. D.: Complications of Smallpox Vaccination, 1968: Results of Ten Statewide Surveys. J. Infect. Dis., *122*:303-309, 1970.
Generalized vaccinia develops in 1 of 100,000 of those revaccinated.

Kempe, C. H.: Studies on Smallpox and Complications of Smallpox Vaccination. Pediatrics, *26*:176-189, 1960.
Sixty-two cases of benign generalized vaccinia, reflecting delay in immune response. Viremia may persist for over six months in otherwise completely well individual.

Töndury, G., Foukas, M., and Scouteris, A.: Prenatal Vaccinia. J. Obstet. Gynec. Brit. Commonw., *76*:47-54, 1969.
Often fatal; not associated with malformations.

Dixon, M. F.: Progressive Vaccinia Complicating Lymphosarcoma. J. Path., *100*:53-67, 1970.
Gangrenous necrotic form seen in children with agammaglobulinemia, in adults with malignant lymphoma. Usually fatal.

Freed, E. R., Duma, R. J., and Escobar, M. R.: Vaccinia Necrosum and Its Relationship to Impaired Immunologic Responsiveness. Amer. J. Med., *52*:411-420, 1972.
Skin tests show these patients are anergic, immunologically defenseless, against heat-inactivated vaccine virus.

Loeffel, E. D., and Meyer, J. S.: Eczema Vaccinatum in Darier s Disease. Arch. Derm., *102*:451-456, 1970.
Mimicked pyoderma; identified by intracytoplasmic (Guarnieri) inclusions in touch biopsy smear.

Lum, G. S., Soriano, F., Trejos, A., and Llerena, J.: Vaccinia Epidemic and Epizootic in El Salvador. Amer. J. Trop. Med. Hyg., *16*:332-338, 1967.
Vaccination of one man followed by accidental contact transfer infection in 22 persons and 450 cows.

Brownstein, M. H., and Datlof, P.: Roseola Vaccinia. Arch. Derm., *97*:422-424, 1968.
Immune exanthem, two weeks after vaccination.

Taylor, W. F., Quaqundah, B. Y., and Black, J. R.: Chronic Localized Non-Progressive Vaccinia During Infectious Hepatitis. Amer. J. Dis. Child., *121*:420-422, 1971.
Persistence for nearly six months related to liver disease.

Marmelzat, W. L.: Malignant Tumors in Smallpox Vaccination Scars. Arch. Derm., *97*:400-406, 1968.
Twenty-four cases of basal cell and squamous cell epithelioma and malignant melanoma originating in smallpox scars.

Reed, W. B., and Wilson-Jones, E.: Malignant Tumors as a Late Complication of Vaccination. Arch. Derm., *98*:132-135, 1968.
Sun exposure on atrophic scarred skin main etiologic factor!

Sehgal, V. N., Rege, V. L., and Vadiraj, S. N.: Inoculation Leprosy Subsequent to Small Pox Vaccination. Dermatologica, *141*:393-396, 1970.
Bacteria as well as virus may enter needle holes.

Joklik, W. R.: The Poxviruses. Bact. Rev., *30*:33-66, 1966.
Comprehensive review. No evidence that pox virus can induce cell to divide.

Wokatsch, R.: Vaccinia Virus. *In* Majer, M., and Plotkin, S. A. (Eds.): *Strains of Human Viruses.* S. Karger, New York, 1972, pp. 241-257.
Vaccinia virus can be inactivated photodynamically! Whole earth catalogue of strains and biologic review.

Becker, Y., and Sarov, I.: Electron Microscopy of Vaccinia Virus DNA. J. Molec. Biol., *34*:655-660, 1968.
Dramatic floral pattern of entire 80 μ long DNA genome from vaccinia.

Padawer, J.: Poxvirus Phagocytosis in Vivo: Electron Microscopy of Macrophages, Mast Cells and Leukocytes. J. Reticuloendothel. Soc., *9*:23-41, 1971.
Virus engulfed by neutrophils, macrophages, eosinophils and mast cells.

Blackman, K. E., and Bubel, H. C.: Origin of the Vaccinia Virus Hemagglutinin. J. Virol., *9*:290-296, 1972.
Circulating antibodies include those against hemagglutinin produced by plasma membrane of vaccinia-infected cell.

Rosenberg, G. L., Farber, P. A., and Natkins, A. L.: In Vitro Stimulation of Sensitized Lymphocytes by Herpes Simplex Virus and Vaccinia Virus. Proc. Nat. Acad. Sci., *69*:756-760, 1972.
Cellular immune response to vaccinia demonstrated by highly specific in vitro technique.

Wheelock, E. F.: Interferon in Dermal Crusts of Human Vaccinia Virus Vaccination Possible Explanation of Relative Benignity of Variolation Smallpox. Proc. Soc. Exp. Biol. Med., *117*:650-653, 1964.
Interferon: broad-spectrum antiviral protein found in vaccination crust. Can suppress vaccination if given subcutaneously.

Grosfeld, J. C. M., and van Ramshorst, A. G. S.: Eczema Vaccinatum. Report of Four Cases by Contact Infection Treatment with Methisazone (Marboran). Dermatologica, *141*:1-10, 1970.
This thiosemicarbazone is the only chemotherapeutic weapon clinically useful to date.

Douglas, R. G., Jr., Lynch, E. C., and Spira, M.: Treatment of Progressive Vaccinia. Use of Methisazone, Vaccinia Immune Serum Globulin, and Surgical Debridement. Arch. Intern. Med., *129*:980-983, 1972.
Patient survived.

Mückter, H., Sous, H., Poszich, G., and Nijssen, J.: Rifampicin Inhibition of Vaccinia Virus in Mice. Arzneim.-Forsch., *21*:1571-1572, 1971.
Antibiotic from *Streptococcus mediterranei* holds promise as new antivaccinial agent.

Finter, N. B.: Interferons: Therapeutic Prospects. *In* Heath, R. B., and Waterson, A. P.: *Modern Trends in Medical Virology 2,* Appleton-Century-Crofts, New York, 1970, pp. 262-283.
Still slender.

Billiau, A., Muyembe, J. J., and De Somer, P.: Interferon-Inducing Polycarboxylates: Mechanism of Protection Against Vaccinia Virus Infection in Mice. Infect. Immun., *5*:854-857, 1972.
Single intraperitoneal injection of polyacrylic acid protects mice for several weeks against I. V. infection with dermotropic strain of vaccinia virus.

Kempe, H. C., Berge, T., and England, B.: Hyperimmune Vaccine Gamma Globulin: Source, Evaluation and Use in Prophylaxis and Therapy. Pediatrics, *18*:177-188, 1956.
Best treatment for generalized vaccinia.

35

Five months ago this man fell on a staircase, abrading his ankle just below the lateral malleolus. The area failed to heal, remaining crusted, very painful and swollen. Despite topical antibiotics and steroids, a **deep 2-centimeter ulcer** *has formed.*

Peripheral pulses, sensation, serum proteins and an ankle roentgenogram were normal.

Biopsy — nonspecific inflammatory changes.

Culture — abundant E. coli.

Leg Ulcer

This is the ulcer of ischemia. Although initiated by trauma, and propagated by infection, this loss of skin tells a story of local arterial insufficiency. The severe pain is the cry of the skin for oxygen and, as we look closely, we can see another sign of arterial insufficiency, namely, a faint reticulate mottling of the skin. This is the livedo that bespeaks a terminal circulation without much vigor. True, the large vessels appear patent, with full pulse, and there has been no evidence of digital gangrene. Furthermore, histologic study of the skin at the edge of the ulcer fails to reveal any evidence of the vascular nature of this insidiously progressive ulceration. Nonetheless, this is a focal ischemic ulcer similar to the decubitus ulcer, in which unrelieved pressure occludes the cutaneous arterial blood supply and leads to necrosis.

This is not the commonplace ulcer of venous stasis. The patient has no evidence of venous incompetence, no varicosities, no history of thrombophlebitis, no preceding edema, and no dermatitis or hyperpigmentation. The ulcer is not at the favored site, just above the internal malleolus. It thus has none of the hallmarks of the venous ulcer.

Nor is there anything to suggest that this ulcer is secondary to a disease of the skin, such as scleroderma, necrobiosis lipoidica or a malignant condition. Nor does a complete medical study of the patient reveal internal disease as a background. It is certainly not the extensive ulceration we see in pyoderma gangrenosum associated with ulcerative colitis. Likewise, the full range of sensory function rules out a trophic or

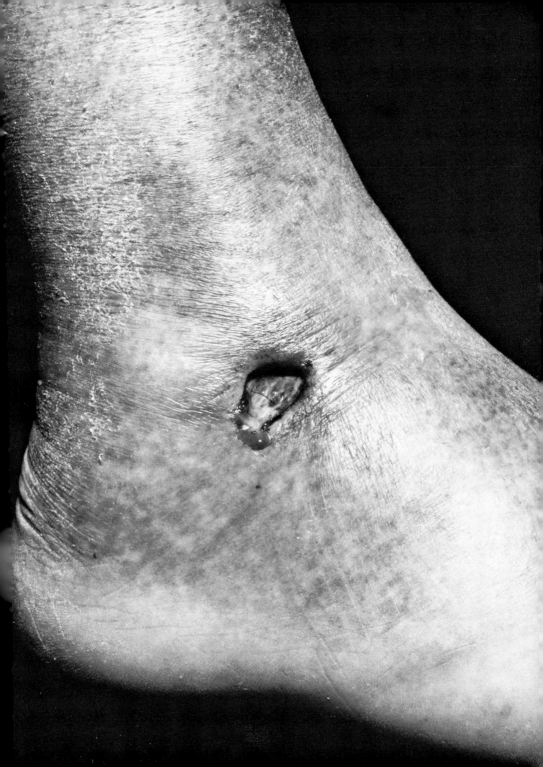

neuropathic ulcer. Nothing in the patient's affect or history alerts us to suspect a factitial lesion, and there is no history of anticoagulant therapy. Assuredly, the biopsy eliminates the possibility of a vasculitic process, and the blood studies remove the sickling trait as well as abnormal proteins and cryoproteins from our diagnostic list. Moreover, no underlying osteomyelitic process could be seen on x-ray. Interestingly, arteriography and venography remain research tools, not commonly employed in clinical practice, although they may be necessary to detect otherwise occult arteriovenous aneurysms, as well as incompetent venous perforators, which at times are responsible for ulceration.

The recitation of causes of leg ulcer can be continued in an almost unending fashion, but the recognition of this as an ischemic arterial ulcer rather than as a venous or stasis ulcer remains of primary importance in the management of this patient.

Our patient's therapy must be centered on improving blood flow to the area. Bed rest is essential to relieve the secondary dependent edema and thereby reduce the occlusive tissue pressures on already compromised arterial vessels. Prolonged sitting in a chair and knee crossing must be avoided, since they favor edema; likewise, propping of the leg above the heart level is contraindicated because of its reductive effect on blood flow. Gradual progressive ambulation comes weeks later with every caveat against further injury. Correction of any nutritional or general medical problems, particularly anemia, is highly desirable. Of equal importance are measures to eliminate the infecting gram-negative bacilli. Until specific susceptibility test data are available from the laboratory it is desirable to employ frequent compressing of the wound with dilute freshly prepared potassium permanganate solutions (1/8000). These can be followed by the topical application of a neomycin cream. The development of bacterial resistance is well known, so that sequential monitoring of the wound pathogens and their sensitivity pattern is often rewarding to the clinician.

The surgical triumphs of arterial grafts as well as venous ligation and stripping are of no avail in this patient, since his problem is not one of large vessel ischemia nor of venous incompetence. Even skin grafting is of questionable value, unless a good supportive granulation tissue base appears. Compressive therapy in the form of casts or elastic supportive hose which is so dramatically helpful in venous ulcers may be of assistance in reducing secondary edema in this patient, but must be used with caution to avoid compromising the local arteriolar supply. Yet there remains the eternal hope of finding a therapeutic short cut. It is this hope that has filled the literature with unfulfilled promises of the benefits of local applications as diverse as gold leaf, raw silk, human amnion and, more recently, hyperbaric oxygen. Much of this therapeutic froth indicates a naïve ignorance of or indifference to the biochemical complexity of the synthesis of even a single collagen fibril. Our mission is to provide a favorable milieu for wound healing, no more, no less.

Both patient and physician must live with the fact that even under optimal care the closing of an ischemic ulcer will be as insidiously slow as its opening was. This is no simple process of re-epithelialization but one of total replacement of an entire organ composed of fat, corium and epidermis. It is a reparative effort that may well call for as many months of therapy as the patient has already had of disease. Like wealth, health often comes but slowly and rarely without effort.

Menendez, C. V.: *Ulcers of the Leg. Cause and Treatment.* Charles C Thomas, Springfield, Illinois, 1967, 73 pp.
The big three common causes: (1) trauma in presence of edema, (2) arterial insufficiency of atherosclerosis and (3) incompetence of perforating veins following phlebitis.

Osmundson, P. J., Fairbairn, J. F., II, Juergens, J. L., Sheps, S. G., Kottke, B. A., and Joyce, J. W.: Ulcers of the Legs. Postgrad. Med., 41:289-300, 1967.
Complete portfolio of Mayo patients with ulcers from arterial ischemia, venous stasis, vasculitis, infections, neoplasms and trauma (at times self-inflicted or due to sensory deficit).

Anning, S. T.: *Leg Ulcers. Their Causes and Treatment.* Little, Brown and Co., Boston, 1954.
Much wisdom in this classic.

Friedman, S. A., and Gladstone, J. L.: The Bacterial Flora of Peripheral Vascular Ulcers. Arch. Derm., 100:29-32, 1969.
In inflamed ischemic ulcers: *Staphylococcus aureus, Escherichia coli, Proteus mirabilis, Aerobacter aerogenes.*

Janssens, P. G.: Skin Ulcers Caused by Acid-Fast Bacteria. In Marshall, J.: *Essays on Tropical Dermatology,* Vol. 2, Excerpta Medica, Amsterdam, 1972, pp. 264-295.
Monographic account of fearsome necrotic ulcers due to atypical Mycobacteria.

Orbach, E. J.: *Candida Albicans,* a Contributing Cause of Torpid Vascular Ulcers of the Lower Extremities. Angiology, 16:664-672, 1965.
All chronic ulcers deserve close microbiologic surveillance.

Grossman, J., Abraham, G. N., Leddy, J. P., and Condemi, J. L.: Crystalalglobulinemia. Ann. Intern. Med., 77:395-400, 1972.
Search for cryoproteins in any patient with an unexplained leg ulcer.

Smith, E. B., and Holder, W. R.: Stasis Ulcer and "Fibrinogen Baltimore." Arch. Derm., 104:221-222, 1971.
Abnormal fibrinogen as a contributing cause.

Fischer, J. A.: Coumarin Skin Necrosis Complicating Thrombophlebitis and Pulmonary Emboli. Case Report. Ann. Surg., 38:451-453, 1972.
Dramatic ulceration due to anticoagulant therapy.

Valtonen, E. J.: Leg Ulcers and Drug Abuse. Lancet, 2:1192-1193, 1970.
A known cause of necrosis: intradermal injection of the unknown.

Gray, H. R., Graham, J. H., Johnson, W., and Burgoon, C. F.: Atrophie Blanche: Periodic Painful Ulcers of Lower Extremities. Arch. Derm., 93:187-193, 1966.
Infarcts due to localized hypersensitivity type vasculitis.

Borrie, P.: Cutaneous Polyarteritis Nodosa. Brit. J. Derm., 87:87-95, 1972.
Manifested by tender painful nodules which may precede ankle ulceration.

Dodd, H., and Cockett, F. B.: *The Pathology and Surgery of the Veins of the Lower Limb.* E. & S. Livingstone Ltd., Edinburgh, 1956, 462 pp.
Ninety per cent of all leg ulcers are venous in origin. A master reference.

Baltaxe, H. A., Meade, J. W., Temes, G. D., Saunders, J., and Mueller, C. B.: Lymphatic and Venous Examination of the Postphlebitic Extremity. Radiology, 91:478-483, 1968.
Incompetence of communicating veins found in all 21 chronic postphlebitic leg ulcers.

Perdrup, A.: The Healing Rate of Leg Ulcers. A Clinical and Statistical Study of 233 Patients Hospitalized with Leg Ulcers. Acta Dermatovener, 52:136-140, 1972.
Slow.

Ger, R.: Surgical Management of Ulcerative Lesions of the Leg. Curr. Probl. Surg., March, 1972, pp. 1-52.
Detailed overview of surgical approach to a problem associated with prolonged convalescence, incapacitating illness, loss of limb or even loss of life.

Ponten, B.: Plastic Surgery Treatment of Chronic Venous Ulcers of the Legs. Scand. J. Plast. Reconst. Surg., 6:74-82, 1972.
Radical excision of ulcer followed later by split-thickness skin graft.

Smith, J. D., Holder, W. R., and Smith, E. B.: Pinch Grafts for Cutaneous Ulcers. South. Med. J., 64:1166-1171, 1971.
Do not graft ischemic ulcers.

Henriksen, S. D., and Gilji, O.: Adhesive Tape. Its Bacteriostatic Effect and Its Use in the Treatment of Ulcus Cruris. Acta Dermatovener., 45:471-478, 1965.
Wound healing effect of adhesive tape is an old observation.

Fisher, A. A.: The Role of Topical Medications in the Management of Stasis Ulcers. Angiology, 22:206-210, 1971.
Avoid contact-sensitizers, since chronic ulcer provides maximal potential for sensitization.

Hallbook, T., and Lanner, E.: Serum-Zinc and Healing of Venous Leg Ulcers. Lancet, 2:780-782, 1972.
Oral zinc sulfate aids in healing of venous leg ulcers if patient is zinc deficient.

From, E., Heydenreich, G., and Siboni, K.: Tetracycline-Resistant Hemolytic Streptococci in Patients with Leg Ulcers. An Argument for Changing The Topical Treatment. Acta Dermatovener., 52:67-70, 1972.
Tailor your antimicrobial therapy to laboratory sensitivity data.

Holm, J., Hofer, P.-A., Lindholm, A., and Littorin, S. H.: Leg Ulcers of Tuberculous Genesis. Report of Fifteen Cases. Acta Clin. Scand., 135:301-309, 1969.
All 15 cured by antituberculous therapy.

Myers, M. B., Rightor, M., and Cherry, G.: Relationship Between Edema and the Healing Rate of Stasis Ulcers of the Leg. Amer. J. Surg., 124:666-668, 1972.
Any therapy which does not improve venous drainage is doomed to failure.

36

Perioral Dermatitis

36

Erythematous papules and pustules *have studded this young woman's chin and lips for the past few years. Treatment has been limited to a variety of topical fluorinated corticosteroids.*

Perioral Dermatitis

Here is a disease with a meteoric career. Less than ten years ago it was first sighted and named. In the ensuing period it has been closely observed, and soon we may anticipate its total disappearance from the medical firmament.

What is this new disease with such a spectacular history? Little more than its forthright name! As can be seen, it is an inflammatory papular rash encircling the mouth. Persistent and erythematous, it may show occasional pustules as well as crusting and fine scaling. An additional feature often seen is a distinctive clear area immediately adjacent to the vermilion border. Virtually a disease of women, it has a nagging chronicity which can be measured in years. Its showcase location invariably calls for a barrage of topical remedies, from abrasive soaps through hypoallergenic cosmetics to corticosteroids. Typically, nothing clears the eruption, but the local steroid therapy is continued, sometimes for years, since its discontinuance evokes a flare. Histologic examination adds little to our understanding, no pathognomonic changes being seen. This is the complete portrait. It does not appear elsewhere on the skin and there are no internal associated medical problems. It is evident that few diseases have been more accurately or better named.

What makes perioral dermatitis a new and different disease? Its unique feature is simply its localization. Seborrheic dermatitis and rosacea may show a lesional resemblance, but they characteristically involve the perinasal, cheek and forehead regions. Acne or acneiform eruptions, especially acne cosmetica, also come to mind, but, again, these processes are not so limited in extent. Contact dermatitis is another on the differential list and may call for patch-testing of the local preparations being used. Most interestingly, candidal infection can produce precisely the changes of perioral dermatitis. Here, the *Candida albicans*

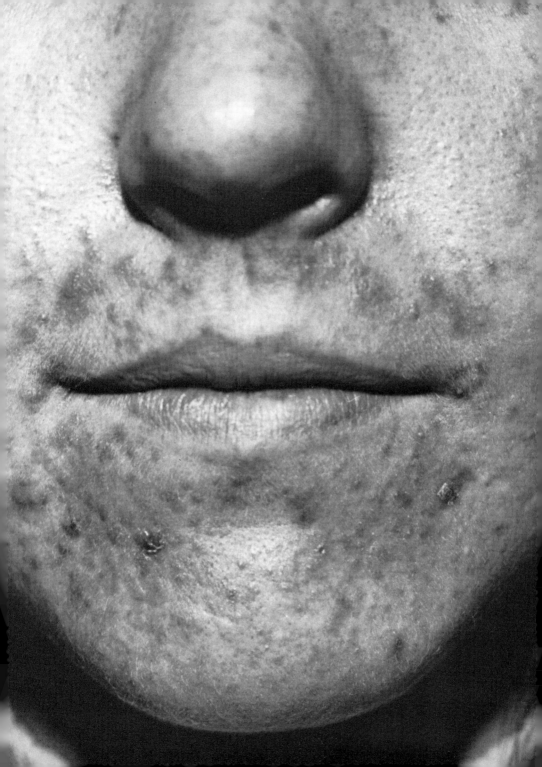

can be suspected on scrapings from the area, confirmed on culture and eliminated by measures such as topical amphotericin B therapy.

What is the pathogenesis of this new coinage, the perioral eruption? Certainly the appearance suggests it could be a variant of rosacea or seborrheic dermatitis. Its location favors an etiologic role for salivary secretions or oral flora. The banal histopathologic findings are uniquely silent, pointing only a finger toward an external cause. And here is where the answer lies. As we focus on new external factors, we perceive the cause—the newly synthesized, highly potent fluorinated cortico-steroids. These are the signal advances of the last decade. It is the obses-sive daily use of these steroid creams which has ushered in this new disease—perioral dermatitis. It is neither an allergic reaction nor a primary irritant phenomenon but rather a pharmacologic effect on the skin itself. The prolonged local use of these steroids in other seborrheic areas can induce rosaceal and erythematous changes as well. Not sur-prisingly, this steroid rosacea develops more often in women, in whom there is a conjunction of long-term daily use and a thin permeable skin structure.

What is the treatment? Total absolute interdiction of topical steroids! This calls for understanding and acceptance by the patient of the fact that such therapeutic withdrawal will produce a flare initially. Some patients have become virtually addicted to their topical steroids and need considerable support during the long three or four months needed for the skin to return to normal. The obverse and equally valu-able side of the page of therapy is systemic tetracycline. This should be given in a dosage of 250 mg. four times a day, preferably before meals and not in conjunction with iron supplements which reduce absorption. This approach almost invariably is associated with a steady return of the skin to its pristine state.

With wider public and medical awareness of this new hazard of the prolonged assiduous use of topical fluorinated steroids, the meteor of perioral dermatitis and steroid rosacea should disappear, just as the "un-dercoat" nail dystrophies and the underarm deodorant zirconium gran-ulomas of yesteryear.

Sneddon, I.: Perioral Dermatitis. Brit. J. Derm., *87*:430-434, 1972.
Experiences with 73 cases prove his thesis that in women long-term application of fluorinated steroids converts banal skin inflammation into picture of perioral der-matitis.

Hjorth, N., Osmundsen, P., Rook, A. J., Wilkinson, D. S., and Marks, R.: Perioral Dermatitis. Brit. J. Derm., *80*:307-313, 1968.
Clinical picture of a common yet new disease: erythematous papulosquamous eruption of chin and upper lip, sparing perivermilion zone.

Marks, R., and Black, M. M.: Perioral Dermatitis. A Histopathological Study of 26 Cases. Brit. J. Derm., *84*:242-247, 1971.
Suggestive of reaction to external irritant; no pathognomonic features; can distinguish from rosacea.

Macmillan, A. L.: Unusual Features of Scabies Associated with Topical Fluorinated Steroids. Brit. J. Derm., *87*:496-497, 1972.
Use of topical fluorinated steroid in infant responsible for fantastic increase in number of itch mite burrows.

Gear, J. H. S.: The Pathogenicity of Demodex Folliculorum. *In Essays on Tropical Dermatology,* Vol. 2, Excerpta Medica, Amsterdam, 1972, pp. 209-215.
(What effect may topical fluorinated steroids have on the pathogenicity of the hair follicle mite, demodex? Vide supra.)

Mullanax, M. G., and Kierland, R. R.: Granulomatous Rosacea. Arch. Derm., *101*:206-211, 1970.
May be perioral in distribution; responds to topical sulfur.

Bradford, L. G., and Montes, L. F.: Perioral Dermatitis and *Candida Albicans.* Arch. Derm., *105*:892-895, 1972.
C. albicans **found in scrapings and on culture in one case; dermatitis cleared with topical anticandidal therapy (nystatin, amphotericin B, and haloprogin).**

Weber, G.: Rosacea-like Dermatitis: Contraindication or Intolerance Reaction to Strong Steroids. Brit. J. Derm., 86:253-259, 1972.
Successful treatment of perioral dermatitis demands complete elimination of strong topical corticosteroids.

Macdonald, A., and Feiwel, M.: Perioral Dermatitis: Aetiology and Treatment with Tetracycline. Brit. J. Derm., 87:314-319, 1972.
Everyone of their 29 patients responded to oral tetracycline given over 3-month period.

37

Hoarseness, thickened everted eyelids *and* **infiltrative plaques of the elbows** *have been the lifelong stigmata of this 60-year-old woman's disease. Her tongue is bound down with the same asymptomatic infiltrative process. General medical studies, including a variety of biochemical parameters, are normal.*

Biopsies — amorphous eosinophilic infiltrates of PAS-positive material in the dermis and in the vocal cords.

Lipoid Proteinosis

Here is a diagnosis that can be made simply by meeting the patient. The thickened eyelid and the husky "hello" can be the basis for instant recognition. Although the diagnosis is just that easy, it is one very rarely made, many dermatologists having spent a lifetime in practice without ever meeting such a patient. But for all its rarity, lipoid proteinosis is an experiment of nature that is fascinating and instructive.

It is a genodermatosis. Indeed, it is felt that the lineage of all those afflicted with this disease in South Africa can be traced back to Jacob Cloete and his sister, Elsje, who migrated there from Germany over 300 years ago. A relatively nondisadvantageous autosomal recessive trait, it has passed down through more than 13 generations. With the aid of consanguinity, it has actually flourished to the extent that one third of all the documented cases in the world are of this South African provenance.

It is more than a genodermatosis. It is a hereditary metabolic disorder, histologically at least as pervasive as the very connective tissue it affects. The singular feature is the deposition of an amorphous protein. It is this anomalous protein, elaborated by fibrocytes, which forms the gross infiltrate in her eyelids, over her elbows and in her tongue. Masses of this same material distort her vocal cords, accounting for her strident voice.

Strangely, physical trauma appears to be a determinant in localization of this atypical protein; for example, the elbows and knees are notably subject to repeated pressure. The tongue, exposed to the daily hazards of mastication, the vocal cords, subjected to the vibrant stimulus of speech, and the rectum under inordinate stretch, might be anticipated to

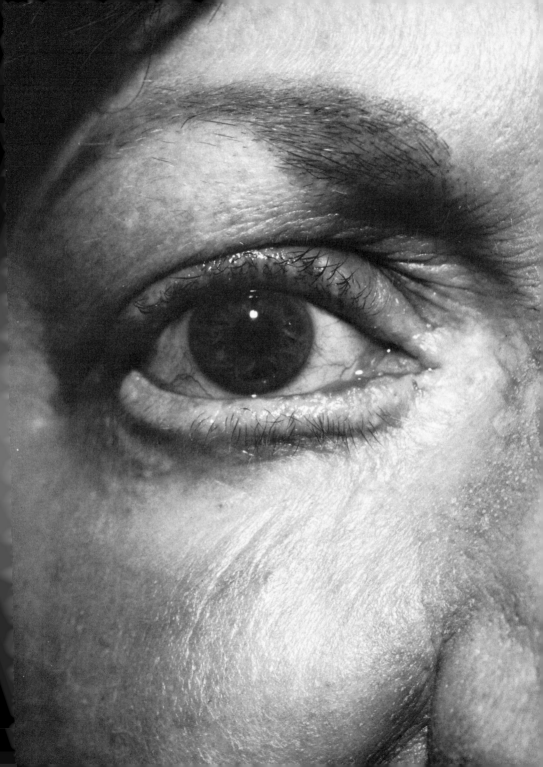

be similar sites of predilection. But other stimuli are operative, since significant deposits are to be found within the brain as well.

Diagnostically, the skin provides a recognizable canvas, with the infiltrates commonly taking on the color of old ivory. In this regard, the protein deposit has an affinity for calcium, sometimes perceived only on electron microscopy as tiny grains. Beading of the eyelid margin is another characteristic as is the pock mark of former infections or resorbed infiltrates. Hair loss is seen at times, not only on the eyelids but also on the scalp, the infiltrative interfering with normal follicular activity. Nail growth as well as dental development may be hampered. Even more typically, xanthomatous-appearing plaques arise and persist on the elbows and knees.

Elsewhere the pathologic deposits are more commonly recognized by their functional effects. The inability of these patients to stick out their tongues, the rasping scratchy voice and the presence of dysphagia all are diagnostic clues. Parotic pain and swelling can indicate ductal obstruction. More seriously, epilepsy, rage attacks, selective memory loss or mental retardation can signal deposits in the caudate nucleus, globus pallidus, amygdaloid nucleus or cerebral cortex. Usually, however, the central nervous system involvement is restricted to an asymptomatic yet significant calcification, seen in a lateral plate as a bean-shaped density above the sella turcica. Actually, the process is bilateral, the calcific deposits localizing in selected nuclei of the brain. No organ of the body is exempt, and an awareness of this systemic potential of lipoid proteinosis adds keenness to any diagnostic appraisal of this patient's future complaints.

Lipoid proteinosis is a local disorder. The blood provides no answers. It is only when we look at the skin under electron microscopy that we begin to sense the story. The fibrocyte normally can respond to the reparative call for new collagen. However, in this disease, the fibrocyte has a presumed enzyme deficit, the resultant product being a functionless hyalin mass of protein rather than the appropriate collagen fibril. Interestingly, in erythropoietic protoporphyria, the fibrocyte is similarly maimed, so that the trauma of light exposure induces a histochemically identical hyalin protein product. These are to be sharply distinguished from the two other classic hyalin deposits of protein, namely, colloid and amyloid. It should be emphasized that, despite its name, lipoid proteinosis is not a disturbance in lipoid metabolism but simply one of protein metabolism. There is no evidence of xanthoma cells, nor does the blood show any lipidemia. Nor is it one of the metabolic errors of mucopolysaccharide formation. In tissue culture the affected fibrocytes show none of the typical inclusions associated with the mucopolysaccharidoses.

Lipoid proteinosis is largely a self-limiting chronic disease and is rarely life threatening. It is not malignant, and most of its harm comes from functional impairment, whether in the respiratory tract, in the nervous system or elsewhere. It is well to recall that severe respiratory infections pose a special threat to these patients with an already compromised airway. Intensive systemic antibiotic therapy, even tracheotomy, may be necessary.

Although we know much about the general nature of this patient's disease, there is little we can do to alter its course. We have neither the tools nor the knack of repairing the molecular machinery of her fibroblasts. Her diagnosis is a gauntlet of challenge for the bioengineers of tomorrow!

Grosfold, J. C. M., Spaas, J., van de Staak, W. J. B. M., and Stadhouders, A. M.: Hyalinosis Cutis et Mucosae (Lipoid Proteinosis Urbach-Wiethe). Dermatologica, *130*:239-266, 1965.
Cardinal signs: beaded thickening of eyelid margins, hoarseness due to vocal cord infiltrates, nonprotrudable tongue and intracranial calcification. References for the 150 cases in world literature.

Newton, F. H., Rosenberg, R. N., Lampert, P. W., and O'Brien, J. S.: Neurologic Involvement in Urbach-Wiethe's Disease (Lipoid Proteinosis). Neurology, *21*:1205-1213, 1971.
Calcification of caudate nucleus, globus pallidum, amygdaloid nucleus (seizures, rage attacks) and hippocampus (selective recent memory loss).

Caplan, R. M.: Visceral Involvement in Lipoid Proteinosis. Arch. Derm., *95*:149-155, 1967.
Hyalin infiltrate appears in virtually every organ of the body, from brain to testis.

Weidner, W. A., Wenzl, J. E., and Swischuk, L. E.: Roentgenographic Findings in Lipoid Proteinosis: A Case Report. Amer. J. Roentgenol., *110*:457-461, 1970.
Classic finding: bean-shaped intracranial calcification in suprasellar area (due to bilateral deposits in temporal lobes).

Heyl, T.: Lipoid Proteinosis in South Africa. Dermatologica, *142*:129-132, 1971.
All cases traced back to autosomal recessive gene brought into continent circa 1650 by a German settler and his sister.

Findlay, G. H., Scott, F. P., and Cripps, D. J.: Porphyria and Lipid Proteinosis. A Clinical, Histological and Biochemical Comparison of 19 South African Cases. Brit. J. Derm., *78*:69-80, 1966.
Sun-sensitive porphyria patients may develop collagenous degeneration resembling infiltrates of lipoid proteinosis, but never hoarseness.

van der Walt, J. J., and Heyl, T.: Lipoid Proteinosis and Erythropoietic Protoporphyria. A Histologic and Histochemical Study. Arch. Derm., *104*:501-507, 1971.

Twenty-two stains attest to histochemical identity of skin deposits in these two conditions.

Rasiewicz, W., Rubisz-Brzezinska, J., and Konecki, J.: Hyalinosis Cutis et Mucosae Urbach-Wiethe. Report of a Case and Results of Histochemical Studies. Dermatologica, *130*:145-157, 1965.

Infiltrate is protein in character, lipids and mucopolysaccharides adventitial.

Fleischmajer, R., Nedwich, A., and Ramos e Silva, J.: Hyalinosis Cutis et Mucosae. A Histochemical Staining and Analytical Biochemical Study. J. Invest. Derm., *52*:495-503, 1969.

Evidence that strongly PAS-positive hyalin material accumulating in boundary areas of upper cutis, perivascular, perifollicular and periglandular zones is a glycoprotein.

Jensen, A. D., Khodadoust, A. A., and Emery, J. M.: Lipoid Proteinosis. Report of a Case with Electron Microscopic Findings. Arch. Ophthal., *88*:273-277, 1972.

Electron microscopy: deposit is a finely granular amorphous material.

Hashimoto, K., Klingmüller, G., and Rodermund, O.-E.: Hyalinosis Cutis et Mucosae. Acta Dermatovener., *52*:179-195, 1972.

Electron microscopy reveals that major portion of hyalin infiltrate in lipoid proteinosis is produced locally as an abnormal product of fibroblasts.

Vukas, A.: Hyalinosis Cutis et Mucosae Regenerative Properties of Tissues Involved in Chronic Pathology. Dermatologica, *144*:168-175, 1972.

Dermabrasion of face helpful in removing some of infiltrate and pock scars.

38

Xeroderma Pigmentosum

38

This 22-year-old woman has had photophobia and sun-sensitive skin since childhood. **Her face, arms and back show thousands of small punctate and irregularly shaped pigmented spots, intermingled with completely achromic white spots.** *Five basal cell epitheliomas are present on her forehead and eyelids.*

Scars are seen on her face, shoulders and back at the sites of basal cell and squamous cell epitheliomas previously removed during the last 12 years. A large skin graft covers the right shoulder where a malignant melanoma was radically excised a year ago.

Xeroderma Pigmentosum

Molecular biology seems so far removed from clinical practice, but here is a disease it has touched. Recognized as a rare fatal inborn sensitivity to sunlight, this disease remained mysterious and incomprehensible for a hundred years. But now, molecular biology has pinpointed the defect to a precise molecular locus. At first recognized only in mutant bacteria, the defect is now known to be in our patient's cells. It consists of an inability to reconstitute the nuclear thread of life, DNA, after it has been altered by ultraviolet light.

Thus, a new concept in medicine has unfolded. This patient's photosensitivity is not due to the absence of melanin, as in the unfortunate albino. It is not due to the peculiar metabolic error of heme metabolism with the consequent accumulation in the skin of photosensitizing porphyrins, as in porphyria. It is not due to the presence of an acquired immune state activated by light, as in contact photosensitivity. Rather, it is a hereditable disease with an enzyme deficiency which becomes clinically manifest only on exposure to ultraviolet radiation.

Xeroderma pigmentosum begins innocently enough. Not present on emergence from the darkness of the birth chamber, this girl's problem began at first as an easily ignored sun sensitivity of her skin. Photophobia and prolonged solar erythema were only later given significance, as freckling and spotty achromia appeared on the sun-exposed areas. The course was insidious but with the inexorable onset of actinic

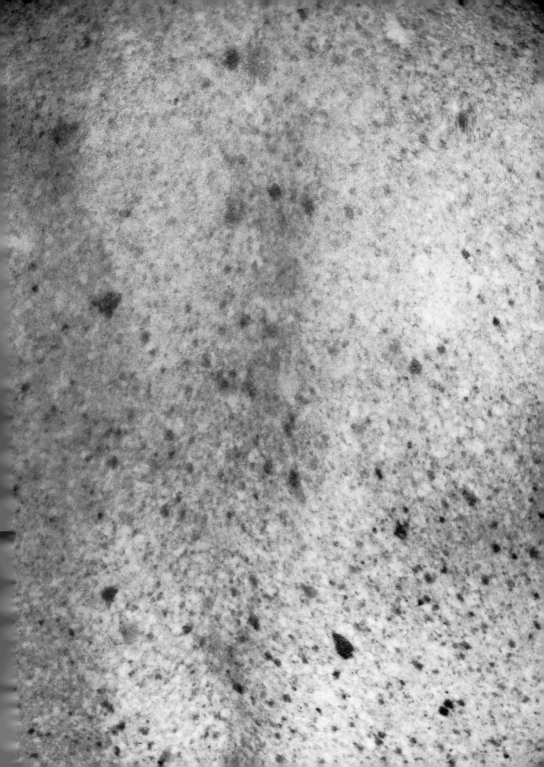

keratoses and basal cell epitheliomas. With sun and time, our patient's exposed skin became the picture of senility and in areas showed the awesome ravages of a radiodermatitis. But recall that she had not been exposed to x-ray but simply to the ultraviolet light we all face daily.

The history is one of an unrelieved sequence of tumors. True, it began somewhat later than usual in childhood, probably because her youth was spent far north of the tropics, and her enzyme deficiency was presumably not total. She has not had the ectropion, entropion or corneal ulcers so characteristic in severe forms. Nonetheless, she has had not only squamous cell epitheliomas but a fearsome malignant melanoma. She has survived well beyond the mean life expectancy of these patients but the prognosis is guarded. The sun still threatens to cause additional tumors, even angio-, fibro-, and lymphosarcomas, since all her cells share the same inability to cope with ultraviolet light.

Her family history gives no clues that her problem is genetic, but she must be acquainted with the fact that it is, and that as an autosomal recessive trait it could be transmitted by her. Should she become pregnant, it is still not possible, practically speaking, to make a prenatal diagnosis, although amniotic cell techniques for this purpose are available on a research level. It is important to note that any sun sensitivity or freckling in her siblings or in any member of her family should be treated with respect, recognizing that in some individuals xeroderma pigmentosum appears late in life.

The diagnosis in our patient is an easy one at this late stage. Even before the tumors had appeared, the history of sun sensitivity, photophobia and a mottled mix of freckling and achromia would have been sufficient. It is a clinical constellation diagnosis, however, since none of the biopsy findings is pathognomonic. One sees simply patchy hypermelaninism and absence of pigment. The changes of premalignant and malignant cells again offer nothing distinctive. Likewise, the thin atrophic skin and solar elastoses observed alert the pathologist only if the age of the patient is recorded and emphasized. Skin testing with appropriate amounts of ultraviolet light in the 280 to 310 nm. range should show a persistent erythema that appears several days after exposure, rather than the normal pattern that occurs after a latent period of 6 to 8 hours. The freckling is diagnostic, since the hyperpigmented spots are set with contrasting white atrophic spots. This is not the typical pattern seen in the syndrome of multiple lentigines. Finally, it should be pointed out that this patient shows none of the features of the DeSanctis-Cacchione variant of xeroderma pigmentosum, in which a related but additional gene defect seems to be responsible for microcephaly, mental retardation, hypogonadism, spasticity and ataxia as well as associated degenerative changes.

The clinical story stops here. To learn more, the molecular biologist has melded the nonclinical techniques of tissue culture, isotopic autoradiography, DNA synthesis and radiobiology. He has found that normally ultraviolet light induces formation of a potentially lethal dimer in the DNA of cells. Normally, this is recognized and enzymatically excised, and new bases are inserted in the DNA, with complete repair. In the xeroderma pigmentosum cell (whether it be the keratinocyte, fibrocyte, lymphocyte or melanocyte) this does not occur. Tissue cultures of these cells thus show no incorporation of isotopically labelled thymidine base on autoradiographs following ultraviolet radiation. Born without the ability to repair the thread of reproductive life, the cell dies or becomes a malignant mutant, presumably owing to a lack of the enzyme endonuclease, which is critically necessary for excision of the dimer. This is the fatal defect of our patient, so lately understood.

The treatment is confinement to darkness. Ideally, our patient must live in an environment as devoid of the sunburn spectrum of light as possible. This calls for living in the north, being out of doors only in the early hours when the rays of sunlight are weak, wearing clothing of sufficient weave to screen light, and using total filter sun screens. Such compulsive living is rarely undertaken, and, indeed, long-term damage may be incurred by sun exposure prior to an awareness of the diagnosis. As a result, tumors appear and must be treated on an individual basis with curettage or excision. Note that there is no defect in wound healing. Topical 5-fluorouracil is useful in the treatment of the actinic keratoses these patients invariably exhibit. X-ray therapy is not to be employed because, although these patients are not directly sensitive to x-ray, their skin is atrophic and therefore abnormally vulnerable.

Extensive radical surgery may be necessary as in the case of patient's malignant melanoma. In others, dermabrasion may serve a prophylactic function by resurfacing the skin with cells not previously exposed to appreciable amounts of ultraviolet light.

Despite all our help and understanding, these patients must go down through life on a lonely dark road.

Reed, W. B., Landing, B., Sugarman, G., Cleaver, J. E., and Melnyk, J.: Xeroderma Pigmentosum. Clinical and Laboratory Investigation of Its Basic Defect. J.A.M.A., *207*:2073-2079, 1969.
The fatal sunlight sensitivity, freckles and skin cancer syndrome.

El-Hefnawi, H., and Mortada, A.: Ocular Manifestations of Xeroderma Pigmentosum. Brit. J. Derm., *77*:261-276, 1965.
Photophobia, conjunctivitis, keratitis and basal and squamous cell epitheliomas in 46 patients.

Lynch, H. T., Anderson, D. E., Smith, J. L., Jr., Howell, J. B., and Krush, A. J.: Xeroderma Pigmentosum, Malignant Melanoma and Congenital Ichthyosis. Arch. Derm., *96*:625-635, 1967.
Sunlight-induced melanoma in the precancerous skin of xeroderma pigmentosum. References on 23 cases.

Reed, W. B., May, S. B., and Nickel, W. R.: Xeroderma Pigmentosum with Neurological Complications. The DeSanctis-Cacchione Syndrome. Arch. Derm., *91*:224-226, 1965.
Xerodermic idiocy: unusual variant with brain, mentality, stature and gonads all diminutive.

Afifi, A. K., Der Kaloustian, V. M., and Mire, J. J.: Muscular Abnormality in Xeroderma Pigmentosum. High Resolution Light-Microscopy and Electron-Microscopic Observations. J. Neurol. Sci., 17:435-442, 1972.
Dysarthria, choreoarthetosis, ataxia with muscular glycogen storage disturbance. Three cases.

Jung, E. G.: New Form of Molecular Defect in Xeroderma Pigmentosum. Nature, *228*:361-362, 1970.
Pigmented xerodermoid: inverse label for tardive form of syndrome appearing after age 35.

Selmanowitz, V. J., Orentreich, N., and Felsenstein, J. M.: Lentiginosis Profusa Syndrome (Multiple Lentigines Syndrome). Arch. Derm., *104*:393-401, 1971.
Not sun sensitive, not precancerous, but sign of cardiovascular problems.

Caputo, R., and Califano, A.: Ultrastructural Changes in the Epidermis of Xeroderma Pigmentosum Lesions in Various Stages of Development. Arch. Derm. Forsch., *241*:364-373, 1971.
Increase in mitoses and irregularities of cell structure reminiscent of cancer.

Cripps, D. J., Ramsay, C. A., and Ruch, D. M.: Xeroderma Pigmentosum: Abnormal Monochromatic Action Spectrum and Autoradiographic Studies. J. Invest. Derm., *56*:281-286, 1971.
Xeroderma pigmentosum — erythema induced best with 293 nm. peaks at 72 hours. Normal — erythema induced best with 250 nm. peaks at 8 hours.

El-Hefnawi, H., Maynard Smith, S., and Penrose, L. S.: Xeroderma Pigmentosum — Its Inheritance and Relationship to the ABO Blood-Group System. Ann. Hum. Genet., *28*:273-290, 1965.
Autosomal recessive.

Parrington, J. M., Delhanty, J. D. A., and Baden, H. P.: Unscheduled DNA Synthesis, Ultraviolet-Induced Chromosome Aberrations and SV_{40} Transformation in Cultured Cells from Xeroderma Pigmentosum. Ann. Hum. Genet., *35*:149-160, 1971.
Ultraviolet irradiation is fatal to xeroderma pigmentosum cells in tissue culture.

Buhl, S. N., Stillman, R. M., Setlow, R. B., and Regan, J. D.: DNA Chain Elongation and Joining in Normal Human and Xeroderma Pigmentosum Cells after Ultraviolet Irradiation. Biophys. J., *12*:1183-1191, 1972.

Ultraviolet irradiation forms dimers between adjacent pyrimidines in DNA, must be repaired by molecular excision; xeroderma pigmentosum cell nucleus incapable of doing this.

Lytle, C. D., Aaronson, S. A., and Harvey, E.: Host-Cell Reactivation in Mammalian Cells. II. Survival of Herpes Simplex Virus and Vaccinia Virus in Normal Human and Xeroderma Pigmentosum Cells. Int. J. Radiat. Biol., *22*:159-165, 1972.

Xeroderma pigmentosum cells likewise lack normal ability to repair ultraviolet irradiation damage induced in herpes simplex virus.

Stich, H. F., San, R. H. C., and Kawazoe, Y.: Increased Sensitivity of Xeroderma Pigmentosum Cells to Some Chemical Carcinogens and Mutagens. Mutat. Res., *17*:127-137, 1973.

Xeroderma pigmentosum cells also lack ability to repair DNA damaged by certain chemical carcinogens.

Robbins, J. H., Levis, W. R., and Miller, A. E.: Xeroderma Pigmentosum Epidermal Cells with Normal UV-Induced Thymidine Incorporation. J. Invest. Derm., *59*:402-408, 1972.

Basic defect in DNA repair resides not only in keratinocytes but also in fibrocytes and lymphocytes. Not present in every patient with xeroderma pigmentosum.

Darzynkiewicz, Z., Chelmickaszorc, E., and Arnason, B. G. W.: UV-Induced DNA Synthesis in Xeroderma Pigmentosum Nuclei in Heterokaryons. Exp. Cell Res., *74*:602-606, 1972.

Correction of xeroderma pigmentosum defect possible in tissue culture: fusion with normal cell to provide the missing repair enzyme, endonuclease.

Regan, J. D., Setlow, R. B., Kaback, M. M., Howell, R. R., Klein, E., and Burgess, G.: Xeroderma Pigmentosum: A Rapid Sensitive Method for Prenatal Diagnosis. Science, *174*:147-150, 1971.

Theoretical, based on recognition by sedimentation constant of damaged DNA of cells cultured from amniotic fluid.

Cleaver, J. E.: Excision Repair: Our Current Knowledge Based on Human (Xeroderma Pigmentosum) and Cattle Cells. Johns Hopkins Med. J., (Suppl.) *1*:195-211, 1972.

Latest review on how xeroderma pigmentosum cells fail to excise critical UVL photo pyrimidine dimers from DNA molecule — by the man who discovered it all.

Muller, W. E. G., Yamazaki, Z., Zahn, R. K., Brehm, G., and Korting, G.: RNA Dependent DNA Polymerase in Cells of Xeroderma Pigmentosum. Biochem. Biophys. Res. Commun., *44*:433-438, 1971.

Suggests tumor development due to presence of oncogenic RNA virus.

de Weerd-Kastelein, E. A., Keijzer, W., and Bootsma, D.: Genetic Heterogenicity of Xeroderma Pigmentosum Demonstrated by Somatic Cell Hybridization. Nature (New Biol.), *238*:80-83, 1972.

Demonstration that separate genes are responsible for skin and central nervous system findings.

Macleod, T. M., and Frain-Bell, W.: The Study of the Efficacy of Some Agents Used for the Protection of the Skin from Exposure to Light. Brit. J. Derm., *84*:266-281, 1971.

Comprehensive study. Recommends a titanium dioxide, zinc oxide, ferric oxide, aluminum silicate, benzophenone cream for xeroderma pigmentosum.

Slater, T. F.: *Free Radical Mechanisms in Tissue Injury.* Pion Ltd., London, 1972.
Carotenes, vitamin C and vitamin E may serve to remove free radicals responsible for tissue damage following irradiation.

Yosipovitch, Z., Sachs, M. I., and Neuman, Z.: Multiple Malignant Tumour Formation in Xeroderma Pigmentosum. Brit. J. Plast. Surg., *18*:314-321, 1965.
Advises prophylactic dermabrasion.

Epstein, E. H., Jr., Burk, P. G., Cohen, I. K., and Deekers, P.: Dermatome Shaving in the Treatment of Xeroderma Pigmentosum. Arch. Derm., *105*:589-590, 1972.
May be necessary to remove large split-thickness sheets of heavily involved skin by means of dermatome, followed by grafting.

Gleason, M. C.: Xeroderma Pigmentosum — Five Year Arrest After Total Resurfacing of the Face. Plast. Reconstr. Surg., *46*:577-581, 1970.
Report of 305 lesions excised in 3 years.

Carter, V. H., Smith, K. W., and Noojin, R. O.: Xeroderma Pigmentosum Treatment with Topically Applied Fluorouracil. Arch. Derm., *98*:526-527, 1968.
Helpful.

39

Darier's Disease

39

This young woman has **greasy, crusted, brownish papules on her face and neck.** *Present since she was age 6, they become more prominent in the summer. Also noted are warty papules of the dorsa of her hands, pitting and punctate hyperkeratosis of her palms and thin, brittle nail plates.*

Topical retinoic acid solution has provided temporary amelioration.

Biopsy — splits in thickened, hyperkeratotic epidermis, and presence of distinctive dyskeratotic cells (corps ronds and grains).

Darier's Disease

You are looking at flaws in the epidermal weave of this patient's outer garment of keratin. The keratinocyte, which so invisibly spins its protective fibrous protein, has been damaged. Crippled but not incapacitated, the cell now elaborates its keratin threads not in their usual orderly strands but as coiled snarled aggregates. It is a picture as disruptive on the ultramicroscopic level as on the clinical.

It is also distinctive. One does not readily forget the dirty brown, waxy keratotic papule which is the primary lesion. It is crumbly and can be rubbed off at times, revealing not only that the intracellular keratin formation is flawed but that the intercellular syncytial attachments of the keratinocytes have been lost. This latent epithelial tear is seen under the microscope as damaged keratinocytes lose their desmosomal attachments and float free in lacunae. It is these cells which are dyskeratotic, with vacuolization and keratin clumping, that produce the pathognomonic cytologic patterning known as "corps ronds and grains."

Not only is the papule unique and diagnostic but the distribution of this disease forms a singular characteristic. It is one predominantly of the face and chest, the hands, the flexural folds and the oral mucosa. From this we have our first clue as to its nature. It occurs at sites of injury. Often in youngsters, a sunburn will usher in the first changes of this chronic disfiguring eruption. In others, seborrheic dermatitis, acne, intertrigo and folliculitis are triggers. Indeed, the follicle is so often involved that keratosis follicularis is a common synonym for the euphon-

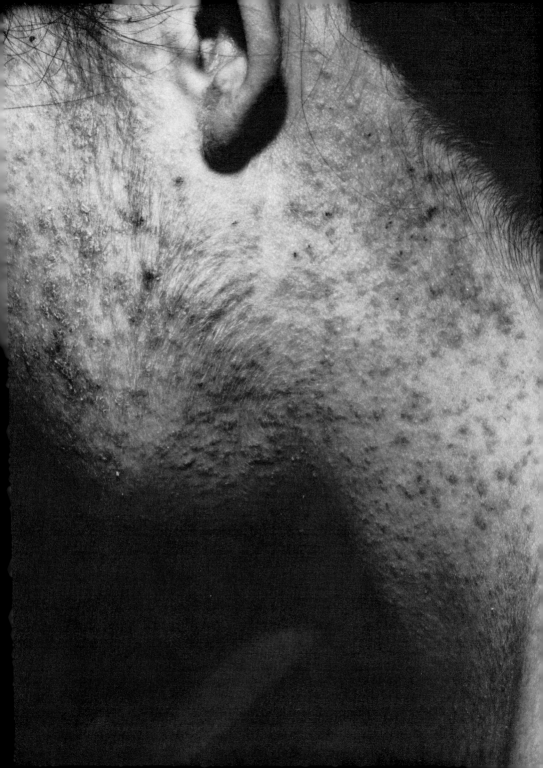

ious eponym of Darier. But lesions can occur at random and do develop in the mucosa. In this nonfollicular site, the resultant leukoplakia-like white papules are often under dentures on the hard palate of edentulous individuals, further pointing to the triggering nature of trauma.

But it is the hands of our patients that present a special subset of remarkably diagnostic signs. The dorsa are covered with fine flat warty papules. The nails are thin and fragile with splintered edges and subungual keratosis. In the palms we read a story of pits and keratotic growths. Surely trauma has to be considered again in the role of an elicitor.

Our second clue as to the nature of this patient's disease comes not from her but from other patients. They recognize that this is a familial trait, and genetic studies confirm it as an autosomal dominant. Our patient's lack of a family history suggests that her problem may be a new mutation, and as such it may be one that could be transmitted to her children.

Our patient's course will continue for years. Papules may come and go, become confluent, be hemorrhagic or leave white atrophic spots. We can assure her that the changes are benign and that they will probably not progress. Only rarely do the lesions become hypertrophic or generalized. The main concern is one of reducing secondary bacterial growth and avoiding superinfection with the vaccinia virus or herpes simplex. She must be instructed to cleanse the skin gently and regularly and to avoid maceration. Malodor is one of the first signs of overgrowth of the surface flora in these moist papules. We must prescribe appropriate topical and systemic antibiotics as needed. Most importantly she must be aware of the frightening risk of exposure to vaccine virus, either directly by vaccination or by contact with someone freshly vaccinated. Her flawed skin is a fertile soil for inoculation and her defenses are likely to be poor. Likewise, the ubiquitous herpes simplex virus must be avoided. Kissing can pose a special hazard for her.

Furthermore, our patient must be aware of the benefits of a lifetime of shade. She must avoid sun bathing and sports such as skiing with high solar exposure and in general must try to walk on the shady side of the street. She must always treat her skin as the delicate sheath it is. Strong soaps, abrasives and even rough clothing are not for her.

The solitary pharmacologic remedy is vitamin A, which has profound yet obscure effects on the keratinocyte. If used orally it should be given in a water-soluble form in massive pharmacologic dosage (e.g.,

Aquasol A, 50,000 units q.i.d.) for a limited time and with an awareness of its toxic effects. In some patients this is of distinctly beneficial but not permanent help. A newer approach is the employment of vitamin A acid (retinoic acid) topically. If irritation can be avoided by using an adequate yet threshold concentration, or by the conjoint use of topical steroids, it may prove to be a helpful measure.

As an intriguing genetic riddle, Darier's disease urges us to learn more of the story of keratinization. Enzyme chemistry must lead the way to better understanding and better therapy.

Lazar, P.: Keratosis Follicularis (Darier's Disease). *In* Demis, D. J., et al. (Eds.): *Clinical Dermatology,* Vol. 1, Harper & Row, New York, 1972, Unit 1-35, pp. 1-7.
Introduction to clinical distinctive, dirty, crusted, warty lesions in seborrheic areas.

Zaias, N., and Ackerman, A. B.: The Nail in Darier-White Disease. Arch. Derm., *107*:193-199, 1973.
Diagnostic: longitudinal subungual red and white streaks with distal subungual keratosis.

Cornelison, R. L., Smith, E. B., and Knox, J. M.: Guttate Leukoderma in Darier's Disease. Arch. Derm., *107*:225-230, 1973.
May see guttate loss of pigment.

Weathers, D. R., Olansky, S., and Sharpe, L. O.: Darier's Disease with Mucous Membrane Involvement. Arch. Derm., *100*:50-53, 1969.
Look for white cobblestone papules on palate and tongue.

Loken, P., and Gundersen, T.: Darier's Disease and Cystic Changes of the Bones. Acta Dermatovener., *48*:162-165, 1968.
Interesting, unusual roentgenologic sign of Darier's disease.

Gottlieb, S. K., and Lutzner, M. A.: Darier's Disease. An Electron Microscopic Study. Arch. Derm., *107*:225-230, 1973.
Essential dyskeratotic change is in keratinocyte: vacuolization, tonofilament condensates, and acantholysis leading to characteristic corps ronds, grains and lacunae.

Leeming, J. A. L.: Acquired Linear Naevus Showing Histological Features of Keratosis Follicularis. Brit. J. Derm., *81*:128-131, 1969.
Linear and zosteriform Darier's disease.

Tanay, A., and Mehregan, A. H.: Warty Dyskeratoma. Dermatologica, *138*:155-164, 1969.
Report of 112 examples of tumors which were histologically but not clinically Darier's disease.

Loeffel, E. D., and Meyer, J. S.: Eczema Vaccinatum in Darier's Disease. Arch. Derm., *102*:451-456, 1970.
Significant complication, mimics pyoderma, identity by intracytoplasmic inclusions on smear, treat with vaccinia immune globulin.

Izumi, A., and Goldschmidt, H.: Herpes Simplex Infection Complicating Darier's Disease. Caused by Type I Herpesvirus Hominis. Arch. Derm., *102*:650-653, 1970.
Another example of susceptibility in Darier's to secondary viral infection.

Higgins, P. G., and Crow, K. D.: Recurrent Kaposi's Varicelliform Eruption in Darier's Disease. Brit. J. Derm., *88*:391-394, 1973.
Example due to Coxsackie virus type A 16.

Liden, S., and Michaelsson, G.: Keratosis Follicularis (Darier's Disease). Acta Dermatovener., *52*:246-247, 1972.
Koebner phenomenon in Darier's disease: elicitation of lesions by irritant reaction following carbon arc lamp treatments, topical dithranol or retinoic acid. Latent period two weeks, duration many months.

Svendsen, I. B., and Albrectsen, B.: The Prevalence of Dyskeratosis Follicularis (Darier's Disease) in Denmark. An Investigation of the Heredity in 22 Families. Acta Dermatovener., *39*:256-269, 1959.
Autosomal dominant with incidence of 1 per 100,000.

Fraser, R. D. B., MacRae, T. P., and Rogers, G. E.: *Keratins. Their Composition, Structure and Biosynthesis.* Charles C Thomas, Springfield, Illinois, 1972, 304 pp.
Provides background music for your thinking on the keratin defect in Darier's disease.

Hollander, M. B.: Ultrasoft X-rays. Williams & Wilkins Co., Baltimore, 1968.
Keratosis follicularis: excellent response to grenz-ray therapy.

Ayres, S., Jr., and Mihan, R.: Keratosis Follicularis (Darier's Disease). Response to Simultaneous Administration of Vitamins A and E. Arch. Derm., *106*:909-910, 1972.
Vitamin A 200,000 units and D-alpha tocopheryl acetate 1,200 units daily gave dramatic help in one case.

Goette, D. K.: Zosteriform Keratosis Follicularis Cleared with Topically Applied Vitamin A Acid. Arch. Derm., *107*:113-114, 1973.
Latest example of dramatic response of Darier's disease to 0.1 per cent retinoic acid in ethyl alcohol-propylene glycol.

Peck, G. L., and Elias, P. M.: Wound Healing in a Patient with Darier's Disease—Preliminary Observations. *In* Maibach, H. I., and Rovee, D. T. (Eds.): *Epidermal Wound Healing.* Year Book Medical Publishers, Inc., Chicago, 1972, pp. 357-363.
Removal of affected skin by curettage or dermatome gives prolonged clinical remission.

40

Incontinentia Pigmenti

40

Streaked, whorled, reticulate hyperpigmentation covers this girl's back. Long linear bands of patchy pigment and fine atrophic scars extend down the backs of her legs. Her left hand shows syndactyly and malformed fingers. Many of her teeth have failed to erupt; others are malformed and conical in shape. In infancy she had a widespread bullous eruption.

Incontinentia Pigmenti

The battle is over. It raged in early infancy and now in adolescence we see only the fading pigmented remains. All we see today is the melanin that an incontinent epidermis dropped down into the dermis many years ago. All we see is the tattoo of incontinentia pigmenti, arranged in swirl-like formations, bespeaking forces that go way back to embryonic days.

This is a battle that begins in utero. It is one that the male fetus rarely if ever wins, miscarriage of males being the ultimate outcome. Only a female such as our patient survives the intrauterine struggle, but not without a mark. Linear groups of bullae are often present at the time of delivery, and new crops come and go for weeks. Nothing remarkable is seen histologically, but the bullae are uniquely filled with eosinophils; the blood shows a dramatic eosinophilia in which virtually every other white cell may be an eosinophil. This aids in distinguishing the process from bullous impetigo, epidermolysis bullosa or herpes simplex and stands in contrast to the bullae of urticaria pigmentosa, which are filled with mast cells. One might think of a bullous drug sensitivity, or dermatitis herpetiformis, but the diagnostic challenge lessens when the secondary stage of irregular linear hyperkeratotic excrescences or reddish plaques evolves. Should ulceration occur, scarring may ensue, suggesting focal dermal hypoplasia. In the scalp such a scar can result in local alopecia and remind one of a pseudopelade. Yet, in a few months the need for a differential diagnosis disappears when the distinctive whorls of melanin hyperpigmentation evolve.

It is from this end stage that the disease derives its name, because histologically melanin can be seen dropping down from the melanocytes

244

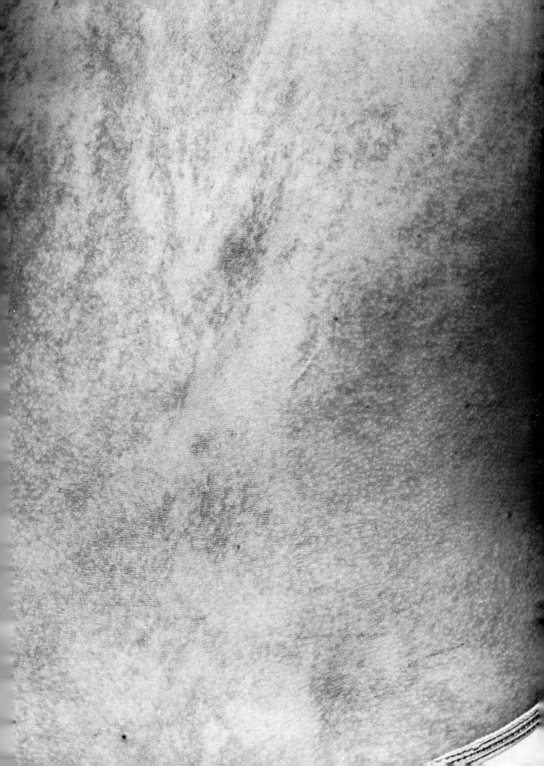

into the dermis, rather than moving outward to be shed with the stratum corneum. Interestingly, this discharge of melanin into the dermis is not restricted to this disease; the same occurs in many diseases with persistent inflammatory pigmentation as in lichen planus or lupus erythematosus. The melanin remains in the dermis, in the scavenger histiocytes, just as an insoluble tattoo pigment. But eventually, years later, it too fades away, most girls entering the nubile period with little trace of their own prenatal problem.

In the absence of a history, our patient's third stage of incontinentia pigmenti might be confused with a systematized melanocytic nevus and also the hypomelanosis of Ito. The systematized nevus is less bizarre in form and extent. More importantly, biopsy discloses melanocytic nevus cells rather than pigment-filled melanophores in the dermis. In the syndrome described by Ito, bizarre whorls of pigment absence occur, so that it is a dramatic negative clinical image of incontinentia pigmenti. There is actually no hyperpigmentation or incontinence of melanin, only an illusory resemblance in patterning.

Our patient's dental changes, syndactyly and osseous malformations are testimony to the fact that incontinentia pigmenti is not simply a skin eruption. It is a serious mesodermal as well as ectodermal dysplastic process. Not only the hair, teeth and nails but the patient's entire growth may be stunted. Microcephaly, mental deficiency, epilepsy and spastic paralysis are additional known neural scars of incontinentia pigmenti. Congenital cardiac disorders and malformation of the central nervous system as well as of the ears, breast and gonads and other birth defects bear witness to the fact that incontinentia pigmenti, lethal to the male fetus, can be cruelly destructive in the female.

Perhaps incontinentia pigmenti gives the best example of *multum in parvo* when it affects the eye, as it does in one of every three of its victims. Strabismus, nystagmus, blue sclerae, corneal opacity, a mass in the anterior chamber, cataracts, retrolental fibroplasia, pseudoglioma, papillitis, chorioretinitis, ophthalmitis, myopia, retinal detachment or optic atrophy may be found. The need for ophthalmologic care is evident.

Behind all these changes are the mysterious moving forces of the gene. As a hereditary disease, incontinentia pigmenti passes from generation to generation as an X-linked dominant trait, ruthlessly wiping out affected males in utero and leaving the affected daughters marked and maimed.

The complexity and heterogeneity of this genetic defect have not been completely unfolded, but observations on sex-linked coloring have revealed a possible mechanism — the dominant x-linked mutant allele. It all begins with the fact that females have two X chromosomes and males have but one. In our patient all her cells initially had both a normal and a mutant X chromosome. At a very early stage, and completely at random, some of the cells inactivated the normal X chromosome, pushing it aside as an effete Barr body. The remaining mutant allele directed the cell progeny, leading to the incontinent melanocyte as an obvious marker cell. By contrast, the other cells, inactivating the mutant allele, remained normal, leaving our patient with the swirling mosaic pattern of normal and abnormal pigmentation that you see now. With only one X chromosome in the male, there is no modulating influence. Should the mutant gene be transmitted, there is no margin of safety. All the cells become wayward, and fetal death is the result.

Our patient has the scars, the end stage of her hereditary disorder. The storm has passed, and we can consider the possibilities of corrective surgery on her hand, restorative orthodontic therapy and ophthalmologic review. The pigment cannot be bleached, or shed, because it lies within the dermis — a true tattoo pigment. Only by the use of dermabrasion, salabrasion or excision might one achieve removal. These procedures are hardly to be considered except under the unusual circumstance of a small cosmetically critical area of involvement. Our patient can be assured that the process will never return although the affected sites may be more sensitive to irritation than normal skin.

She should know that each year brings her closer to the time when the melanin in the dermis will have faded out completely. More importantly, she must know and understand that her malady is caused by an ineluctably dominant genetic trait. For her, pregnancy will offer only a 50 per cent chance of bearing a normal baby. These are bad odds for a bad disease.

Gordon, H., and Gordon, W.: Incontinentia Pigmenti: Clinical and Genetical Studies of Two Familial Cases. Dermatologica, *140*:150-168, 1970.
In infant girls: look for streaks of bullae, followed by bands of warty growth, leaving whorls of pigment.

Surana, R. B., and Scott, R. B.: Incontinentia Pigmenti (Bloch-Sulzberger Syndrome). Report of a Negro Infant with Typical Skin Lesions, Alopecia and Delayed Atypical Dentition. Clin. Pediat., *8*:286-289, 1969.
Marked eosinophilia occurs regularly during initial bullous phase.

Adam, J. E., and Richards, R.: Ichthyosis Hystrix. Epidermolytic Hyperkeratosis; Discordant in Monozygotic Twins. Arch. Derm., *107*:278-282, 1973.
Mimics second stage of incontinentia pigmenti.

Jelinek, J. E., Bart, R. S., and Schiff, G. M.: Hypomelanosis of Ito ("Incontinentia Pigmenti Achromians"). Report of Three Cases and Review of Literature. Arch. Derm., *107*:596-601, 1973.
A negative image of the pigmented tertiary stage of incontinentia pigmenti.

Schmidt, H., Hvidberg-Hansen, J., and Christensen, H. E.: Incontinentia Pigmenti with Associated Lesions in Two Generations. Acta Dermatovener., *52*:281-287, 1972.
Associated ophthalmologic findings: corneal opacities, cataracts, iris malformations, uveitis, chorioretinitis, optic atrophy, squint, nystagmus.

Hoggins, G. S.: Partial Anodontia in Incontinentia Pigmenti. Brit. J. Oral Surg., *4*:111-115, 1966.
Dental defects: anodontia, delayed eruption, hypoplasia, spaced malformed conical teeth.

Holmes, L. B., Moser, H. W., Halldorsson, S., Mack, C., Pant, S. S., and Matzilevich, B.: *Mental Retardation. An Atlas of Diseases with Associated Physical Abnormalities.* The Macmillan Co., New York, 1972, pp. 362-363.
Of 145 patients, 43 had neurologic problems: hemiparesis, spastic tetraplegia, seizures, mental deficiency.

O'Doherty, N. J., and Norman, R. M.: Incontinentia Pigmenti (Bloch-Sulzberger Syndrome) with Cerebral Malformation. Dev. Med. Child Neurol., *10*:168-174, 1968.
Autopsy findings included small cavities in central white matter, atrophy of cerebral gyri and neuronal loss in cerebellum.

Wong, C. K., Guerrier, C. J., MacMillan, D. C., and Vickers, H. R.: An Electron Microscopical Study of Bloch-Sulzberger Syndrome (Incontinentia Pigmenti). Acta Dermatovener., *51*:161-168, 1971.
Melanin-releasing dendrites of melanocytes extend into dermis through gaps in basement membrane.

McCrary, J. A., and Smith, J. L.: Conjunctival and Retinal Incontinentia Pigmenti. Arch. Ophthal., *79*:417-422, 1968.
Good histologic pictures of incontinence of pigment: melanin dropping down into subepithelial area.

Kidd, R. L., and Wilgram, G. F.: Incontinentia Pigmenti. Arch. Derm., *105*:767-767, 1972.
Merkel cell; a dendritic analogue of melanocyte and Langerhans cell, found in amazing numbers in epidermal basal layer. Role?

Curban, G. V., and Zamith, V. A.: A Quantitative Study of Mast Cells in Incontinentia Pigmenti. Brit. J. Derm., *79*:690-692, 1967.
Increased.

McKusick, V. A.: Genetics and Dermatology, or If I Were to Rewrite Cockayne's Inherited Abnormalities of the Skin. J. Invest. Derm., *60*:343-359, 1973.
Delightfully erudite introduction to 220-page symposium on cutaneous genetics today. A master reference.

Curth, H. O., and Warburton, D.: The Genetics of Incontinentia Pigmenti. Arch. Derm., *92*:229-235, 1965.
A dominant trait seen only in girls, since it is lethal to males in utero.

Lyon, M. F.: Chromosomal and Subchromosomal Inactivation. Ann. Rev. Genet., 2:31-52, 1968.

Classic genetic analysis of how X-linked mottled coloration develops in female mice: chance inactivation of the normal member of X Chromosomal pair in one group of cells, and of the mutant in another.

Carney, R. G., and Carney, R. G., Jr.: Incontinentia Pigmenti. Arch. Derm., 102:157-162, 1970.

Our patient's chances with pregnancy: 50 per cent chance of normal boy or girl; 25 per cent chance of daughter with disease; 25 per cent chance of dead male fetus.

Simonsson, H.: Incontinentia Pigmenti, Bloch-Sulzberger Syndrome, Associated with Infantile Spasms. Acta Paediat. Scand., 61:612-614, 1972.

ACTH treatment resulted in disappearance of convulsions.

41

Four months ago this 24-year-old man developed a small ulcer on his left calf. Despite local treatment, this ulcer evolved into a **group of inflamed and painful, crusted, seropurulent, phagedenic ulcers.** *Additional necrotic ulcers were present on his left shoulder and right hip. Multiple cultures revealed no specific pathogenic bacteria.*

Biopsy — nonspecific inflammatory ulceration.

For the past 6 years, the patient has had proven ulcerative colitis that required steroids and azulfidine for control of diarrhea and hemorrhaging.

Pyoderma Gangrenosum

This patient has ulcers, not only of the skin but of the bowel as well. We can inform him that they are directly related. Worsening of his colitis should induce further progression of these phagedenic skin lesions. Conversely, improvement of his colitis should favor involution of this pyoderma. Most dramatic of all, a colectomy should result in spontaneous healing and ultimate replacement of these necrotic sores by thin white scars.

However, this amazing conjunction of skin and gut ulceration is no simple one. Only a few patients with ulcerative colitis ever develop pyoderma gangrenosum, and the presence of pyoderma gangrenosum does not invariably herald ulcerative colitis. Nonetheless, over half the patients with unexplained, progressive, necrotic ulcers of this type have obvious ulcerative colitis. About 10 per cent more have regional ileitis. In some of the others, occult, possibly focal, yet definite colitis is present, to be found only by careful gross microscopic and radiologic observation. In a few, clinical colitis appears much later than the skin ulceration.

In the remainder of cases, further study of the patient or the skin itself may erase the initial diagnosis of pyoderma gangrenosum. Thus, all patients with pyoderma gangrenosum without colitis should be examined carefully for a post-thrombophlebitic gangrene, iododerma or a

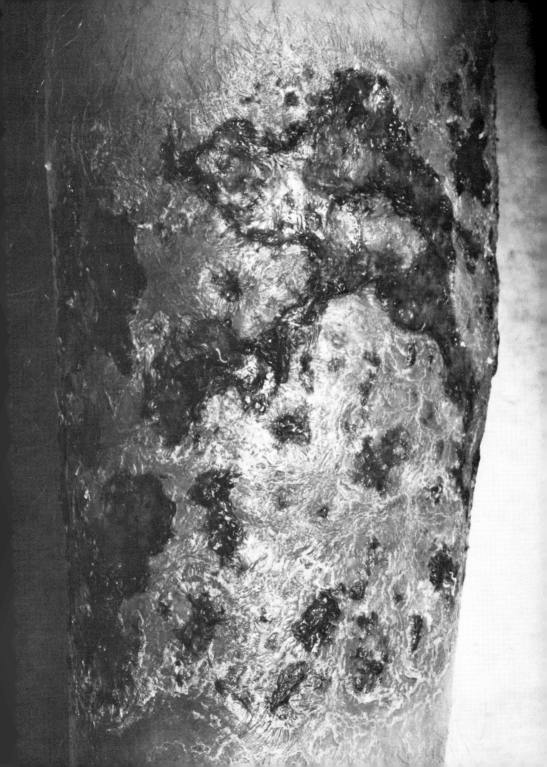

factitial component. One should search the biopsy specimen for evidence of allergic vasculitis. Laboratory study should be directed toward detecting diabetes, sickle cell anemia, leukemia, multiple myeloma or systemic lupus erythematosus. The microbiology team should be alerted to the need to explore for atypical mycobacteria, amebae, blastomycetes and Sporotrichum, as well as virulent bacterial pathogens.

Although any chronic unexplained ulcer becomes pyoderma gangrenosum in a patient with ulcerative colitis, we recognize that there is a characteristic clinical picture of pyoderma gangrenosum. It is this entity as we see it here that always demands continuous study of the patient until evidence of colitis or ileitis is found. It is the pattern of rapidly extending ulceration, often beginning on the extremity after insignificant trauma such as venipuncture or an insect bite. It is the presence of multiple ulcers which are chronic, phagedenic and often brutally painful. It is this picture which finds its ultimate explanation in the bowel.

Despite our perception that these ulcers are the clinical equivalents and indeed derivatives of ulcerative colitis, we can distinguish little else in the fog of data about us. These patients do have immune changes. Some show paraproteinemia, others show cryoglobulins, and a few show elevated or depressed gamma globulins. A new subset has been described with cutaneous anergy. Others are hyperreactive, developing new ulcers from bacterial skin tests in a fashion reminiscent of the Shwartzman phenomenon. Most of these patients are also reactive to iodides, either orally or topically. From all this we vaguely sense a disturbed immune state and a sharply compromised capacity to cope with the bumps, bruises and bites of everyday living. Possibly bacterial antigens of enteric origin are circulating in these patients to be deposited at the sites of trauma and capillary leakage. Such antigens could account for the spreading ulcers, the arthritis and the erythema nodosum found at times with ulcerative colitis. However, only with continued study will the morning fog of our early tentative experiences with this disease lift.

In a disease in which every nuance may reflect the status of the colonic problem, therapy centers on treating the ulcerative colitis. The azulfidine and steroids this patient is taking are absolutely essential. In this instance the dose must be raised above routine dose levels, as for example to 8 grams of azulfidine and 100 mg. of prednisone daily, or their equivalents. Many patients do well with Avlosulphon (200 mg. a day), coupled with triamcinolone acetonide injections (40 mg. I. M.). Immunosuppressants provide another new avenue for attack and in the intractable, totally resistant patient, colectomy may be not only necessary, but absolutely curative.

The ulcers per se are a sign that every effort must be made to reduce trauma to a minimum. Skin testing must be done with circumspection, and the patient must be made aware of the hazard of minor damage to the skin. Should he show any medical problems such as anemia or an elevated blood sugar, corrective measures are essential.

These ulcers, covered with a necrotic sphacelous crust, are swarming with astronomical numbers of microflora. Most of these can be removed by virtually continuous open compresses with potassium permanganate (1/8,000) or silver nitrate (1/200). Frequent gentle debridement is an invaluable additional aid. Recalcitrant ulcers may respond also to intralesional triamcinolone acetonide suspension given in large quantity over a period of days. It should be injected at multiple sites around the entire perimeter. Allografting, necessary at times, can succeed only when the ulcer base is clean and relatively sterile. With months of care these geometric phagedenic ulcers should fade into thin healthy white scars as the diarrhea and hemorrhages terminate.

As a final point, it is interesting that just as the vesicles of dermatitis herpetiformis give us a skin window through which to perceive the gluten enteropathy of the small bowel, so do the ulcers of pyoderma gangrenosum swing open for us a view of the large bowel enteropathy of ulcerative colitis. Other windows must surely appear as we learn more about the skin and what's within.

Perry, H. O.: Pyoderma Gangrenosum. South. Med. J., *62*:899-908, 1969.
    Profile on 62 patients: rapidly growing painful necrotic ulcers, associated in over half with ulcerative colitis.

Forman, L.: The Skin and the Colon. Trans. St. Johns Hosp. Derm. Soc., *52*:139-162, 1966.
    Reflective wisdom on the nature of the skin signs of ulcerative colitis: dermatitis vegetans, erythema nodosum and pyoderma gangrenosum.

Sluis, I.: Two Cases of Pyoderma (Ecthyma) Gangraenosum Associated with the Presence of an Abnormal Serum Protein (B_2A-paraprotein). Dermatologica, *132*:409-424, 1966.
    Detailed literature sweep: triggered by trivial trauma; inhabited by bacterial polyglot; flared by iodides.

Apted, J. H., Buntine, D., and Newell, A. C.: Pyoderma Gangrenosum. Med. J. Aust., *2*:423-425, 1971.
    May precede diagnosis of ulcerative colitis.

Stathers, G. M., Abbott, L. G., and McGuinness, A. E.: Pyoderma Gangrenosum in Association with Regional Enteritis. Arch. Derm., *95*:375-380, 1967.
May precede diagnosis of regional enteritis.

Perry, H. O., and Winkelmann, R. K.: Bullous Pyoderma Gangrenosum and Leukemia. Arch. Derm., *106*:901-905, 1972.
May precede diagnosis of leukemia.

Thompson, D. M., Main, R. A., Beck, J. S., and Albert-Recht, F.: Studies on a Patient with Leucocytoclastic Vasculitis "Pyoderma Gangrenosum" and Paraproteinaemia. Brit. J. Derm., *88*:117-125, 1973.
May develop with vasculitis.

Cream, J. J.: Pyoderma Gangrenosum with a Monoclonal IgM Red Cell Agglomerating Factor. Brit. J. Derm., *84*:223-226, 1971.
Associated with gammopathy suggestive of multiple myeloma.

Stroud, J. D.: Sporotrichosis Presenting as Pyoderma Gangrenosum. Arch. Derm., *97*:667-670, 1968.
Pathogenic organism found on biopsy.

Lazarus, G. S., Goldsmith, L. A., Rocklin, R. E., Pinals, R. S., de Buisseret, J.-P., David, J. R., and Draper, W.: Pyoderma Gangrenosum, Altered Delayed Hypersensitivity and Polyarthritis. Arch. Derm., *105*:46-51, 1972.
Four pyoderma gangrenosum patients with cutaneous anergy and arthritis but no colitis.

Delescluse, J., de Bast, C., and Achten, G.: Pyoderma Gangrenosum with Altered Cellular Immunity and Dermonecrotic Factor. Brit. J. Derm., *87*:529-532, 1972.
Lesions reproduced (1) in patient by intradermal streptococcal antigen, and (2) in guinea pig by intradermal injection of patient's serum.

Kaplan, I.: Pyoderma Gangrenosum, Peptic Ulcer and a $625,000 Damage Award. J.A.M.A., *190*:942-943, 1964.
$475,000 finally paid by railroad which failed to clear stagnant pool which bred the insect which bit the defendant which induced pyoderma gangrenosum which led to amputation.

Comaish, J. S., and Cunliffe, W. J.: Absorption of Drugs from Varicose Ulcers. A Cause of Anaphylaxis. Brit. J. Clin. Pract., *21*:97-98, 1967.
Anaphylaxis from bacitracin: any ulcer is an open pathway to the systemic circulation.

Gardner, L. W., and Acker. D. W.: Triamcinolone and Pyoderma Gangrenosum. Arch. Derm., *106*:599-600, 1972.
Confirmation of effectiveness of multiple peripheral intralesional injections of triamcinolone acetonide/lidocaine.

Dominguez Soto, L.: Diaminodiphenylsulfone and Steroids in the Treatment of Pyoderma Gangrenosum. Int. J. Derm., *9*:293-300, 1970.
Systemic steroids coupled with sulfone produced healing in 1 to 3 months.

Maldonado, N., Torres, V. M., Mendez-Cashion, D., Perez-Santiago, E., and de Costas, M. C.: Pyoderma Gangrenosum Treated with 6-Mercaptopurine and Followed by Acute Leukemia. J. Pediat., *72*:409-414, 1968.
Immunosuppression with 6-mercaptopurine resulted in healing.

Crawford, S. E., Sherman, R., and Favara, B.: Pyoderma Gangrenosum with Response to Cyclophosphamide Therapy. J. Pediat., 71:255-258, 1967.

Immunosuppression with either cyclophosphamide (Cytoxan) or azathioprine (Imuran) produced healing.

Ridenhour, G., and Stephenson, H. E., Jr.: Pyoderma Gangrenosum Successfully Treated with Aqueous Silver Nitrate (0.5%) Steroids and Skin Autografts. Ann. Surg., 168: 905-910, 1968.

Silver nitrate combats secondary Pseudomonas overgrowth.

Shatin, H.: How I Treat Pyoderma Gangrenosum. Postgrad. Med., 49:251-253, 1971.

Treatment of colitis is essential!

42

These **eccrine sweat droplets** *appeared in this man's shaved ax-illa* **in response to a few minutes of mental arithmetic.** *For years as a salesman, this patient has suffered from excessive sweat-ing in the axillary area. The armpits of his shirt and suit coat become drenched when he is under tension, especially in a warm, humid environment. A variety of commercial antiperspirants have been of little help.*

Biopsy — normal eccrine and apocrine glands.

Hyperhidrosis

You are looking at sweat. This is the secretion which has made it possible for man to spread over the surface of the earth, to till the land in the summer sun, to survive the torrid equatorial day, to combat the dead-ly fevers of infection. This is the watery fluid which cools by evaporating and which gave primitive man one of his great adaptive advantages — thermal homeostasis. But for our patient in an air-conditioned twenti-eth-century world, this local outpouring of sweat is nothing more than a source of embarrassment.

He comes for help. Not only are his emotions evident to all, but the dry cleaning bill for his salt-stained coats mounts up. The armpits of his shirts and coats rot and disintegrate, if not from the sweat, from contact with destructive metallic antiperspirant compounds. He himself is sub-ject to contact dermatitis from sweat-leached dyes and finishes. Should the hyperhidrosis be localized to the soles, maceration, odor, contact shoe dermatitis and rotting shoes are to be expected. On the palms, such localized hyperhidrosis results in the social disadvantage of a cold, clammy handshake, and can seriously cripple one who has to do skilled digital operations such as typing, playing the piano or repairing watches. In the crural area, such hyperhidrosis is commonly followed by disabling intertrigo and dermatitis which may mask the primary cause, sweating. It is apparent that localized hyperhidrosis can be as great a burden as generalized anhidrosis. It deserves medical attention.

Let us examine the problem. The sweat glands responsible for this problem are the garden variety eccrine ones. Spaced all over the body,

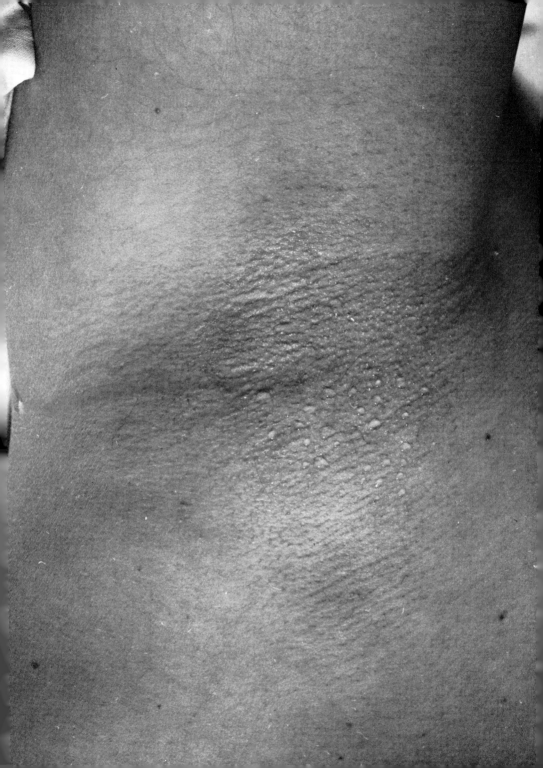

they number over 2 million, but here just a few thousand are intensely active. The microscope gives us no clue as to why. On biopsy of this man's axillary tissue we see normal eccrine and apocrine glands in normal number. Incidentally, the apocrine group is of no concern here, for these are reservoir glands squeezing out small milky droplets and never in large volume. As we survey the eccrine glands of this man's axilla by special histochemical stains, nerve stains and electron microscopy, we find an entirely normal picture. The same cholinergic fibers can be shown to envelop these glands and the normhidrotic glands elsewhere. The same salt-secreting clear cells are found in the coils of these glands as in the normhidrotic glands. The answer is not to be found in form but in function.

We learn far more by noting that this problem of episodic sweating is triggered by emotional stress, by the pressure of making a sale or by mental strain. There is no hyperhidrosis during total relaxation, such as taking a nap, but even the unexpected ring of a phone can bring a new surge of sweating. It is a problem that appeared as he passed from the tranquility of childhood to the stormy stresses of adolescence. We come to realize that neither his stress nor his basic response of sweating is abnormal. Nearly all individuals show localized sweating in the axilla, as well as on the palms and soles in response to fright, pain or tension. Some have argued that it aids in our flight to escape, a better grip, a smoother motion. But no matter what the reason it is not thermoregulatory, and although the very same eccrine glands can respond to both stimuli via the same autonomic nerves, in the one case the control is cortical, in the other, hypothalamic. In our patient, it is the response to cortical control that is so grossly exaggerated. Presumably this reflects a sensitivity of this population of eccrine glands to the mediating acetylcholine. Supporting this view of end-organ supersensitivity is the observation that the sweating response to the stimulus or a warm environment first becomes evident in the axillae in these individuals.

What can be done? In our experience, tranquilizers and sedatives to ablate the cortical factor have little place in the life of a vibrantly successful salesman. If we race to the other end of the circuit, we have the choice of employing an atropine compound to block adenoneural transmission. Whether it be tincture of belladonna or propantheline, the side effects of blurred vision, dry mouth and difficult voiding often are more obvious to the patient than the anticipated reduction in sweat. Suppression of the supersensitive sweat gland by these oral anticholinergics can call for a sympathetic blockage too drastic to be practical, but only a trial will tell. The topical use of these agents, however, is more encouraging but still experimental, since no commercial product is yet available in the United States. Surgical sympathectomy would seem the permanent answer, but present skills cannot consistently section the autonomic fibers coursing to the axillae. It does remain the best treatment, however, for the rare case of disabling palmar hyperhidrosis. The glandular end organ itself can be destroyed by radiotherapy, but to do this requires a dosage which can lay the skin itself to waste. For some, it can be an open invitation to develop the same radiodermatitis with all its ugly sequelae as we saw when x-ray was used to treat hirsutism.

What should be done? Dr. Harry Hurley and I have developed two effective approaches to this problem: one is surgical, the other is a new antiperspirant system. The surgical approach arose from our serendipitous discovery that we could permanently alleviate axillary hyperhidrosis by simply excising a large block of this hyperhidrotic skin. The unobvious became the obvious. It was appealing in that the procedure could be done under local anesthesia, with primary closure and without subsequent limitation of motion. It was successful in that it has been widely employed in the ten years since we first described it. Look again at our patient, and you can see that the simple bilateral excision of a 3-centimeter ellipse from his axillary vault would be beneficial.

Our second approach is new; indeed, unpublished. Although topical axillary antiperspirants have long enjoyed the favor of the public, they provide virtually no relief for the hyperhidrotic. Nearly all are based on the principle of achieving closure of the eccrine pore by the use of an astringent metallic salt, such as an aluminum or zirconium compound. On the sole, the alternate use of the protein denaturants formaldehyde and, more recently, glutaraldehyde has been successful, although sensitization and staining remain drawbacks. The axillae, however, have remained uniquely resistant to topical agents, the best commercial products reducing sweat production only by half.

In contrast we have discovered that the following simple yet trinary system will provide virtually total suppression of axillary hyperhidrosis. Just before retiring at bedtime the patient applies a 20 per cent solution of aluminum chloride hexahydrate in absolute ethyl alcohol to the axilla and closely covers the area with Saran Wrap. All three steps are critical; elimination of any one results in failure. The solution must be applied to the dry axilla during a period of sweat gland rest. The pH of the aluminum chloride solution must be less than 1.0, and a water vapor-impermeable film (e.g., vinyl vinylidene chloride) must be kept in close apposition by clothing or otherwise, without tape. The Saran Wrap is removed in the morning, and the area is washed free of the acidic salt. After two successive nights of therapy our patient may expect virtually absolute protection for a week. Even without further treatment a diminishing yet gratifying anhidrotic effect should persist for a month. Routinely, treatment one night a week gives the patient the assurance of an essentially dry armpit under any emotional or thermal stress.

Have him try it. He'll like it.

Hurley, H. J., and Shelley, W. B.: Axillary Hyperhidrosis: Clinical Features and Local Surgical Management. Brit. J. Derm., *78*:127-140, 1966.
Details on the socially embarrassing sweat sign of stress and strain, and its alleviation by local excision of skin.

Cunliffe, W. J., Johnson, C. E., and Williamson, D. M.: Localized Unilateral Hyperhidrosis—A Clinical and Laboratory Study. Brit. J. Derm., *86*:374-378, 1972.
Enlarged eccrine glands responding to thermal, not emotional, stress; blocked by topical anticholinergic agent.

McGibbon, B. M., and Paletta, F. X.: Further Concepts in Gustatory Sweating. Plast. Reconstr. Surg., *49*:639-642, 1972.
Due to regeneration of aberrant parasympathetic fibers in greater auricular nerve sheath.

Jenkinson, D. M.: Comparative Physiology of Sweating. Brit. J. Derm., *88*:397-406, 1973.
Present only in skin of mammals, sweat glands protect against (1) high temperature, (2) frictional damage, (3) accumulation of waste products, (4) bacteria and (5) extinction of species.

Wolf, J.: Configuration of Orifices of the Sweat Ducts on the Surface of the Horny Layer of the Skin of Man. Folia Morph., *18*:14-20, 1970.
Orifices—so clear on ridges of palms—are invisible elsewhere owing to slitlike lumen.

Juhlin, L., and Shelley, W. B.: A Stain for Sweat Pores. Nature, *213*:408-408, 1967.
Five per cent *o*-phthalaldehyde in xylene, applied topically.

Johnson, C., Dawber, R., and Schuster, S.: Surface Appearances of the Eccrine Sweat Duct by Scanning Electron Microscopy. Brit. J. Derm., *83*:655-660, 1970.
Ducts are patent but inconspicuous until outer surface of terminal spiral is removed by Scotch Tape stripping.

Willis, I., Harris, D. R., and Moretz, W.: Normal and Abnormal Variations in Eccrine Sweat Gland Distribution. J. Invest. Derm., *60*:98-103, 1973.
New silicone elastomer provides permanent record of sweating pattern.

Nicolaidis, S., and Sivadjian, J.: High-Frequency Pulsatile Discharge of Human Sweat Glands: Myoepithelial Mechanism. J. Appl. Physiol., *32*:86-90, 1972.
High-speed photographic techniques showed pulsatile expulsion of sweat in 12 to 21 bursts per second.

Ito, T., and Shibasaki, S.: Electron Microscopic Study on Human Eccrine Sweat Glands. Arch. Histol. Jap., *27*:81-115, 1966.
Good micrographs of axillary eccrine secretory coils with myoepithelium enspiraling basal (clear) and superficial (dark) cells.

Goodall, M.: Innervation and Inhibition of Eccrine and Apocrine Sweating in Man. J. Clin. Pharm., *10*:235-246, 1970.
Eccrine gland actuated by cholinergic fibers; inhibited by atropine and analogues.

Dobson, R. L., and Sato, K.: The Stimulation of Eccrine Sweating by Pharmacologic Agents. *In* Montagna, W., et al. (Eds.): *Advances in Biology of Skin*, Vol. XII, Meredith Corporation, New York, 1972, pp. 447-475.
Details on how cholinergic drugs stimulate secretory activity by increasing permeability of basal membrane of clear cell to sodium which activates sodium pump.

Dobson, R. L., and Sato, K.: The Secretion of Salt and Water by the Eccrine Sweat Gland. Arch. Derm., *105*:366-370, 1972.
In turn, clear cells pump sodium into intercellular canaliculus leading to lumen; followed by flow of water to maintain osmotic equilibrium.

Cage, G. W.: Eccrine and Apocrine Secretory Glands. *In* Fitzpatrick, T. B., et al. (Eds.): *Dermatology in General Medicine*. McGraw-Hill Book Co., New York, 1971, pp. 103-109.
Sodium chloride and some water reabsorbed in part while passing up duct.

Johnson, H. L., and Maibach, H. I.: Drug Excretion in Human Eccrine Sweat. J. Invest. Derm., *56*:182-188, 1971.
Significant amounts may be excreted.

Cullen, S. I.: Management of Hyperhidrosis. Postgrad. Med., *52*(Nov.):77-79, 1972.
Equanil or Valium may be helpful in reducing emotional sweating.

Zahejsky, J., and Rovensky, J.: A Comparison of the Effectiveness of Several External Antiperspirants. J. Soc. Cos. Chem., *23*:775-789, 1972.
On forearm, formaldehyde most effective.

Papa, C. M.: Mechanisms of Eccrine Anhidrosis. III. Scanning Electron Microscopic Study of Poral Occlusion. J. Invest. Derm., *59*:295-298, 1972.
Demonstration of cast of amorphous material clogging sweat duct orifice in formalin-induced anhidrosis.

Juhlin, L., and Hansson, H.: Topical Glutaraldehyde for Plantar Hyperhidrosis. Arch. Derm., *97*:327-330, 1968.
Stains, but 10 per cent solution very useful.

Sato, K., and Dobson, R. L.: Mechanism of the Antiperspirant Effect of Topical Glutaraldehyde. Arch. Derm., *100*:564-569, 1969.
Due to poral closure.

MacMillan, F. S. K., Reller, H. H., and Snyder, F. H.: The Antiperspirant Action of Topically Applied Anticholinergics. J. Invest. Derm., *43*:363-377, 1964.
Application of 0.05 per cent benzoylscopalamine reduced thermal axillary sweating 95 per cent three hours after a single application.

Frankland, J. C., and Seville, R. H.: The Treatment of Hyperhidrosis with Topical Propantheline — A New Technique. Brit. J. Derm., *85*:577-581, 1971.
Aerosol anticholinergic used successfully for plantar hyperhidrosis.

Grice, K., Sattar, H., and Baker, H.: Treatment of Idiopathic Hyperhidrosis with Iontophoresis of Tap Water and Poldine Methosulphate. Brit. J. Derm., *86*:72-78, 1972.
Iontophoresis of anticholinergic valuable for palms and soles but not axilla.

Levit, F.: Simple Device for Treatment of Hyperhidrosis by Iontophoresis. Arch. Derm., *98*:505-507, 1968.
Ten minutes of tap water iontophoresis once a month controlled palmar and plantar hyperhidrosis.

Smith, R. O., Hemenway, W. G., Stevens, K. M., and Ratzer, E. R.: Jacobson's Neurectomy for Frey's Syndrome. Amer. J. Surg., *120*:478-481, 1970.
Microsurgical division of Jacobson's nerve under tympanic membrane cures gustatory hyperhidrosis resulting from parotic gland surgery.

Greenhalgh, R. M., Rosengarten, D. S., and Martin, P.: Role of Sympathectomy for Hyperhidrosis. Brit. Med. J., *1*:332-334, 1971.
Cervical sympathectomy recommended for palmar hyperhidrosis. Not consistently reliable for axillary hyperhidrosis.

Weaver, P. C., and Copeman, P. W. M.: Simple Surgery for Axillary Hyperhidrosis (Two Cases). Proc. Roy. Soc. Med., *64*:607-608, 1971.
Cites death of two girls as result of sympathectomy for axillary hyperhidrosis.

Skoog, T., and Thyresson, N.: Hyperhidrosis of the Axillae. A Method of Surgical Treatment. Acta Chir. Scand., *124*:531-538, 1962.
Radical plastic excision of axillary skin gives good results.

Gillespie, J. A., and Kane, S. P.: Evaluation of a Simple Surgical Treatment of Axillary Hyperhidrosis. Brit. J. Derm., *83*:684-689, 1970.
Success in 24 patients, employing Hurley-Shelley procedure.

Harry, R. G.: Harry's Cosmeticology, 6th ed., Ralph G. Harvey Chemical Publishing Co., Inc., New York, 1973, 824 pp.
Modern formulas for antiperspirants.

CTFA Cosmetic Ingredient Dictionary 1973. The Cosmetic, Toiletry & Fragrance Association, Washington, D.C., 1973.
How to find your way through the 5000 ingredients used in cosmetics.

Frain-Bell, W.: Anidrotics. Practitioner, *202*:79-87, 1969.
Good general review: cannot justify long-term use of systemic anticholinergic drugs.

43

Necrobiosis Lipoidica

43

This **indurated geographic plaque** *has been slowly enlarging and extending over the right shin of this 50-year-old woman for the past seven years. The lesion* **shows fine scaling, reddish brown borders and a glossy atrophic center, distinctly yellow and patterned with numerous spidery telangiectatic vessels.** *A similar tender, dusky red plaque of but three months' duration is seen on the left shin.*

Patient had a thyroidectomy five years ago. She denies any personal or family history of diabetes mellitus.

Glucose tolerance — normal.

Biopsy — hyalinized disrupted collagen, histiocytic inflammatory response.

Necrobiosis Lipoidica

Look for diabetes when you see this remarkable picture. The sharp border, the shiny yellow atrophy and the telangiectasis are the brush strokes we have come to attribute to diabetes. The pretibial localization in a middle-aged woman, the chronicity and indifference to therapy all add authenticity to our attribution. And yet, in this patient we can find no other evidence of diabetes mellitus.

Our patient is the one in three who shows an unquestioned clinical and histologic picture of necrobiosis lipoidica diabeticorum, but without systemic diabetes. To make note that she has violated the rule of association, diabeticorum is deleted from the diagnostic label. We still should watch for and wait for diabetes to appear, since some of these individuals develop the cutaneous change while they are in a prediabetic state. As stress testing advances it may be possible to detect diabetes in earlier stages or even in forms other than the classic alteration in carbohydrate metabolism. Nevertheless, today we are obliged to view our patient's seven-year problem as only conceptually related to diabetes.

Indeed, even in the diabetic, the relationship of this skin change to this disease is obscure. Whereas individuals with necrobiosis lipoidica diabeticorum commonly have frank diabetes, individuals with diabetes rarely have necrobiosis — as few as three in a clinic population of a

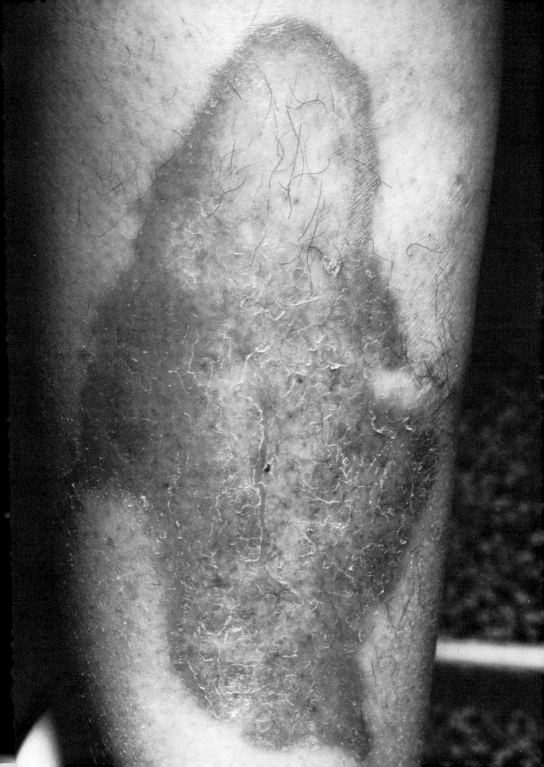

thousand diabetics. Furthermore, unlike the vascular lesions of the eye and kidney which develop in juvenile diabetics with a frequency several hundredfold greater, necrobiosis lesions cannot be correlated with the duration, the severity of the patient's diabetes or the response to treatment.

Nevertheless, a diabetes-related vascular occlusive process in the dermal vessels is viewed by many as the critical factor in necrobiosis lipoidica. Trauma to these vessels in the corium, already compromised by diabetic microangiopathy, is presumed to result in cellular death, collagen breakdown and all the reactive inflammatory change we see histologically. Under this schema, our patient may have an angiopathy of occult diabetes or other origin, with identical gross and microscopic changes as a result of the insult of local trauma. Unfortunately, current techniques of functional assessment of the cutaneous vasculature are inadequate to our needs for these patients. Certainly the appearance of lesions over the noncushioned shin speaks loudly for a coetiologic role for the accidental bruises and bumps of ambulation.

Additional awareness of the role of the vessels in necrobiosis lipoidica comes from a study of some of its clinical variants, especially those occurring on the face in nondiabetics. Here, essentially only the histiocytic granulomatous infiltrate is present, and destruction is limited to the elastic tissue. Necrobiosis and atrophy are absent as is obvious vascular change. Conversely, study of biopsy specimens from diabetic patients with necrobiosis lipoidica show more vascular occlusion and more swelling and loss of collagen structure as a rule than those from nondiabetic patients such as ours. However, it is not a distinguishing feature which permits recognition of the presence or absence of diabetes on the reading of a specific slide. In any event, the presence of occlusive vascular disease, whatever its cause, appears to correlate with necrobiotic change per se.

Lesions may appear anywhere on the body and at times pose a diagnostic challenge. Granuloma annulare and rheumatoid nodule bear some gross and microscopic resemblance, being closely related necrobiotic processes. Granuloma annulare with its ringed lesions and discrete foci of necrobiosis is a dermal change often of the dorsa of the hands and feet. In contrast, the rheumatoid nodule with its massive necrobiosis is deeper, occurring largely in the subcutaneous tissue. Hair loss may be the presenting sign when the atrophic necrobiosis affects the scalp. Sarcoidosis enters the differential especially for facial lesions when the necrobiotic changes are minimal and the prominent finding is epithelioid granulomas. Xanthomatous infiltrates may be suggested by the yellow color, but the atrophic appearance as well as the characteristic telangiectasis of necrobiosis lipoidica makes a distinction easy. Under the microscope, fat stains reveal the "lipoidica" yellow as extracellular lipid. In this patient, we are actually looking at a classic clinical example of necrobiosis lipoidica, well defined and easy to diagnose by simple inspection. It is still remarkable how many indistinct obscure papular, nodular and plaque versions occur. Only by histologic study do these variants become identifiable.

The course of necrobiosis lipoidica is exquisitely chronic, being measured in years. Some patients may develop recalcitration ulceration from trauma. Only one in six lesions resolves to a noninflammatory scar, all being resistant to therapy.

Our patient must be instructed as to the medical nature of her problem: the absence of malignant sequelae, the permanence of her cosmetic defect and the grave hazards of local trauma and injury. Blindly walking into a chair can initiate a new lesion. Although dark hose or leg make-up may virtually hide the change, it is well to try high-potency corticosteroid creams under Saran Wrap as an initial therapeutic approach. However, the best results are usually achieved by multiple direct intralesional injections of a triamcinolone acetonide suspension (10 mg. per ml.). Scarring is not averted, but inflammatory progression and pain are reduced and eliminated. Ulcerative lesions are treated conservatively with compresses and topical antibiotic creams. Rarely surgical excision and grafting are advisable. Strangely, control of any diabetes present is not associated with obvious cutaneous improvement.

Necrobiosis lipoidica diabeticorum must remain a fascinating cutaneous sign of diabetes mellitus. Its presence should alert us to search for frank diabetes, latent diabetes, the prediabetic state or diabetic angiopathy.

Muller, S. A., and Winkelmann, R. K.: Necrobiosis Lipoidica Diabeticorum. A Clinical and Pathological Investigation of 171 Cases. Arch. Derm., *93*:272-281, 1966.
  Primary reference source on this chronic atrophic change, usually pretibial, in a diabetic and best treated with intralesional steroid.

Bauer, M., and Levan, N. E.: Diabetic Dermangiopathy. A Spectrum Including Pigmented Pretibial Patches and Necrobiosis Lipoidica Diabeticorum. Brit. J. Derm., *83*:528-535, 1970.
  Relates necrobiosis to occlusive diabetic angiopathy, which may precede any problem in handling glucose.

Wilson-Jones, E.: Necrobiosis Lipoidica Presenting on the Face and Scalp. Trans. St. Johns Hosp. Derm. Soc., *57*:202-220, 1971.
Seminal paper of dissent pointing out that necrobiosis occurs in only 2 in 1000 diabetics, is not related to severity or duration of diabetes and that the facial form may occur in absence of vascular change.

Muller, S. A., and Winkelmann, R. K.: Atypical Forms of Necrobiosis Lipoidica Diabeticorum. Arch. Path., *81*:352-361, 1966.
Differential diagnosis includes granuloma annulare, morphea and sarcoidosis.

Mehregan, A. H., and Altman, J.: Miescher's Granuloma of the Face. A Variant of the Necrobiosis Lipoidica-Granuloma Annulare Spectrum. Arch. Derm., *107*:62-64, 1973.
Non-atrophic, non-necrobiotic.

Feldman, F. F.: Granuloma Annulare and Necrobiosis Lipoidica in the Same Patient. Arch. Derm., *98*:677-678, 1968.
Unusual clinical association of the histologically similar conditions.

Muller, S. A., and Winkelmann, R. K.: Necrobiosis Lipoidica Diabeticorum. Histopathologic Study of 98 Cases. Arch. Derm., *94*:1-10, 1966.
Palisading granuloma around necrobiotic foci; occlusive vascular changes of wall thickening and endothelial proliferation; most closely resembles granuloma annulare and rheumatoid nodule.

Lukasiak, B., Wnorowski, J., and Rozanski, J.: Capillaroscopic Changes in the Course of Necrobiosis Lipoidica. Polish Med. J., *8*:230-237, 1969.
Serpentine constricted nail fold capillaries.

Marten, R. H., and Dulake, M.: Hydrocortisone in Necrobiosis Lipoidica Diabeticorum. Brit. J. Derm., *69*:395-399, 1957.
Injectable steroids helpful.

Nylen, B. O., and Skoog, T.: Surgical Treatment of Necrobiosis Lipoidica. Acta Dermatovener., *38*:366-371, 1958.
Excise and graft large ulcers.

44

Epidermolysis Bullosa

44

Vesicular and bullous *lesions regularly form* **at sites of minor friction** *in this 18-month-old baby girl. Occasionally* **hemorrhagic***, the blisters may become* **crusted** *or infected, but they heal without scarring. They were first noted when she was only 3 days old and have been returning, usually appearing on the palms, soles, knees, elbows, neck and diaper area. Rarely, erosions develop intraorally. There is no family history of a similar problem.*

Epidermolysis Bullosa

Every step in life is a hazard for this little girl. Every embrace or hug is a threat to her. Every pull or push is a peril. All this because she has epidermolysis bullosa, a hereditary fragility of her cellular sheath, the epidermis.

The simple twirling of an eraser pencil top on her skin will reproduce her disease. For this is not the ordinary delicate skin of infancy, but a skin which is ultra-delicate. Long thought to be pemphigus because the epidermis could be rubbed off in the manner of Nikolsky, epidermolysis bullosa now stands as a separate yet rarely seen mountain range of disease. It can be sharply distinguished from those diseases which are uniquely bullous when they appear in infancy. It is not bullous impetigo, although secondary infection may supervene. It is not congenital lues, as a serologic test for syphilis will attest. There are none of the concomitant signs that would suggest the bullae of urticaria pigmentosa, incontinentia pigmenti, epidermolytic hyperkeratosis (ichthyosiform erythroderma) or acrodermatitis enteropathica. Photosensitivity and drug reactions can be excluded by the history. Onset within hours after birth speaks against a diagnosis of juvenile dermatitis herpetiformis. No, despite the absence of a family history, this is an example of a hereditary disease. This is epidermolysis bullosa arising apparently as a mutation.

But what peak in the mountain range of epidermolysis bullosa is this? As clinicians, we can sight it clearly as epidermolysis bullosa simplex. It is the simple type, since there is none of the scarring, milia, nail dystrophy or mutilation seen in the dystrophic types. True, there is mucosal involvement and sporadic hemorrhaging, but this is trivial and

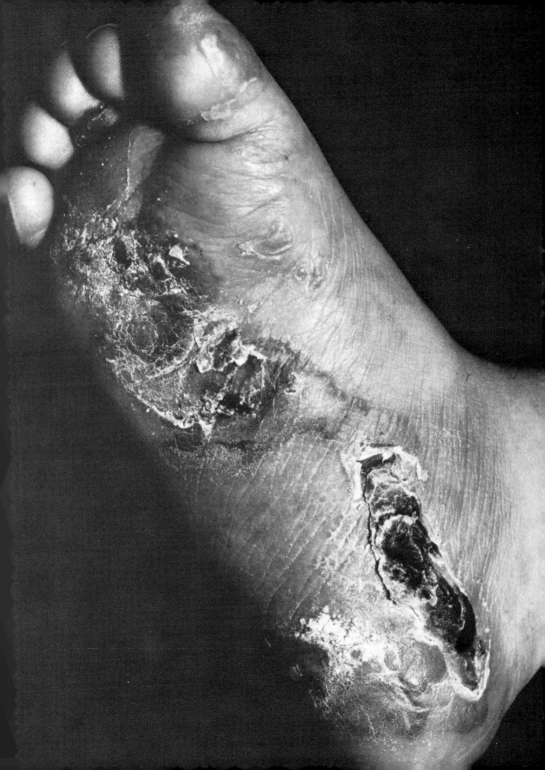

not the major silhouette we see in the dystrophic form. Involvement of the palms and soles as well as the benign course militates against thinking of this as the fulminant lethal type, although that too is nonscarring. Nor is this the acquired nonhereditary epidermolysis bullosa of adult life.

Histologic examination of a fresh, preferably induced blister will reveal a basement membrane floor and a complete epidermal roof. However, only electron microscopy of early lesions permits assured distinction of the various types of epidermolysis bullosa. This simplex version shows rupture precisely within the lower-most basal cell layer of the epidermis. In the lethal form the separation is *between* the basal cells and the basement membrane. In the dystrophic examples the separation is still lower, being between the basement membrane and the dermis. Such a deeper cleft helps explain the scarring that occurs in this form. Indeed, it conjures a totally different disease, one of dermal or collagen origin. Such has been the basis for the winds of change in nomenclature. Many now favor this peak being renamed dermolytic bullous dermatosis. All this comes from the fine inspiration of newer insight but is disturbing to the old school. In any event our patient has a more superficial and a truly epidermolytic process.

Genetic distinctions can be made as well. Although seemingly this girl's lesions arose as a de novo mutation, epidermolysis bullosa simplex is basically an autosomal dominant trait, there being a 50 per cent chance of inheritance from the affected parent. Dystrophic epidermolysis bullosa may be either dominant or recessive, the latter characteristically being the more severe mutilating destructive form. The lethal type is only recessive, so seemingly innocent in its encoded state, so dreadful when it emerges from a consanguineous or chance union. Usually such infants live for only a few months.

But what we learn from the chemistry of this range of diseases is most fascinating. Apparently, when the basal cells of our patient are physically stressed, their intracellular lysosomes in turn release their bag of autolytic enzymes, with resultant lysis of the basal cell layer. The enzymatic nature of this epidermolytic bulla formation can be dramatically underscored by simply chilling the skin. Under these circumstances, frictional torque no longer produces the anticipated separation of the epidermis from the basement membrane by lysis of the basal cells. Conversely, heating the skin accelerates this whole autolytic process, markedly reducing the force necessary to induce a blister.

Interestingly, frictional blisters in normal individuals as well as in those who have a lowered threshold for bullae of the hands and feet (Weber-Cockayne syndrome) arise not in the basal area but in the midepidermis. Presumably similar autolytic enzymes may be released also but at a different stage in keratinocyte maturation. In the lethal form the separation occurs at the point of contact between the epidermis and its basement membrane. It has been theorized that here the cement substance may be inadequate, leading to separation in response to frictional forces. In the case of the subepidermal bulla, i.e., the dystrophic scarring form of epidermolysis bullosa, it has been postulated that there is enzymatic destruction of the fine dermal collagen strands which moor the epidermal basement membrane. Supporting this view is the finding of increased collagenase in the lesions of just this type of epidermolysis bullosa. Understandably such collagenase implies that this is a dermolytic rather than epidermolytic bullous dermatosis. Further study is necessary before the collagenase can be given a firm pathogenic role, since it could be a secondary change.

Treatment of our little tot calls for a studied avoidance of frictional stresses. Suspension in the weightless world of the astronauts would be a theoretical ideal. But in this real world, her clothing, her shoes and her wraps must be as soft as possible. Her food must be chosen as well with a view to avoiding mechanical and thermal trauma to the mucosa. She should not be lifted and bounced in normal baby fashion. Soft carpeting, padded covering for furniture and objects in her way will prevent many a blister. A cool environment, avoidance of overheating and open, well-ventilated shoes are rewarding ways of critically reducing the activity of the temperature-dependent autolytic enzymes basically responsible for the epidermal separation. As she grows older, she must learn to derive her enjoyment from spectator sports. The racing, running and rough and tumble of sibling contacts are not for her.

The parents should acquire the skill of opening tense bullae by actually clipping away part of the insensitive roof with a fine iris scissors. Cool compresses with Burow's solution are helpful and can be followed by the application of a topical antibiotic ointment or Lassar's zinc oxide paste. Topical steroid creams and ointments also are valuable in speeding healing. A gentle daily bath, without benefit of a washcloth, is another essential. If neglected, secondary pyodermas will surely supervene, requiring appropriate systemic antibiotic therapy. Often cultures are necessary to make other than a preliminary assessment in this regard.

This is not the therapy of a day, a week or a year; it is for a lifetime. But it is a routine that will become less rigorous as this naturally fragile sheath of infancy gives way to the more sturdy epidermis of childhood and, in time, to that of early adulthood. Indeed, one may regularly anticipate a significant improvement at the time of puberty. This may seem eons away to the parents, but they must find some edge of comfort in the awareness that their daughter does not have a lethal disease, nor one to contract her life span. Nor will it scar, mutilate or deform.

Like burns, epidermolysis bullosa comes in several degrees. It helps to know that this is a first-degree one.

Pearson, R. W.: The Mechanobullous Diseases (Epidermolysis Bullosa). *In* Fitzpatrick, T. B., et al. (Eds.): *Dermatology in General Medicine*. McGraw-Hill Book Co., New York, 1971, pp. 621-643.
A marvelous survey of all aspects of hereditable pathologic blistering from physical trauma.

Gedde-Dahl, T., Jr.: *Epidermolysis Bullosa. A Clinical, Genetic and Epidemiological Study.* Johns Hopkins Press, Baltimore, 1971, 180 pp.
Definitive monographic Norwegian study of 53 cases illustrating the four types: (1) dominant nonscarring simplex, (2) dominant scarring dystrophic, (3) recessive mutilating dystrophic, and (4) recessive nonscarring lethal.

Sehgal, V. N., Shamsuddin, N. I., and Tyagi, S. P.: Epidermolysis Bullosa Simplex in Five Consecutive Generations. Aust. J. Derm., *11*:42-45, 1970.
Benign nonscarring variant, worse in summer, improves at puberty.

Becker, M. H., and Swinyard, C. A.: Epidermolysis Bullosa Dystrophica in Children. Radiology, *90*:124-128, 1968.
Severe scarring deforming type with esophageal strictures.

Wechsler, H. L., Krugh, F. J., Domonkos, A. N., Scheen, S. R., and Davidson, C. L., Jr.: Polydysplastic Epidermolysis Bullosa and Development of Epidermal Neoplasms. Arch. Derm., *102*:374-380, 1970.
Scars in dystrophic form may develop metastasizing squamous cell epitheliomas.

Bergenholtz, A., and Olsson, O.: Epidermolysis Bullosa Hereditaria. I. Epidermolysis Bullosa Hereditaria Letalis. A Survey of the Literature and Report of 11 Cases. Acta Dermatovener., *48*:220-241, 1968.
Neonatal onset, spares palms and soles; death occurs within a few months.

McKusick, V. A., and Wells, R. S.: Genetics in Relation to the Skin. *In* Fitzpatrick, T. B., et al. (Eds.): *Dermatology in General Medicine*. McGraw-Hill Book Co., New York, 1971, pp. 1089-1098.
A pedigree from the Amish showing how consanguinity brings out fatal recessive form of epidermolysis bullosa.

Reddy, A. R. R., and Wong, D. H. W.: Epidermolysis Bullosa. A Review of Anaesthetic Problems and Case Reports. Canad. Anaesth. Soc. J., *19*:536-548, 1972.
A special look at how to protect these patients during the rigors of general anesthesia.

Roenigk, H. H., Ryan, J. G., and Bergfeld, W. F.: Epidermolysis Bullosa Acquisita Report of Three Cases and Review of All Published Cases. Arch. Derm., *103*:1-10, 1971.
Nonhereditary, adult onset, associated with systemic disease.

Muller, S. A., Sams, W., Jr., and Dobson, R. L.: Amyloidosis Masquerading as Epidermolysis Bullosa Acquisita. Arch. Derm., *99*:739-747, 1969.
Trauma induces blisters and hemorrhage.

Akers, W. A., and Sulzberger, M. B.: The Friction Blister. Milit. Med., *137*:1-7, 1972.
In normal skin.

Comaish, J. S.: Epidermal Fatigue as a Cause of Friction Blisters. Lancet, *1*:81-83, 1973.
Fatigue rather than wear, heat, enzymes, pressure, stretching or ischemia is the chief mechanism in friction blister formation.

Arndt, K. A., Mihm, M. C., and Parrish, J. A.: Bullae: A Cutaneous Sign of a Variety of Neurologic Diseases. J. Invest. Derm., *60*:312-320, 1973.
Due to pressure-induced ischemia from prolonged immobilization.

Pearson, R. W.: Studies on the Pathogenesis of Epidermolysis Bullosa. J. Invest. Derm., *39*:551-575, 1962.
Electron microscopy reveals blister may form just above (simplex), exactly at (lethal) or just below (scarring) the epidermal basement membrane.

Jarrett, A.: *The Physiology and Pathophysiology of the Skin.* Academic Press, New York, 1973, pp. 1-356.
The latest on epidermal physiology.

Pierce, G. B.: The Origin of Basement Membrane: *In* Montagna, W., et al. (Eds.): *The Dermis.* Appleton-Century-Crofts, New York, 1970, pp. 173-194.
Just as fibroblasts synthesize collagen in response to injury, so do epithelial cells synthesize basement membrane in response to injury.

Pearson, R. W.: Some Observations on Epidermolysis Bullosa and Experimental Blisters. *In* Montagna, W., and Lobitz, W. C., Jr. (Eds.): *The Epidermis.* Academic Press, New York, 1964, pp. 613-626.
Blister formation in epidermolysis bullosa simplex, due to friction-triggered disintegration of basal cells, prevented by cooling skin.

Eisen, A. Z.: Human Skin Collagenase: Relationship to the Pathogenesis of Epidermolysis Bullosa Dystrophica. J. Invest. Derm., *52*:449-453, 1969.
In dystrophic recessive form, collagenase level increased.

Lazarus, G. S.: Collagenase and Connective Tissue Metabolism in Epidermolysis Bullosa. J. Invest. Derm., *58*:242-248, 1972.
Collagenase elevation in dystrophic clinical lesion viewed as secondary phenomenon, since not seen in tissue culture.

Keller, L.: Silver Nitrate Therapy in Epidermolysis Bullosa Hereditaria of the Newborn. J. Pediat., *72*:854-865, 1968.
Compresses 0.5 per cent silver nitrate to reduce secondary infection.

de Brito Caldeira, J., and Lacerda e Costa, M. H.: Epidermolysis Bullosa Hereditaria. Clinical Trial with Fluocinonide FAPG[R] 0.05% in Five Cases. Acta Dermatovener., *52*(Suppl. 67):88-90, 1971.
Topical steroids somewhat helpful.

Akers, W. A., Leonard, F., Ousterhaut, D. K., and Cortese, T. A.: Treating Friction Blisters with Alkyl-α-Cyanoacrylates. Arch. Derm., *107*:544-547, 1973.
Rapidly polymerizing glue used as dressing for denuded friction blister.

Smith, E. G., and Michener, W. M.: Vitamin E Treatment of Dermolytic Bullous Dermatosis. Arch. Derm., *108*:254-256, 1973.
Help for dystrophic epidermolysis bullosa from 1600 I. U. daily.

Purdy, M. J., and Fairbrother, G. E.: Case Report: Epidermolysis Bullosa Acquisita. Aust. J. Derm., *13*:27-30, 1972.
Therapy: Dapsone.

Swinyard, C. A., Swenson, J. R., and Rees, T. D.: Rehabilitation of Hand Deformities in Epidermolysis Bullosa. Arch. Phys. Med. Rehab., *49*:138-144, 1968.
In dystrophic type, fingers may be lost in cutaneous cocoon, unless finger exercises, Telfa dressings and antibiotics employed.

Schuman, B. M., and Arciniegas, E.: The Management of Esophageal Complications of Epidermolysis Bullosa. Amer. J. Dig. Dis., *17*:875-880, 1972.
In dystrophic type, stenotic scarred esophagus may have to be replaced by colon.

Severin, G. L., and Farber, E. M.: The Management of Epidermolysis Bullosa in Children. Effective Topical Steroid Treatment. Arch. Derm., *95*:302-309, 1967.
Tender loving care 24 hours a day: let clothing, food and handling be gentle.

45

Secondary Syphilis

For the past six weeks this 22-year-old student has had a **scaling papular eruption of the palms and soles**, *an annular scaling plaque of the scrotum and a mucous patch on the hard palate.*

Darkfield examination of the palmar lesions—negative.

VDRL serologic test for syphilis—reactive.

Secondary Syphilis

You can read much in this man's palm. You can read that he has a serious systemic contagious disease. You can sense that just beneath those scales, the infectious agent has poured out of the circulation through capillaries and into the epidermis, eventually lodging within the keratinocyte. You are aware that a droplet of fluid from a scraped lesion may harbor this agent. You have learned that the agent is a live organism, so unbelievably thin that it remains completely invisible under the microscope until it is revealed as a motile coiled thread, reflecting light in darkfield illumination. This is the spirochete *Treponema pallidum.* You know that these palmar lesions are the result of an immune struggle between the patient and this parasite. As such, your palm-reading can be supported or refuted by a variety of diagnostic immunologic tests which trace their ancestry back to Wassermann.

You can translate these palm lesions into numerous other systemic immune lesions, since he may have concurrent symptomatic or asymptomatic hepatitis, iritis, periostitis, nephritis or even meningitis. You can confidently predict that his palm and skin lesions as well as any associated malaise, and lymphadenopathy, will magically disappear in a few months—and all this without treatment! But as a fortune teller you must also reveal that without treatment at this time, not only does he remain a threat to his intimate or sexual contacts, but he has two chances in five of having the disease reappear many years later, this time with vengeance. Not only may it then involve the skin with ulcerative gummatous nodules, but also it may come as a dreaded aneurysmal dilatation of an aorta scarred as a result of the endarteritis obliterans of its vasa vasorum. Or it may come as the destruction of the posterior columns of

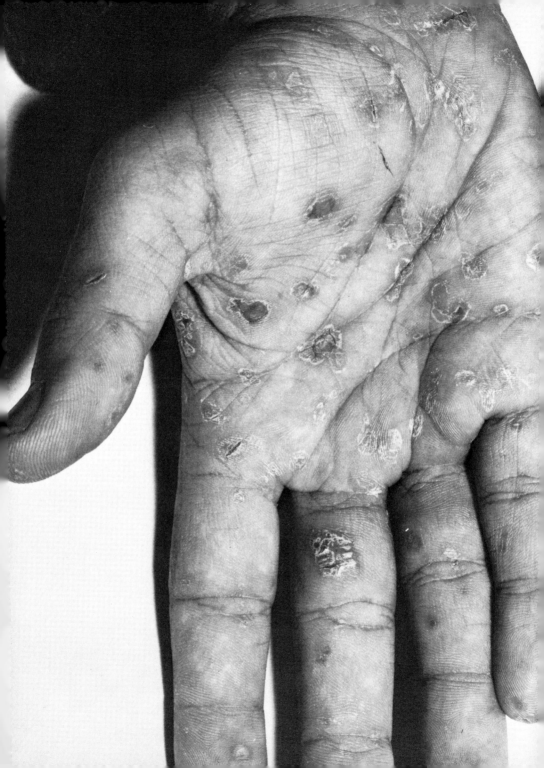

the spinal cord with the lightning pains, the ataxia and the sensory defects of tabes dorsalis. Or it may insidiously present as general paresis with the progressive psychosis, convulsions and dementia of a brain itself being gradually destroyed. All this can be the irreparable result of ignoring or not recognizing the present early warning signals of these palms.

You see in these palms the disease of kings and their poets, of mothers and their unborn infants, of prostitutes and their clients. You see in these palms the disease which down through the centuries literally fashioned the sexual mores and private lives of mankind. You see a disease man first conquered in the early dawn of our age of antibiotics. This man has syphilis. You can read it in his palms.

Not all the cutaneous lesions of early syphilis can be read as easily. Many are merely suggestive, others mimic known disease and all are conditioned by the skin site at which they appear. Thus, on the scalp, hair loss may be the only sign. It need not be in the characteristic moth-eaten alopecic patterning but simply diffuse. The face is a site for annular lesions, especially in blacks. The oral mucosa commonly shows only a nonspecific erosion, the mucous patch. It resembles an aphthous ulcer, and should it be laryngeal, the patient complains of hoarseness. The trunk may show no more than an ephemeral morbilliform rash, the sign of spirochetes within the endothelium of the fine dermal vasculature. An associated lymphadenopathy may suggest a viral infection such as rubella and mislead unless the serologic test for syphilis is secured routinely. On the trunk, the pattern may be papulosquamous, at times suggesting an atypical pityriasis rosea or drug eruption. On the extremities, it can easily mimic psoriasis or lichen planus. In the vulvar or perianal area, moist flat warty papules, the extremely contagious condylomata lata, are another sign of early syphilis, the lesion again being modified by the skin site. Complete inspection of the patient is necessary; otherwise, one can easily miss the split papule of a toe web or the fine scaling area on the back of the scrotum. Nevertheless, very few findings are specific, so that anything from anxiety to xerosis may be suspect and merit blood serologic tests.

Our suspicions of syphilis are heightened not only by skin and mucosal lesions but by the mild constitutional signs of spirochete intolerance seen in about half the patients. These include headaches, arthralgias, lymphadenopathy, splenomegaly, fever and a variety of vague yet organ-directed complaints. The need for serologic studies becomes greater when the patient is in the active sexual age group, is a homosexual or gives a history of a possible primary chancre-like lesion of the genitalia or elsewhere.

A biopsy of a suspect lesion is only modestly helpful. If there is a vasculitic process and plasma cells are present in abundance, a stain for spirochetes should be done. Far more valuable is the darkfield examination of serous exudate from an abraded lesion. This is invariably positive in the moist erosive infectious lesions of the genitalia. In the dry keratotic papule, only with persistent skilled efforts, which include Scotch Tape stripping and suction, does the diagnostic spirochete appear. For the oral lesion the presence of numerous saprophytic harmless spirochetes renders darkfield examination useless unless specific immunofluorescent staining is employed.

At this stage, serologic tests for syphilis are almost invariably positive and are our main laboratory support. The practical inexpensive routine test is the VDRL, a nontreponemal flocculation procedure. An analogue is the Kolmer test, which assesses complement fixation. For more sensitivity and specificity we can turn to the treponemal tests. The FTA-ABS has served for the last ten years as a valuable immunofluorescent procedure. The ultimate in specificity is the TPI test, which is based on the fact that the serum from a syphilitic will immobilize living treponemes.

It is evident that a high degree of sophistication has been brought to our understanding of the immune state in the varying stages of syphilis and its application to diagnostic testing. We understand that no one has natural immunity to *Treponema pallidum*. Only several weeks after the inoculation of spirochetes—and this occurs only under favorable moist conditions—does the body begin to reject this organism. It is then that the initial site of entry, whether it be on the penis, cervix or elsewhere, shows an inflammatory reaction, leading to mucosal or epidermal erosion, the primary chancre. It is at this time, nearly three weeks after exposure, that the blood serum first shows antibodies to treponemes and, curiously, even to related lipoidal antigens which can be extracted from tissue. These latter are the nontreponemal antigens used in the VDRL and Kolmer tests. As the weeks pass, the antibody titer climbs, usually to levels at which quantitative testing reveals that the serum can be diluted 32-fold or more and will still give a reaction. The active elaboration of these antibodies is associated with plasma cell as well as lymph node hyperplasia. If the condition is not treated, the serologic tests remain positive for years, gradually diminishing in titer. With involvement of the central nervous system, the cerebrospinal fluid follows suit, showing a positive STS. With treatment, there is a rapid fall in titer, often within six months, to a very low level (2 dils) or negativity. It is felt that the persistence of a positive test may reflect the persistence of a few spirochetes in the plasma cells or in such sanctuaries as the aqueous humor of the eye or the cerebrospinal fluid. With relapse or reinfection, titers again rapidly climb, allowing us to monitor events rather precisely. With complete return of the serologic tests to nonreactivity, the patient loses all resistance and is back in his pristine state. Only with the continued presence apparently of traces of the spirochetal antigen can the patient maintain resistance to reinfection.

As in all testing procedures, specificity and sensitivity are parameters of great concern. The fact that some patients who do not have and never have had syphilis show positive serologic tests for syphilis is of special concern. These are the so-called biologic false positives (BFP). They may be temporary, are often of low titer, and are usually associated with the nontreponemal antigen tests. Nevertheless, they deserve attention. In the authentic chronic BFP reaction, the TPI test must be found to be negative on two occasions a month apart. Such a BFP reaction seems to reflect the presence of antibodies to the patient's own tissues, the autoimmune state. Further studies may reveal such autoimmune states as systemic lupus erythematosus, rheumatoid disease or viral infection. The picture is not simple, however, since a wide spectrum of other disease states may be uncovered, including leprosy as well as narcotic addiction.

Penicillin is still the treatment of choice, after 30 years. For centuries before that mercury rubs were used, because mercury kept the spirochete out of the epidermis. This in turn was replaced by the "magic bullet" of arsenic, which had to be machine-gunned in for years and which killed some patients as well as the spirochete. Today, in contrast, penicillin acts quietly and effectively, killing the spirochete within hours and rendering the patient noninfectious virtually overnight. Yet a significant number of patients do experience within hours after penicillin a temporary flare or the first appearance of cutaneous signs, as well as fever and an influenza-like syndrome. This Herxheimer reaction could very well be an immune response due in part to the release of antigen from the treponemes which are lysed. The patient should be instructed concerning the possibility of such a flare and its ordinarily benign nature in early syphilis. If a therapeutic dose of 0.03 unit per ml. is maintained for 14 days, the disease is cured in over 95 per cent of the patients with early syphilis. This can be achieved assuredly by two intramuscular injections of 2.4 million units of benzathine penicillin G, the second being given after a one-week interval. For late syphilis, a third injection is given a week later.

The patient should have a quantitative VDRL serologic followup every 3 months for the first year and again at two years. Spinal fluid examination and re-treatment are recommended for those who fail to show a negative test by this time or for any who develop a rising titer. For the persistently serofast patient, guidance and an explanation that the positive test does not indicate the presence of either clinical disease or infectiousness must be provided. He must further understand that additional treatment and followup is not only unnecessary but undesirable.

For those who are allergic to penicillin, 2 grams of either erythromycin or tetracycline is to be taken orally each day for 15 days. In this regard, note that tetracycline is to be avoided in pregnant women because of its adverse effects on the fetus.

Prompt epidemiologic followup of this patient's contacts and in turn of their contacts is necessary to guard their health and effect a quasi-cordon sanitaire to limit further spread. Often this can best be done by a professional team such as provided by the Public Health Service.

Syphilis is a disease that must be treated early if it is to be treated well. Ask for it in the history, look for it in the skin, check for it in the blood. Don't let it hide from you until it's too late.

Drusin, L. M.: The Diagnosis and Treatment of Infectious and Latent Syphilis. In Symposium on Venereal Diseases, Med. Clin. N. Amer., 56:1055-1222, 1972.
Secondary syphilis: look for scalp hair loss, annular lesions of face, mucous patches in mouth, macular eruption of trunk, flat warts of genitalia, or papules of palms and soles.

King, A., and Nicol, C.: *Venereal Diseases*, 2nd ed., Bailliére, Tindall, Cassell, London, 1969, 319 pp.
A friendly, lucid book showing the whole picture of early and late acquired syphilis, as well as congenital, cardiovascular and neurosyphilis.

Stokes, J. H., Beerman, H., and Ingraham, N. R.: *Modern Clinical Syphilology Diagnosis, Treatment Case Study*, 3rd ed. W. B. Saunders Co., Philadelphia, 1944, 1332 pp.
The magnum opus on the great pox: everything the *Treponema pallidum* can do from the chancre to the grave.

Willcox, R. R.: The Treponematoses. *In* Simons, R. D. G. P., and Marshall, J. (Eds.): *Essays on Tropical Dermatology*. Excerpta Medica Foundation, Amsterdam, 1969, pp. 35-47.

Engrossing story of the evolutionary climb of treponemes up from slime to animals to man, and their mutational course from pinta to yaws to syphilis as civilization reduced opportunities for intimate skin contact to sexual encounters.

Kingsbury, D. H., Chester, E. C., and Jansen, G. T.: Syphilitic Paronychia: An Unusual Complaint. Arch. Derm., *105*:458-458, 1972.
Associated with papulosquamous syphilid of the palms and darkfield positive condylomata lata.

Mikhail, G. R., and Chapel, T. A.: Follicular Papulopustular Syphilid. Arch. Derm., *100*:471-473, 1969.
A cutaneous sign that urges you to watch for neurosyphilis.

Hartsock, R. J., Halling, L. W., and King, F. M.: Luetic Lymphadenitis: A Clinical and Histologic Study of 20 Cases. Amer. J. Clin. Path., *53*:304-314, 1970.
Immune defense response to entrapped spirochetes.

Parker, J. D. J.: Uncommon Complications of Early Syphilis Hepatitis, Periostitis, Iritis with Papillitis and Meningitis. Brit. J. Vener. Dis., *48*:32-36, 1972.
Four cases to remind you that syphilis is more than skin deep.

Hudson, E. H.: Diagnosing a Case of Venereal Disease in Fifteenth Century Scotland. Brit. J. Vener. Dis., *48*:146-153, 1972.
Urbane, scholarly work of detection: before Columbus, syphilis was considered a form of leprosy.

Sparling, P. F.: Diagnosis and Treatment of Syphilis. New Eng. J. Med., *284*:642-653, 1971.
Laboratory diagnosis:
Lesion — Darkfield visualization of spirochetes.
Serum — (1) VDRL (Venereal Disease Research Lab) test for nonspecific antibodies; (2) FTA-ABS specific immunofluorescent treponemal antibody test; (3) TPI ultraspecific *Treponema pallidum* immobilization test.

Catteral, R. D.: Systemic Disease and the Biologic False Positive Reaction. Brit. J. Vener. Dis., *48*:1-12, 1972.
Complete survey of perplexing problem of positive tests for syphilis revealed to be false by negative TPI: often sign of autoimmune disease, e.g., systemic lupus.

LeClair, R. A., Montague, T. S., and Keetin, L. M.: Biologic False-Positive Reactions for Syphilis as Measured by the Treponema Pallidum Immobilization Test. J. Med., 3:264-269, 1972.
Half were in pregnant women and narcotic addicts.

Jeerapaet, P., and Ackerman, A. B.: Histologic Patterns of Secondary Syphilis. Arch. Derm., *107*:373-377, 1973.
Plasma cell infiltrate seen in 23 of 27 cases; spirochetes seen with silver stain in 9 of 27.

Metz, J., and Metz, G.: Elektronenmikroskopischer Nachweis von Treponema pallidum in Hautefflorescenzen der unbehandelten Lues I und II. Arch. Derm. Forsch., *243*:241-254, 1972.
Spirochete found between and within keratinocytes as well as within plasma cells in secondary lesions.

Smith, E. B., Bartruff, J. K., and Blanchard, V.: Skin Biopsy in Cases of Secondary Syphilis. Brit. J. Vener. Dis., *46*:426-426, 1970.
Immunofluorescent staining revealed no antigen-antibody complex in vessel walls.

Schmidt, H., and Goldschmidt, E.: Demonstration of Motile Treponemes in Aqueous Humour in Secondary Syphilis. Brit. J. Vener. Dis., *48*:400-401, 1972.
Only 0.25 micron wide, the spirochete can go anywhere and hide.

Dunlop, E. M. C.: Persistence of Treponemes After Treatment. Brit. Med. J., *2*:577-580, 1972.
Apparently some few spirochetes can even hide from penicillin in aqueous humor and CSF. 131 references.

Ovcinnikov, N. M., and Delektorskij, V. V.: Current Concepts of the Morphology and Biology of Treponema Pallidum Based on Electron-microscopy. Brit. J. Vener. Dis., *47*:315-328, 1971.
Persistence of spirochetes in plasma cells may explain persistently positive STS.

Fulford, K. W. M., and Brostoff, J.: Leucocyte Migration and Cell-Mediated Immunity in Syphilis. Brit. J. Vener. Dis., *48*:483-488, 1972.
In secondary syphilis, treponemal antigen can induce lymphocyte transformation, but discordant immune deficit revealed by failure to induce migration inhibitory factor.

Magnuson, H. J., Thomas, E. W., Olansky, S., Kaplan, B. I., DeMello, L., and Cutler, J. C.: Inoculation Syphilis in Human Volunteers. Medicine, *35*:33-82, 1956.
Unable to infect if volunteer had untreated latent syphilis.

WHO Scientific Group: Treponematosis Research. Technical Report 455, World Health Organization, Geneva, 1970, 91 pp.
Major obstacle: inability to grow *T. pallidum* **in laboratory. Superb summation.**

Frye, W. W.: The Importance of Contact Investigation in the Control of Syphilis. Med. Clin. N. Amer., *48*:637-651, 1964.
All sexual contacts of infectious patients deserve a discrete medical alert!

Hatos, G.: Evaluation of 460 Cases of Treated Syphilis. Med. J. Aust., *2*:415-420, 1972.
Thirty-six per cent of secondary syphilis appeared in homosexuals.

Ackerman, A. B., Goldfaden, G., and Cosmides, J. C.: Acquired Syphilis in Early Childhood. Arch. Derm., *106*:92-93, 1972.
Not only by rape, pederasty and sexual play, but also by breast feeding, kissing and handling.

Chambers, R. W., Foley, H. T., and Schmidt, P. J.: Transmission of Syphilis by Fresh Blood Components. Transfusion, *9*:32-34, 1969.
An unfortunate way of acquiring the disease.

Miller, J. N.: Development of an Experimental Syphilis Vaccine. Med. Clin. N. Amer., *56*:1217-1220, 1972.
Not yet for man.

Clark, E. G., and Danbolt, N.: The Oslo Study of the Natural Course of Untreated Syphilis: An Epidemiologic Investigation Based on a Re-study of the Boech-Bruusgaard Material. Med. Clin. N. Amer., *48*:613-623, 1964.
Over 60 per cent of untreated syphilitics went through life with little or no inconvenience from disease. A classic.

Schroeter, A. L., Lucas, J. B., Price, E. V., and Falcone, V. H.: Treatment for Early Syphilis and Reactivity of Serologic Tests. J.A.M.A., *221*:471-476, 1972.
Treat with 2.4 million units of benzathine penicillin G given I.M. and follow serologically with serial quantitative VDRL tests. Tetracycline and erythromycin suitable alternates.

Ovcinnikov, N. M., and Delektorskij, V. V.: Effects of Crystalline Penicillin and Bicillin-1 on Experimental Syphilis in the Rabbit. Electron Microscope Study. Brit. J. Vener. Dis., *48*:327-341, 1972.

Within six hours, penicillin causes lysis of extracellular treponemes but not the intracellular ones.

Velasco, J. E., Miller, A. E., and Zaias, N.: Minocycline in the Treatment of Venereal Disease. J.A.M.A., *220*:1323-1325, 1972.

Minocycline, 100 mg. b.i.d. for 15 days, efficacious in treating 5 cases of secondary syphilis.

Putkonen, T., Salo, O. P., and Mustakallio, K. K.: Febrile Herxheimer Reaction in Different Phases of Primary and Secondary Syphilis. Brit. J. Vener. Dis., *42*:181-184, 1966.

Febrile episode regularly seen after penicillin treatment if syphilis present for over one month.

46

Miliaria

*This obese hospitalized patient developed a temperature of 102°
because of a bacterial infection.* **Numerous tense clear vesicles
of varying sizes** *were subsequently noted over her back and arms.*

Miliaria

Look again! That is not sweat. That is trapped sweat. Those are
vesicles within the stratum corneum, each one distended with sweat.
This is miliaria crystallina. The ostia of the sweat ducts have closed over
and now sweat is pouring *into* instead of *onto* the skin. You see the resultant asymptomatic pellucid vesicles. Since a brisk stroke with a towel will
wipe them away, once recognized they are usually ignored.

But in the lower left you see a few erythematous papules. These,
too, are a form of miliaria. This is miliaria rubra, a sibling in the family
of sweat retention dermatitides. Here the trapped sweat is escaping
deeper into the living epidermis, producing the prickling and redness
vividly known as prickly heat. This is an important commonly seen
disease of high environment temperatures, whether it be in the tropics,
in a ship's hold or in a malfunctioning space lab.

Few diseases are as well understood as this environmental one of
miliaria. Subject to experimental dissection in man, it has been found to
be a disease of the functioning sweat gland unit. As such it does not
occur in patients with congenital absence of sweat glands, nor in the
nonsweating plaques of tuberculoid leprosy or sympathectomized skin.
Not only do we know that it is a disease of the sweat gland unit, but we
can define the following three pathogenetic determinants.

(1) First, miliaria occurs only in glands in which egress of sweat is
blocked. The nature of this blockage is usually inapparent, not only to
the clinician but to the pathologist. The sweat pore, except on the palms
and soles, is somewhat of a misleading abstraction. Even the scanning
electron microscope fails to disclose a beaker-like ductal orifice. Actually
the terminal duct lies on its side, hidden under a cap of keratin until uncovered by Scotch-Tape stripping. Although the biophysical nature of

the occlusive change is as hidden as the duct itself, we do know that the precipitating cause is prolonged presence of unevaporated sweat on the skin. It is thus a disease more of the humid tropics than the hot day desert country. In susceptible subjects several days of wet sweaty skin is invariably followed by poral closure of sweat glands in such areas as the antecubital and popliteal fossae. This can best be experimentally reproduced by simply inducing total vapor occlusion of the skin with Saran Wrap. This produces the macerated skin of tropical heat and humidity and within 48 hours leads to the poral occlusion requisite for miliaria.

Much has been written to explain just how the prolonged sweating or Saran Wrap maceration induces the poral closure. Some view the hydration itself as causal, yet prolonged immersion of skin in water produces dermatitis, not poral closure. Others view the salt of sweat as a factor. Certainly bathing in salt water seems to accentuate miliaria, and the sweat of patients with miliaria has a greater salt concentration than that of the nonmiliarial group. Another group stresses the pathogenicity of the enormous bacterial overgrowth that occurs in macerated skin. However, at least in experimental miliaria there is no singular cause. Any of a variety of minor nonspecific injuries to the epidermis can trigger poral closure. This correlates with the clinical finding of miliaria limited to areas of simple friction, such as an area rubbed by a belt. A mild sunburn can be the antecedent to the efflorescence of miliaria crystallina in a person on the tennis court. It fits, too, with the observation that the more delicate skin of infants is the more susceptible to miliaria and that the resistant skin of the palms and soles is not a site for miliaria. The absence of a protective lipoidal mantle also seems to favor miliaria; conversely, the face that is well endowed with a continuous supply of sebum is usually exempt from miliaria.

(2) The second and at once the simplest pathogenetic determinant of miliaria is the secretion of sweat. The appearance of the lesions is totally dependent on the production (and, in turn, abnormal escape) of sweat. Atropinize an area of miliaria, and the vesicles, erythema and itching rapidly fade, leaving only the inapparent poral closure to be followed later by a fine postinflammatory scaling. Increase the sweating rate, and you will accentuate the signs and symptoms of miliaria. It is truly a sweat-actuated disease.

(3) The third sine qua non and final determinant of miliaria is ductal rupture. The clinical picture reflects the level at which such rupture occurs. Thus, our patient's asymptomatic miliaria crystallina is indicative

of a ductal tear or leak into the inert stratum corneum. Miliaria rubra, i.e., prickly heat, occurs when the ductal rupture is within the innervated cellular sheath of the living epidermis. A third form, rarely seen except in the tropics, miliaria profunda, is associated with rupture farther down the duct, with extravasation into the dermis. This is dermal, so that the sweat retention appears as a nonfollicular papular eruption. It occurs below the itch organ of the epidermis and thus is also essentially asymptomatic.

Although the levels of sweat escape are as evident histologically as clinically, the reason for the rupture is elusive. We do know that individual and ethnic factors are important. Actually individual gland susceptibility is important, since, as we see in our patient, only a small fraction of the sweat gland units show miliarial change. It is in these specific glands only that the rupture or ductal escape of sweat is occurring. Indeed, the other glands may be covering the skin with so much sweat that it is hard to remember that miliaria is a sweat retention disease. However, the key factor may be the presence or absence of intraductal bacterial growth. In some instances the immense overgrowth of staphylococci and other organisms which occurs in sweaty skin may enter the sweat pore, prior to occlusion. These trapped bacteria elaborate toxins or proteases which lead to loss of integrity of the sweat duct. Even pustule formation (miliaria pustulosa) as seen in infants may occur, as well as pustular miliaria secondary to various dermatitides. The pathogenetic role of bacteria is supported by both their abundant presence in the wet soil of miliarial skin and the fact that pyodermas can predispose to miliaria. Furthermore, the use of topical antibiotics distinctly reduces the severity of miliaria.

Without doubt, the best medicine for miliaria is air conditioning. With a drop in environmental temperature, the sweat gland turns off, the extravasated sweat is reabsorbed and within hours the patient feels and looks better. This is one disease for which we turn to the engineer rather than to the pharmacist. Even without the blessings of air conditioning much can be done to reduce the internal as well as external heat load and thereby the intensity of miliaria. A fan, cooler clothing, a swim and resting all help.

Little can be done with topical or systemic therapy, although every cool wave ushers in new faith in the remedy used at the time. We usually recommend a neomycin-betamethasone valerate lotion. Atropine-like compounds are of little help systemically, and may aggravate the thermal intolerance already present. Cholinergic drugs are understandably interdicted. To prevent further extension, harsh soaps, detergents and irritant topical agents must be avoided. It is tempting to assume that a keratolytic such as salicylic acid will peel open the occluded sweat pore, but in practice the chance of further irritation and additional closures is often greater than the benefits of induced desquamation. Occlusive ointments, protective as they may seem, are generally poorly tolerated, with the patient complaining of increased pruritus. Simple elimination of sweating by cooling the patient is the sovereign cure.

Once the gland remains at rest, the epidermis and the blocked acrosyringium restore themselves completely to normal within two weeks. Conversely, should the sweating persist, more glands may become involved, leading to serious thermoregulatory deficits. The patients become asthenic as the miliarial anhidrosis spreads from unit to unit. When these susceptible units remain involved for prolonged periods, the superficial miliarial element may fade, leaving only a widespread deep tropical anhidrosis. Such patients can no longer work without fear of heat collapse. This diagnosis is generally obvious when one sees a patient under severe thermal stress remain bone dry except for the face. Exempt from miliaria, as well as the postmiliarial anhidrosis, the face continues to sweat profusely in a vain attempt to compensate for the loss of up to 90 per cent of the body's evaporative cooling system.

Miliaria is a remarkable disease—it is one of the few we know precisely how to recognize, how to elicit, how to prevent and how to cure.

Leeming, J. A. L.: Miliaria. *In* Marshall, J. (Ed.): *Essays on Tropical Dermatology,* Vol. 2, Excerpta Medica, Amsterdam, 1972, pp. 169-182.
   Magnificent complete critical review of what is known and not known about the sweat retention lesions of miliaria.

Rochmis, P. G., and Koplon, B. S.: Iatrogenic Miliaria Crystallina Due to Bethanechol. Arch. Derm., *95*:499-500, 1967.
   Cholinergic drug induced profuse sweating and miliaria crystallina.

Lobitz, W. C., Jr.: Pustular Miliaria: Sweat Retention Phenomenon Complicating Common Dermatoses. J.A.M.A., *148*:1097-1100, 1952.
   Important pustular variant of miliaria seen in hot environments.

Sulzberger, M. B., and Herrmann, F.: *The Clinical Significance of Disturbances in the Delivery of Sweat.* Charles C Thomas, Springfield, Illinois, 1954, 212 pp.
   Secondary sweat retention accounts for much of the pruritus of atopic and other lichenoid dermatitides. Monographic.

Shelley, W. B., Horvath, P. N., and Pillsbury, D. M.: Anhidrosis. An Etiologic Interpretation. Medicine, *29*:195-224, 1950.
Sweat retention anhidrosis may occur in absence of clinical signs.

O'Brien, J. P.: A Study of Miliaria Rubra, Tropical Anhidrosis and Anhidrotic Asthenia. Brit. J. Derm. Syph., *59*:125-158, 1947.
An inspiring classic by a lone pathologist assigned to the tropics during World War II.

Hambrick, G. W., and Blank, H.: The Microanatomy of Miliaria Crystallina. J. Invest. Derm., *26*:327-336, 1956.
Photo of sweat retention vesicle within stratum corneum, with duct emptying into central point of the base.

Hindson, T. C.: A Comparison of Experimentally Produced Prickly Heat and Hypohidrosis in Gurkha and British Troops. J. Invest. Derm., *52*:543-544, 1969.
Ninety per cent of British troops susceptible to miliaria, but only 45 per cent of Nepalese.

Shelley, W. B.: Experimental Miliaria in Man. V. The Effect of Poral Closure on the Secretory Function of the Eccrine Sweat Gland. J. Invest. Derm., *22*:267-271, 1954.
Series of studies showing that minor nonspecific epidermal injury can produce poral occlusion and subsequent sweat retention lesions.

Sulzberger, M. B., and Harris, D. R.: Miliaria and Anhidrosis. III. Multiple Small Patches and the Effects of Different Periods of Occlusion. Arch. Derm., *105*:845-850, 1972.
Area of skin occluded by Saran Wrap for 48 hours, then stimulated to sweat, developed miliaria; skin returns to normal in 2 weeks.

Willis, I.: The Effects of Prolonged Water Exposure on Human Skin. J. Invest. Derm., *60*:166-171, 1973.
Dermatitis but not miliaria produced by continuous exposure to water for 3 days, despite increase in bacterial population.

Loewenthal, L. J. A., Politzer, W. M., and Wyndham, C. H.: The Salt Excretion of Miliaria Subjects. S. Afr. Med. J., *38*:315-319, 1964.
Higher concentration of salt in sweat of miliarial group; may play etiologic role.

Christophers, E., and Plewig, G.: Formation of the Acrosyringium. Arch. Derm., *107*:378-382, 1973.
The anatomy and physiology of the target unit in miliaria.

Johnson, C. E., and Shuster, S.: The Use of Partial Sweat Duct Occlusion in the Elucidation of Sweat Duct Function in Health and Disease. J. Soc. Cos. Chem., *24*:15-29, 1973.
Capacity of duct to reabsorb water limited despite increase at times of occlusion. Excess produced by secretory coil escapes from acrosyringium to produce miliarial signs.

Griffin, T. B., Maibach, H. I., and Sulzberger, M. B.: Miliaria and Anhidrosis. The Relationships Between Miliaria and Anhidrosis in Man. J. Invest. Derm., *49*:379-385, 1967.
Severity and duration of hypohidrosis and miliaria directly related.

Sulzberger, M. B., and Griffin, T. B.: Induced Miliaria, Post-miliarial Hypohidrosis, and Some Potential Sequelae. Arch. Derm., *99*:145-151, 1969.
Experimentally produced sweat-retention heat collapse.

Stoughton, R. B.: Suppression of Miliaria Rubra (Prickly Heat) by a Topical Anticholinergic Agent. J. Invest. Derm., *42*:287-287, 1964.
No sweat, no miliaria.

Hindson, T. C., and Worsley, D. E.: The Effects of Administration of Ascorbic Acid in Experimentally Induced Miliaria and Hypohidrosis in Volunteers. Brit. J. Derm., *81*:226-227, 1969.
Recovery speeded by a gram a day.

Lyons, R. E., Levine, R., and Auld, D.: Miliaria Rubra. A Manifestation of Staphylococcal Disease. Arch. Derm., *86*:282-286, 1962.
Finds antibiotic lotion helpful.

Stillman, M. A., Hindson, T. C., and Maibach, H. I.: The Effect of Pretreatment of Skin on Artificially Induced Miliaria Rubra and Hypohidrosis. Brit. J. Derm., *84*:110-116, 1971.
Lanolin, steroids, antibiotics and acid buffers each afforded a measure of prophylaxis.

Lobitz, W. C., and Dobson, R. L.: Miliaria. Arch. Environ. Health, *11*:460-464, 1965.
Therapy — remove patient from thermal stimulus to sweating.

47

Dermatomyositis

47

Nine months ago this 84-year-old woman developed large wide-spread plaques of erythema and edema, as well as an insidious muscle weakness. The skin changes now range from the **distinctive purplish red inflammatory change on her upper eyelids** *to blotchy maculopapular lesions over the knuckles (Gottron's papules). The finger tips show paronychial erythema, telangiectasia and a markedly hyperkeratotic cuticle.*

Serum glutamic oxaloacetic acid transaminase level was elevated (55 units per ml.). Biochemical parameters, chest x-ray, upper and lower G.I. series, sigmoidoscopy, intravenous pyelogram and otolaryngologic and gynecologic surveys failed to reveal evidence of malignancy.

Skin biopsy — edema, collagen degeneration.

Muscle biopsy — inflammatory myopathy.

Dermatomyositis

This is not the eyeshadow of cosmetics, but rather the shadow of malignancy or death itself. You are looking at the diagnostic sign of dermatomyositis, heliotrope erythema of the upper eyelids. It is the sign which points to a strange connective tissue disease which involves the muscles as well as the skin. It tells of a route of progressively worsening myopathy. It bespeaks of both malignancy and death. It is a sign that demands both study and treatment.

Dermatomyositis is an elusive disease and difficult to characterize. Its skin changes are protean. It may come as the malar flush of lupus erythematosus, authentic even to being aggravated by sunlight. It may appear as scleroderma of the fingers, with Raynaud's phenomenon and calcinosis (sclerodermatomyositis). It may present as a poikiloderma vasculare atrophicans, as bullae or ulcers, as nonspecific alopecia or as psoriasis or lichen planus. It may take the guise of a necrotizing vasculitis or a follicular hyperkeratosis.

Not only are the skin changes elusive but the muscle patterns are as well. The muscle weakness may not seem especially unusual for an octogenarian or in one who has been sick. It may be accompanied by an

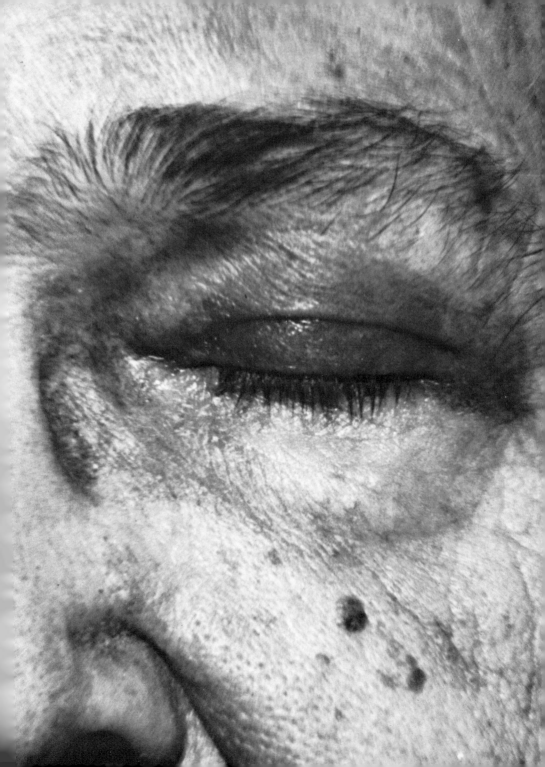

arthralgia which blinds us to the primary nature of the weakness. It may mimic the clinical picture of myasthenia gravis, trichinosis or thyrotoxicosis. It may present with pain or tenderness of the muscle or neither of these. It may elude the surgeon's biopsy knife, or even the light microscope, changes being evident only on electron microscopy. Indeed, it may even occur without skin changes, and as such we simply call it polymyositis.

But the most elusive feature of the disease is malignancy. It is not an essential feature of the diagnosis nor is it even present in the childhood form of dermatomyositis. Yet, as the patient ages, malignancy in one form or another can be identified in as many as one half these patients. Should it be a solid circumscribed tumor, excision is associated with remission or improvement. We know that an immune state exists, since these patients show positive skin tests specifically to an extract of their tumor. Moreover, circulating antibodies can be demonstrated and the tumor extract will induce blast formation in the patient's lymphocytes. But the relationship of dermatitis, myositis and malignancy remains obscure. Only now has a new clue appeared, namely, the repeated demonstration that virus-like particles are consistently present as inclusions in the endothelial cells of the skin of all these patients. Thus, as in lupus erythematosus and malignancy itself, a viral etiology is being tentatively suggested. Footnoting this is the fact that the blood-borne larvae of trichinosis preferentially lodge in the eyelids as well as in muscle. Thus, we have a small but interesting correlate to suggest a viremic origin for both the heliotrope eyelid and the myasthenia of dermatomyositis. Indeed, the sharply delimited heliotrope we see in our patient's lid could be telling us that the underlying orbicular muscle itself is a primary site of involvement.

Elusive as dermatomyositis is, how do we make a diagnosis? What gives us a degree of diagnostic confidence? First, in the skin there are three pathognomonic signs. The best known is the unique violaceous erythema of the upper eyelids. There is often associated periorbital edema, demonstrated in our patient by the paranasal depression at the site where her glasses rest. The second observation of importance relates to the skin over joints. Edematous erythematous plaques over the large joints and atrophic scaling lesions over the small phalangeal joints are typical of dermatomyositis. The third singular and significant skin change is on the finger tips. Periungual erythema with telangiectasia and hyperkeratotic cuticles greatly strengthen one's clinical assurance in the diagnosis of dermatomyositis.

A biopsy of the skin does not reveal a pathognomonic picture, showing instead a variety of nonspecific inflammatory changes. It is only when the research probe of electron microscopy is added that one finds the new precise evidence of dermatomyositis in the form of virus-like endothelial inclusion particles.

The second diagnostic area of study is the hidden one of the muscle. The secret here is to be aware of the patient's weakness and to recognize it as the specific disease it is. In the early stages it is easy to dismiss it as the asthenia of age, malaise or flu. Listen to the patient, watch her, note the proximal nature of the muscle groups involved, palpate for tender doughy muscles and take biopsy specimens as well as electromyograms. Biopsy will show muscle degeneration, and the myogram deviations will show primary myopathy. Finally, look to the serum for elevation of the muscle enzymes. The best indicator of this is glutamic oxaloacetic acid transaminase (SGOT), although lactic dehydrogenase (LDH) and creatine phosphokinase (CPK) may be monitored as well, especially for therapeutic appraisal.

But the most important diagnostic step of all is the search for malignancy. Every adult patient with dermatomyositis deserves hospitalization with a rigorous, detailed screen for occult malignancy of any type, be it a reticulosis or a malignant melanoma. Inspection and palpation of the skin, the breast, the testis and the prostate is only the starting point. Radiologic spying must include the chest, the G.I. tract, the kidney, the bones and the skull. Endoscopic maneuvers in the bronchi, sigmoid and upper G.I. tract may be appropriate. The otolaryngologist, the gynecologist and the hematologist must join as co-sleuths. Appropriate blood and urinary studies help close the gap but at times the patient may yield her secret only to an exploratory laparotomy.

If the malignancy search-and-destroy mission fails, prednisone is the treatment par excellence. Although seemingly it does not shorten the course of the disease, one to be measured in years, it provides immeasurable help to the patient along the way. Large oral doses are initially required, but these can be slowly tapered at regular two- to four-week intervals as deemed appropriate by review of the clinical and SGOT findings. Triamcinolone and dexamethasone are to be avoided, since they have a record of inducing steroid myopathy. The patient must be observed for the usual side effects of steroids, particularly hypokalemia and its associated weaknes, which can easily pass for the primary disease. Cytotoxic drugs such as cyclophosphamide, methotrexate, and azathioprine may be employed also in the treatment of dermatomyositis, being of special value for those intolerant of steroids. Valuable adjunctive treatments include bed rest, nasogastric feedings, mechanical respiratory aids and physical therapy in the later stages. Ultraviolet light and excessive sun exposure should be avoided because of the possibility of inducing a cutaneous flare.

The prognosis of dermatomyositis is not easily given. Always a serious chronic yet rare disease, it may still undergo spontaneous remission and is generally less threatening to children. In contrast is the inexorably slowly fatal course in the older person, especially one not responding quickly to systemic steroids. It is not a disease known to be transmissible and only sporadic examples of familial incidence are recorded. If death comes, it may result from an underlying malignancy, recognized or unrecognized. It may result from pulmonary disease, with the contributing factors of an intrinsic pulmonary fibrosis, super-infection associated with prolonged steroid therapy or aspiration pneumonia as a consequence of the dysphagia from loss of function of the striate muscle of the upper esophagus. Myocarditis can also be a rare cause of death.

Despite this, we can remind ourselves that disease, about which we read and write in medical texts and journals, is often in its most florid, newsworthy form. There are many milder, less noteworthy versions which quietly come and go. Let us hope that our patient's shadow comes from one of these.

Mills, J. A.: Dermatomyositis. *In* Fitzpatrick, T. B., et al. (Eds.): *Dermatology in General Medicine.* McGraw-Hill Book Co., New York, 1971, pp. 1518-1525.
A distinguished overview.

Degos, R., Civatte, J., Belaich, S., and Delarue, A.: The Prognosis of Adult Dermatomyositis. Trans. St. Johns Hosp. Soc., *57*:98-104, 1971.
Survey of rare association of dermatitis and muscle weakness which may herald malignancy.

Sullivan, D. B., Cassidy, J. T., Petty, R. E., and Burt, A.: Prognosis in Childhood Dermatomyositis. J. Pediat., *80*:555-563, 1972.
Disease not indicative of tumor in children but presents same violaceous heliotrope discoloration of upper eyelid.

Findlay, G. H., Whiting, D. A., and Simson, I. W.: Dermatomyositis in the Transvaal and Its Occurrence in the Bantu. S. Afr. Med. J., *43*:694-697, 1969.
Failure to diagnose can result from failure to palpate girdle muscles.

Wong, K. O.: Dermatomyositis: A Clinical Investigation of Twenty-Three Cases in Hong Kong. Brit. J. Derm., *81*:544-547, 1969.
Nasopharyngeal malignancy most common concomitant finding in Chinese.

Laubenheimer, R.: An Unusual Case of Dermatomyositis. Wis. Med. J., *68*:351-351, 1969.
Associated with metastatic carcinoma of breast discovered 17 years after radical mastectomy.

Rapaport, A. H., and Omenn, G. S.: Dermatomyositis and Malignant Effusions: Rare Manifestations of Carcinoma of the Prostate. J. Urol., *100*:183-187, 1968.
Here, a cutaneomuscular sign of prostatic malignancy.

Beck, P.: Myelomatosis Presenting as Dermatomyositis. Brit. Med. J., *1*:747-748, 1968.
In this instance, the sign of plasmacytoma.

Katz, A., and Digby, J. W.: Malignant Melanoma and Dermatomyositis. Canad. Med. Assoc. J., *93*:1367-1369, 1965.
Dermatomyositis preceded appearance of metastatic malignant melanoma by three months.

Connor, B.: Mycosis Fungoides with Dermatomyositis. Proc. Roy. Soc. Med., *65*:251-252, 1972.
In search for malignancy, don't forget to look at skin.

Gotoff, S. P., Smith, R. D., and Sugar, O.: Dermatomyositis with Cerebral Vasculitis in a Patient with Agammaglobulinemia. Amer. J. Dis. Child., *123*:53-56, 1972.
Dermatomyositis always demands complete systemic workup.

Grünebaum, M., and Salinger, H.: Radiologic Findings in Polymyositis-Dermatomyositis Involving the Pharynx and Upper Oesophagus. Clin. Radiol., *22*:97-100, 1971.
Weakness in deglutition indicates involvement of striate muscle of upper esophagus; distinct from problem in scleroderma, in which abnormality is in smooth muscle of lower esophagus.

Kessler, E., Weinberger, I., and Rosenfeld, J. B.: Myoglobinuric Acute Renal Failure in a Case of Dermatomyositis. Israel J. Med. Sci., *8*:978-983, 1972.
Rare transient acute renal failure due to myoglobin from areas of myositis.

Janis, J. F., and Winkelmann, R. K.: Histopathology of the Skin in Dermatomyositis. A Histopathologic Study of 55 Cases. Arch. Derm., *97*:640-650, 1968.
Usually nonspecific inflammation with mucin deposition or poikilodermatous change of epidermal atrophy, basal cell degeneration, vasodilatation.

Jablonska, S., Jakubowicz, K., Biczysko, W., and Dabrowski, J.: Studies on Ultrastructure of Muscles in Dermatomyositis and Other Collagenoses with Secondary Involvement of the Muscular System. Acta Med. Pol., *12*:187-190, 1971.
Muscle shows degenerative inflammatory change, although at times seen only under electron microscopy.

Landry, M., and Winkelmann, R. K.: Tubular Cytoplasmic Inclusion in Dermatomyositis. Mayo Clin. Proc., *47*:479-492, 1972.
Diagnostic change in endothelial cells found in skin biopsy from each of 10 cases of dermatomyositis.

Brundin, A.: Pulmonary Fibrosis in Scleroderma and Dermatomyositis. Scand. J. Resp. Dis., *51*:160-170, 1970.
Usually need pulmonary function tests to detect pulmonary fibrosis occurring in dermatomyositis.

Jablonska, S.: Diagnostic Criteria of Dermatomyositis. Polish Med. J., *5*:1472-1483, 1966.
Best laboratory correlate of disease; elevated serum glutamic oxaloacetic transaminase.

Alexander, S., and Forman, L.: Dermatomyositis and Carcinoma. A Case Report and Immunological Investigation. Brit. J. Derm., *80*:86-89, 1968.
Three cases with rising titer of complement-fixing antibodies specific for their own malignancy.

Winkelmann, R. K., Jordon, R. E., and de Moragas, J. M.: Immunofluorescent Studies of Dermatomyositis. Dermatologica, *145*:42-47, 1972.
Pattern was nonspecific.

Alexander, S., and Stimmler, L.: Antibodies to Hair Follicles and Striated Muscle in a Case of Juvenile Dermatomyositis. Arch. Dis. Child., *46*:363-365, 1971.
Fluorescent antibodies found around patient's follicles and at A bands of serum-treated striate muscle of rat.

Winkelmann, R. K., Mulder, D. W., Lambert, E. H., Howard, F. M., and Diessner, G. R.: Course of Dermatomyositis-Polymyositis: Comparison of Untreated and Cortisone-Treated Patients. Mayo Clin. Proc., *43*:545-556, 1968.
Systemic steroid in full dosage reduces morbidity and accelerates healing, but remissions occur just as often in untreated patients.

Malaviya, A. N., Many, A., and Schwartz, R. S.: Treatment of Dermatomyositis with Methotrexate. Lancet, *2*:485-488, 1968.
Good response in 4 cases.

Tannenberg, W.: Dermatomyositis. Arch. Derm., *105*:771-772, 1972.
Azathioprine is another excellent immunosuppressant drug for this disease.

Fink, U., and Begemann, H.: Clinical Studies with L-Asparaginase in Dermatomyositis. *In* Rentchnick, P. (Ed.): *Recent Results in Cancer Research. 33*:329-330, Springer-Verlag, New York, 1970.
Rapid clinical improvement in one case.

Swenson, W. M., Witkowski, L. J., and Roskelley, R. C.: Total Colectomy for Dermatomyositis. Amer. J. Surg., *115*:405-407, 1968.
Dramatic help from colectomy to relieve obstipation.

Allan, R. N., Dykes, P. W., Harris, O. D., and Oates, G. D.: Dermatomyositis Associated with Hepatic Secondaries from Carcinoma of the Colon. Gastroenterology, *62*:1227-1231, 1972.
Resolution of dermatomyositis associated with resection of lobe of liver containing residual metastatic lesion.

48

Urticaria Pigmentosa

48

Brownish-red macular and papular lesions have been present on the trunk *and upper arms of this woman for the past ten years. When vigorously rubbed, the lesions rapidly become pruritic, erythematous and swollen. No other abnormalities were disclosed on general medical study.*

Biopsy — toluidine blue stain revealed numerous metachromatic mast cells in dermis.

Urticaria Pigmentosa

These lesions give us a lesson in pharmacology. Each one is a cluster of cells which specifically manufactures and stores large quantities of histamine. Each one is ready to release its granules of histamine when rubbed or traumatized. Each one but scratched can produce for us all the local effects of histamine — itching, erythema and urticaria.

This lesson in pharmacology is not lost on the diagnostician who recognizes urticaria pigmentosa as one of the most distinctive of the dermatologic disorders. It is another disease for which the diagnosis is at one's finger tips. Whether the lesion is a macular stain, a patch of papules or an isolated nodule, the simple scratch-induced histamine release gives a flash diagnosis. Thus, the histamine release sign (Darier) can erase from our differential such entities as fixed drug eruption, nevi, papular urticaria and lichen planus. In the infant, with the associated bullous lesions of fragile skin, it can sort out incontinentia pigmenti and epidermolysis bullosa. Furthermore, it is this histamine sign which clinically identifies such atypical examples as yellow lesions in infancy (xanthelasmoidea) and nonpigmented lesions of the soles. It is a sign of proved clinical worth and one that fails us only when a lesion has been repeatedly traumatized to the point of histamine depletion. In such an instance, the local area may remain indifferent to scratching for as long as two weeks while the granules are being reconstituted and histamine stores are being replenished by the action of histidine decarboxylase on histidine.

The lesson in pharmacology continues as we find in many of these patients' complaints an ever-widening spectrum of histamine effects.

304

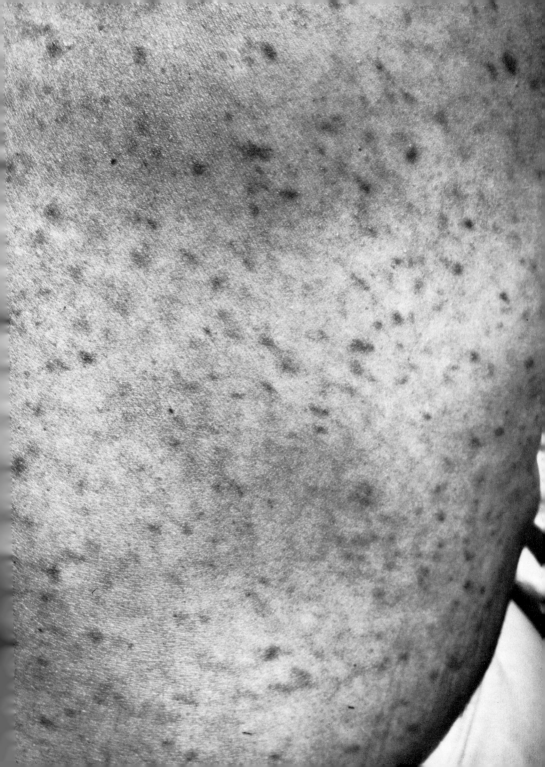

Many of these are of a vascular nature such as flushing, headache, tachycardia, vertigo, faintness, dyspnea and even shock. The flushing is especially noteworthy, appearing not only as a result of stroking a lesion but also in response to psychic stress. It can also be triggered by temperature elevation, spicy foods, alcohol, exercise or histamine liberator drugs such as codeine or aspirin. This histamine flush is to be distinguished from the serotonin flush of carcinoid. Despite the fact that both may be triggered by the same factors and both involve the flush area of the upper body, carcinoid flushing has a more cyanotic hue. Furthermore, it can be specifically elicited by epinephrine and is associated with elevated 5-hydroxyindoleacetic acid levels in the urine.

The histaminemia of urticaria pigmentosa may further be reflected by the gastric distress of hyperchlorhydria. Many patients have only an ill-defined abdominal discomfort, but others show the nausea, vomiting and epigastric pain of the histamine-induced peptic ulcer which can develop. The effects of histamine on the smooth muscle and mucosal glands of the respiratory tract may also be apparent in the rhinorrhea, dyspnea, wheezing and tightness in the chest experienced by some patients.

Not only do these aggregates of mast cells synthesize and release histamine, but they also produce and discharge in their granules another powerful pharmacologic agent, the anticoagulant heparin. It is this acidic heparin which is responsible for the unique metachromatic staining of the mast cell granules routinely seen with basic dyes such as toluidine blue. Interestingly, the histamine component is not visualized unless fluorescent staining is employed. In the case of heparin, the clinical evidence of release is not so apparent as with histamine. Bleeding and purpuric or hemorrhagic changes are seen only occasionally, and it is the unusual patient in whom the blood coagulogram reveals heparinemia. Nevertheless, degranulation of the mast cell is regularly associated with heparin release. Thus, local control of flow within the microvasculature is achieved in large degree through the mast cell.

Even on gross examination, we sense in this patient a vascular relationship for the mast cell. The lesions appear in a shadowy reticulate patterning reminiscent of livedo reticularis. As we look more closely some of the macules show telangiectatic vessels, the hallmark of a special adult form of urticaria pigmentosa, known to the cognoscenti as telangiectasia macularis eruptiva perstans. The vascular relationship is further strengthened as we look under the microscope and find that mast cells virtually ensheath all the fine vessels. Incidentally, a biopsy provides the ultimate diagnostic answer, since the hyperplasia of mast cells is absolutely pathognomonic of mastocytosis. It shows us further that the pigmentation is melanin in nature, presumably a postinflammatory response of the melanocytes to the repeated urtication.

As knowledge has grown, the name urticaria pigmentosa has been replaced by mastocytosis to indicate the systemic nature of this disease. Despite the fact that the skin alone gives us a full awareness of the pharmacologic nature of this disease, these mysterious unexplained overgrowths of mastocytes may actually occur in the fine arborescent vascular tree of any organ. Our sensing system is primitive, often limited to a search for gross infiltrates. These may be detected as lymphadenopathy, hepatomegaly, splenomegaly or radiologic deficits in the bone or gastrointestinal tract. Thus, bone pain in these patients merits radiologic study, but it is obvious that the vast majority of lesions must be too small to detect. In the laboratory, we can monitor the extent of involvement by measuring the degree of histaminuria which results from a codeine challenge. Urinary acid mucopolysaccharides and serum histamine are similar parameters, suitable as monitors. Examination of the blood and bone marrow for mast cells, a coagulogram for heparin, and a Schilling test for gastrointestinal malabsorption may be valuable as well. Otherwise, we remain content with our diagnosis of cutaneous mastocytosis recognizing that the process may be or may become systemic. We should also realize that, although our patient's process has been stationary for years, it could become progressive. In fact, on rare occasions these neoplastic mast cells become malignant, producing a mast cell leukemia.

Since this disease may be viewed as one of hyperplasia of histaminocytes, the treatment par excellence would appear to be antihistaminics. Yet these compounds have all proved to be disappointing. Acting competitively for the histamine receptor sites, they apparently are no match for the massive quantities of histamine which pour out of these mast cell granules. No topical or systemic drug is known which has a consistently beneficial effect on mastocytosis. Nevertheless, we favor the use of hydroxyzine because of its ameliorative effect on dermographism, a commonly associated finding. In infants with diffuse cutaneous mastocytosis with bullae, systemic steroids may also be indicated for a short term.

For the average patient, more important than medication are the explanatory caveats against the drugs which release histamine. These patients should not take aspirin, nor should they be given codeine or polymyxins. Anesthetics and cytotoxic drugs would have to be given with caution. Even the topical use of a salicylic acid ester in a sun screen or the penetrant vehicle dimethyl sulfoxide itself can provoke histamine release. Their enormously hyperplastic system of mast cells can send these patients into histamine shock if it is activated physically, chemically or immunologically. The hot bath, the vigorous rubdown, overexertion, alcohol, spicy foods can each evoke the torments of generalized itching as well as hives. The trauma of surgery poses a special threat, and most alarming of all are allergic reactors of the immediate type. Should this patient become sensitized, the antigen from a simple beesting could combine with her IgE-coated mast cells to release a potentially lethal load of histamine.

It is evident that our patient provides us with a remarkable vignette of histamine disease.

Sagher, F., and Even-Paz, Z.: *Mastocytosis and the Mast Cell.* Year Book Medical Publishers, Inc., Chicago, 1967, 427 pp.
A stunning encyclopedic account of urticaria pigmentosa: the story of a cell and its pharmacodynamics in disease.

Selye, H.: *The Mast Cells.* Butterworth & Co., Ltd., London, 1965, 498 pp.
A fabulous information retrieval system for 2500 articles on these cells and how they elaborate histamine and heparin.

Schacter, M.: Histamine and Antihistamines. *In* International Encyclopedia of Pharmacology and Therapeutics, Section 74, Pergamon Press, New York, 1973, pp. 1-188.
Background on histamine and how it is released.

Orkin, M., Good, R. A., Clawson, C. C., Fisher, I., and Windhorst, D.: Bullous Mastocytosis. Arch. Derm., *101*:547-564, 1970.
Urticaria pigmentosa: pigmented lesions which urticate on stroking; often a bullous disease in infants.

Burgoon, C. F., Graham, J. H., and McCaffree, D. L.: Mast Cell Disease. A Cutaneous Variant with Multisystem Involvement. Arch. Derm., *98*:590-605, 1968.
Diffuse skin involvement and enlarged liver, spleen and lymph nodes indicative of widespread mast cell infiltrates. Guarded prognosis.

Bakos, L., Storck, R., and Netto, E. S.: Congenital Macular Urticaria Pigmentosa Complicated by Massive Nodular Mastocytosis with Systemic Involvement. Brit. J. Derm., *87*:635-641, 1972.
One man's 37 years of mastocytosis.

Selmanowitz, V. J., Orentreich, N., Tiangco, C. C., and Demis, D. J.: Uniovular Twins Discordant for Cutaneous Mastocytosis. Arch. Derm., *102*:34-41, 1970.
Forty intrafamilial patients in literature.

Barer, M., Peterson, L. F. A., Dahlin, D. C., Winkelmann, R. K., and Stewart, J. R.: Mastocytosis with Osseus Lesions Resembling Metastatic Malignant Lesions in Bone. J. Bone Joint Surg., *50A*:142-152, 1968.
Usually epiphyseal location, sclerotic halo around discrete lytic focus.

McKee, W. D., Cochrane, C. G., and Farr, R. S.: A Clinical Study of an Unusual Case of Asthma Associated with Urticaria Pigmentosa. J. Allerg., *37*:38-47, 1966.
Asthmatic attacks associated with episodic flushing and bulla formation.

Broitman, S. A., McCray, R. S., May, J. C., Deren, J. J., Ackroyd, F., Gottlieb, L. S., McDermott, W., and Zamcheck, N.: Mastocytosis and Intestinal Malabsorption. Amer. J. Med., *48*:382-389, 1970.
Associated with gluten sensitivity and mast cell infiltrate in small bowel.

Fromer, J. J., Jaffe, N., and Paed, D.: Urticaria Pigmentosa and Acute Lymphoblastic Leukemia. Arch. Derm., *107*:283-284, 1973.
Urticaria pigmentosa may rarely lead to mast cell, myeloid, lymphoblastic or monocytic leukemia.

Diamond, J. H., and Gross, L.: Urticaria Pigmentosa Complicated by Polycythemia Vera. Report of a Case. Blood, *27*:253-257, 1966.
Mastocytosis resembles myeloproliferative disorders.

Cohen, A. H., and Vogel, J. M.: Systemic Mastocytosis and Multiple Carcinomas. Mt. Sinai J. Med., *39*:365-370, 1972.
Urticaria pigmentosa, a possible correlate of carcinoma of colon, liver and nasopharynx.

Möller, H.: Pigmentary Disturbances Due to Drugs. Acta Dermatovener., *46*:423-431, 1966.
Detailed tabulation of pigmented macules which do not urticate on stroking.

Tennenbaum, J. L., and Lowney, E.: Localized Heat and Cold Urticaria Rare Phenomena Occurring in the Same Individual. J. Allerg. Clin. Immunol., *51*:57-59, 1973.
Details on wheals which do not pigment.

Kobayasi, T., and Asboe-Hansen, G.: Degranulation and Regranulation of Human Mast Cells. An Electron Microscopic Study of the Whealing Reaction in Urticaria Pigmentosa. Acta Dermatovener., *49*:369-381, 1969.
Mast cells in skin lose their granules within one minute of stroking area.

Kobayasi, T., and Asboe-Hansen, G.: Remarkable Cytoplasmic Structures in Mast Cells of Urticaria Pigmentosa. Acta Dermatovener., *50*:3-8, 1970.
Enormous overgrowth of endoplasmic reticulum then occurs as cell is reforming granules.

Hakanson, R., Owman, C., Sjöberg, N.-O., and Sporrong, B.: Direct Histochemical Demonstration of Histamine in Cutaneous Mast Cells: Urticaria Pigmentosa and Keloids. Experientia, *25*:854-855, 1969.
Staining with *o*-phthalaldehyde reveals histamine in mast cell.

Greaves, M. W., and Sondergaard, J.: Urticaria Pigmentosa and Factitious Urticaria Direct Evidence for Release of Histamine and Other Smooth Muscle-contracting Agents in Dermographic Skin. Arch. Derm., *101*:418-425, 1970.
In urticaria pigmentosa, skin perfusate contained histamine.

Keller, R. T., and Roth, H. P.: Hyperchlorhydria and Hyperhistaminemia in a Patient with Systemic Mastocytosis. New Eng. J. Med., *283*:1449-1450, 1970.
Histamine level elevated in plasma and urine.

Lagunoff, D.: The Mechanism of Histamine Release from Mast Cells. Biochem. Pharm., *21*:1889-1896, 1972.
Histamine can also be released without loss of granules or heparin.

Ishizaka, K., and Ishizaka, T.: Mechanisms of Reaginic Hypersensitivity: A Review. Clin. Allerg., *1*:9-24, 1971.

Histamine released by allergen making contact with immunoglobulin E-coated mast cell.

Newcomb, R. W., and Nelson, H.: Dermographia Mediated by Immunoglobulin E. Amer. J. Med., *54*:174-180, 1973.
IgE fixes to mast cells in skin sensitizing them to release histamine following physical trauma.

Perelmutter, L., Liakopoulu, A., Bernstein, I. L., and Phills, J. A.: Some Comments on the Rat Mast Cell Test. J. Allerg. Clin. Immunol., *51*:60-61, 1973.
Exposure of rat mast cells to immunoglobulin E in patient's serum and then to allergen induces specific degranulation.

Csaba, G., and Richter, T.: Attempt to Produce Animals Devoid of Mast Cells. Acta Biol. Acad. Sci. Hung., *22*:467-470, 1971.
Unsuccessful.

Vaidya, A. B., Wustrack, K. O., and Levine, R. J.: Failure of Epinephrine to Provoke Flushing in Patients with Systemic Mastocytosis. Ann. Intern. Med., *74*:711-713, 1971.
By contrast, epinephrine flushing is a provocative diagnostic test for carcinoid syndrome.

Orkin, M.: Mastocytosis in Animals. Arch. Derm., *96*:381-385, 1967.
Most common in dog.

Macdonald, A.: Cutaneous Mastocytosis: An Unusual Radiation Dermatitis. Proc. Roy. Soc. Med., *64*:29-30, 1971.
Urticaria pigmentosa locally induced by 2400 R given postoperatively.

Sahihi, T., and Esterly, N. B.: Atypical Diffuse Cutaneous Mastocytosis. Amer. J. Dis. Child., *124*:133-135, 1972.
Urticaria pigmentosa patients should avoid aspirin, codeine and polymyxin B, as well as brisk toweling.

49

Seborrheic Dermatitis

49

Following a cerebrovascular accident three years ago, this 57-year-old man developed a **pruritic scaling, erythematous eruption of the scalp and eyebrows as well as of the paranasal and beard areas.**

Seborrheic Dermatitis

Here the diagnosis does not rest on clinical appearance of the lesion. The scales and erythema are so commonplace and nondescript as to occur in a myriad of dermatitides. Nor does the diagnosis rest on what can be found by looking at the lesion with a magnification of a hundred-, a thousand-, or even a hundred-thousandfold. The histologic picture remains a monotonously banal, nonspecific, inflammatory one. Neither does the diagnosis rest on laboratory studies. There is no pathogenic organism to be found, although the skin swarms with saprophytes enjoying the environmental delights of abundant scales, sebum and moisture. No, the diagnosis of seborrheic dermatitis is made by standing back and perceiving an absolutely distinctive symmetrical distribution pattern. It is the dermatitis of the seborrheic areas.

No more characteristic site exists than the scalp. Here, it is everyman's disease—dandruff. It may remain rather hidden under the hairs localized to this area, doing little more than causing itch, but always producing its telltale flakes of excess stratum corneum. Punctate excoriations may testify to the pruritus and secondary bacterial infection as well as eczematization with oozing, and crusting may ensue. One must be alert to the fact that a contact sensitivity reaction to hair tonic or even a topical medicament may simulate seborrheic dermatitis. In these instances patch-testing is invaluable. Another disease commonly entering the differential list is psoriasis. Should the plaques be discrete and thick, one has little difficulty in recognizing them as psoriasis, despite the patient's complaint of dandruff. However, in some the picture is a blend, and the clinician grudgingly calls it "seborrhiasis."

In our patient the condition has extended to the face, with the characteristic involvement of the eyebrows and paranasal area. Moreover, his

312

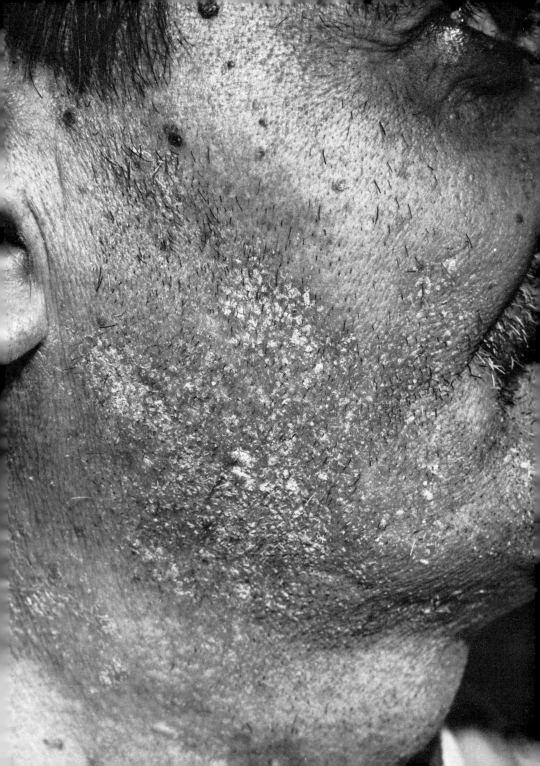

bearded area is a major locus for erythema and scaling. Were it to extend further, we would anticipate the same type of inflammatory change across the nose and cheeks, as well as on the eyelids and in the ear canal. A butterfly facial distribution always suggests the possibility of lupus erythematosus, but appropriate laboratory maneuvers can usually distinguish the common benign seborrheic dermatitis from the rare, serious lupus. At times, photosensitivity must be ruled out also.

On the chest, the imprint of seborrheic dermatitis is a presternal plaque which may be virtually reproduced on the back in the interscapular area. The now obvious predilection of seborrheic dermatitis for the high-density pilosebaceous sites is highlighted by its appearance in the pubic region. Finally, it is a disease of skin in apposition: the axillae, the crural folds, the gluteal cleft, the submammary region and the umbilicus. In these intertriginous sites the appearance is more inflammatory, and often we can scarcely distinguish it from intertrigo or psoriasis, were it not for the associated findings. At times, tinea and candidiasis must be ruled out by KOH examination. Often one area alone may be the cause of complaint, but a look for bilateral symmetry as well as muted evidence of seborrheic scaling in other typical sites may result in an assured diagnosis of seborrheic dermatitis. Likewise, in evaluating generalized exfoliative dermatitis it may be possible to distinguish seborrheic dermatitis as the antecedent by a good history of the original sites of involvement.

Although the cause of seborrheic dermatitis remains unknown, there are several clues. The most remarkable is the relationship with sebum. Not only does the distribution templet reveal that this is a disease of the areas rich in sebaceous glands, but the incidence of the disease correlates with periods of seborrhea or increased excretion of sebum. Thus, the seborrheic cradle cap of infancy is self-limited, receding as the early wave of maternal hormonal stimulant to the sebaceous gland fades. Seborrheic dermatitis does not reappear until the androgens of adolescence activate their seborrhea. But most striking of all is the joint appearance of seborrhea and seborrheic dermatitis which develops with parkinsonism or with brain disease, as in our patient. In these instances the pituitary is exerting a direct stimulating effect on the sebaceous gland, apparently via the melanocyte-stimulating hormone or a related peptide. But we do not know how, or even if, the seborrhea is inducing the seborrheic dermatitis.

Many investigators support the view that the sebum favors the growth of surface microflora that, in turn, liberate irritating free fatty acids which induce a low-grade epidermal inflammatory response. These are not the flora susceptible to systemic antibiotics but rather the saprophytic staphylococci and such yeasts as the often implicated *Pityrosporon ovale*. Certainly individuals with seborrheic dermatitis do seem predisposed to the bouillabaisse of opportunistic organisms which arise in the moist intertriginous zones. In this respect they seem to lack an essential means of defense. Possibly drugs such as gold or pyridoxine antagonists that can induce seborrheic dermatitis do so by interfering with host resistance. Be that as it may, the most striking piece of evidence to support this view that seborrheic dermatitis results fundamentally from a defect in defense against surface flora comes from a recent discovery. It has been found that severe generalized seborrheic dermatitis in infants (Leiner's disease) is associated with a defect in immune complement. Temporary correction of this complement defect by plasma transfusions is associated with remission in the seborrheic dermatitis. In this we may see a clue as to the fundamental nature of the seborrheic diathesis which underlies this chronic relapsing disease.

Despite the central role of sebum in the pathogenesis of this seborrheic dermatitis, our means for reducing sebum flow are limited. The gland remains independent of peripheral neural control, not yielding to adrenergic blockage, anticholinergics or even sympathectomy. L-dopa is only occasionally helpful in suppressing the seborrhea of parkinsonism and is useless in normals. The sebocyte, hastening only to the sound of androgens and MSH, transforms itself from a basal cell deep within the gland to a droplet of oil on the surface in a mere eight days. Like the keratinocyte it remains independent, autonomous and indifferent to our topicals.

Our best therapeutic maneuver is to wash away the oil and thereby protect the patient. Frequent shampooing and washing is the first law of therapy for seborrheic dermatitis. Like dental hygiene it is an injunction that must last, not for a week or two, but forever. When hospitalized, patients with the seborrheic diathesis often experience flare early in their stay, because of the difficulty of washing carefully and regularly. Likewise, we have seen that the failure to wash one side of the face can induce the anomaly of a unilateral seborrheic dermatitis. Much of the effectiveness of the medicated shampoo is due to the surfactant rather than the medicament. What we cannot inhibit, we must wash away!

Rest is a second simple but essential element of therapy. A nap a day can keep the scurf away is more than a jingle. Many individuals with seborrheic dermatitis are driving, competitive and fatigued. In the medical field, obstetricians with their endless irregular hours seem especially prone. All need rest, recreation and reassurance. A vacation is wonderful medicine for them. Sunlight is an adjunctive of merit, as are all the rules of hygiene. A balanced diet, with weight reduction for those with seborrheic intertrigo of pendulous folds, should be encouraged. For a few, vitamin B supplementation may be beneficial. Many deserve general medical review with special attention to uncovering drug sensitivity, diabetes mellitus or any factor which could lower general resistance.

In the pharmacopeia we find a mammoth repertoire for seborrheic dermatitis, and over-the-counter sales are in the hundreds of millions of dollars. Yet the "big five" remain: corticosteroids, antibiotics, tar, sulfur and salicylic acid. Each has a special niche. The corticosteroids allay the secondary inflammatory response and are used in vehicles to match local requirements. These may range from an aerosol spray for the scalp to a propylene glycol solution for the groin. On the face, they are to be applied sparingly, in low-dose nonfluorinated form, for short periods to minimize the chances of inducing an acneiform eruption, rosacea or perioral dermatitis. Invariably they are superior when applied in conjunction with antibiotics to suppress the invariant proliferation of bacteria and yeasts. Here, Vioform, nystatin, gramicidin and amphotericin B are incorporated with success. Tar has an anti-eczematous effect, and sulfur among other roles must surely reduce the microflora. Salicylic acid aids in debriding the keratin scaling which is sequential to the inflammatory insult. These agents may be compounded in a variety of vehicles, usually in concentrations of a few per cent. For the scalp, selenium sulfide shampoo is especially valuable. In the intertriginous areas, Castellani paint remains a sovereign remedy to suppress secondary microfloral overgrowth. Only a few patients with seborrheic dermatitis require systemic corticosteroids and antibacterial agents.

Like dry skin and warts, seborrheic dermatitis remains a common annoyance for man. It can follow him literally from the cradle to the casket. We should know more about it.

Parrish, J. A., and Arndt, K. A.: Seborrheic Dermatitis of the Beard. Brit. J. Derm., *87:*241-244, 1972.
Critical introduction to a disease that has eluded investigators better than they have eluded it.

Ackerman, A. B.: A Clinical Concept of Seborrheic Dermatitis. Med. Times N. Y., *95*:16-28, 1967.
The distribution is the diagnosis: scalp, central face, presternal, interscapular, intertriginous.

Tager, A., Berlin, C., and Schen, R. J.: Seborrheic Dermatitis in Acute Cardiac Disease. Brit. J. Derm., *76*:367-369, 1964.
Often flares in hospitalized patients.

Alexander, S.: Loss of Hair and Dandruff. Brit. J. Derm., *79*:549-552, 1967.
No clear relationship.

Bettley, F. R., and Marten, R. H.: Unilateral Seborrheic Dermatitis Following a Nerve Lesion. Arch. Derm., *73*:110-115, 1956.
Possibly due to failure to wash affected side.

Pinkus, H., and Mehregan, A. H.: The Primary Histologic Lesion of Seborrheic Dermatitis and Psoriasis. J. Invest. Derm., *46*:109-116, 1966.
Stresses passage of leukocytes into epidermis.

Beare, J. M., Cheeseman, E. A., and Mackenzie, D. W. R.: The Association Between Candida Albicans and Lesions of Seborrhoeic Eczema. Brit. J. Derm., *80*:675-681, 1968.
Infantile seborrheic dermatitis: special self-limiting form commonly colonized by *C. albicans* and bacteria.

Roia, F. C., and Vanderwyk, R. W.: Resident Microbial Flora of the Human Scalp and Its Relationship to Dandruff. J. Soc. Cos. Chem., *20*:113-134, 1969.
Thirty yeasts, 143 molds, 44 bacteria and 8 actinomycetes found growing in dandruff of 28 adult patients.

Gosse, R. M., and Vanderwyk, R. W.: The Relationship of a Nystatin-Resistant Strain of Pityrosporon Ovale to Dandruff. J. Soc. Cos. Chem., *20*:603-613, 1969.
Neomycin-nystatin induced 63 per cent reduction in dandruff; subsequent application of resistant *P. ovale* followed by 88 per cent increase.

Norn, M. S.: Demodex Folliculorum Incidence and Possible Pathogenic Role in the Human Eyelid. Acta Ophthal., *Suppl. 108*:1-85, 1970.
No role discerned in seborrheic blepharitis for this mite which lives in the hair follicles of 14 per cent of teen-agers and 100 per cent of the elderly. Fascinating study.

Ebling, F. J.: Steroid Hormones and Sebaceous Secretion. *In* Briggs, M. H., (Ed.): *Advances in Steroid Biochemistry and Pharmacology,* Vol. 2. Academic Press, New York, 1970, pp. 1-39.
Androgens increase; estrogens decrease.

Kirschner, M. A., and Schneider, G.: Suppression of the Pituitary-Leydig Cell Axis and Sebum Production in Normal Men by Medroxyprogesterone Acetate (Provera). Acta Endocr., *69*:385-393, 1972.
This progesterone agent suppresses androgen production and thereby the secretion of sebum.

Burton, J. L., Shuster, S., Cartlidge, M., Libman, L. J., and Martell, U.: Lactation, Sebum Excretion and Melanocyte-Stimulating Hormone. Nature, *243*:349-350, 1973.
Seborrhea of parkinsonism due to excessive production of pituitary hormone, MSH.

Burton, J. L., Libman, L. J., Cunliffe, W. J., Wilkinson, R., Hall, R., and Shuster, S.: Sebum Excretion in Acromegaly. Brit. Med. J., *1*:406-408, 1972.
Greatly increased.

Bullough, W. S., and Laurence, E. B.: Chalone Control of Mitotic Activity in Sebaceous Glands. Cell Tissue Kinet., *3*:291-300, 1970.
Demonstration of specific chalone inhibition of sebaceous gland mitotic activity.

Archibald, A., and Shuster, S.: A Non-Endocrine Control of Sebum Secretion. Arch. Derm. Forsch., *246*:175-180, 1973.
Ether-ethanol removal of sebum from rat stimulates gland to greater activity.

Sarkany, I., and Gaylarde, P.: A Method for Demonstration of the Distribution of Sebum on the Skin Surface. Brit. J. Derm., *80*:744-746, 1968.
Plaster of Paris replica of skin surface stained with osmium tetroxide.

Pochi, P. E., Downing, D. T., and Strauss, J. S.: Sebaceous Gland Response in Man to Prolonged Total Caloric Deprivation. J. Invest. Derm., *55*:303-309, 1970.
Fast for a month and watch your sebum secretion decrease 40 per cent.

Anderson, A. S., and Fulton, J. E.: Sebum: Analysis by Infrared Spectroscopy. J. Invest. Derm., *60*:115-120, 1973.
Crystal of thallium bromide-iodide enables determination of free fatty acids and fatty esters, as well as amount of sebum.

Karunakaran, M. E., Pochi, P. E., Strauss, J. S., Valerio, E. A., Wotiz, H. H., and Clark, S. J.: Androgens in Skin Surface Lipids. J. Invest. Derm., *60*:121-125, 1973.
Probable source: apocrine sweat.

Troller, J. A.: Model System for the Investigation of Dandruff. J. Soc. Cos. Chem., *22*:187-198, 1971.
Views seborrheic dermatitis as the result of release of free fatty acid in sebum as result of lipolysis by microflora, in particular *Pityrosporon ovale.*

Freinkel, R. K., and Shen, Y.: The Origin of Free Fatty Acids in Sebum II Assay of the Lipases of the Cutaneous Bacteria and Effects of pH. J. Invest. Derm., *53*:422-427, 1969.
Low pH reduces amount of irritant fatty acids formed on skin surface by lipases of *C. acnes* **and** *S. albus.*

Parish, L. C.: L-Dopa for Seborrheic Dermatitis. New Eng. J. Med., *283*:879-879, 1970.
Only 3 of 18 patients with parkinsonism showed marked improvement with reduction in sebum production.

Kohn, S. R., Pochi, P. E., Strauss, J. S., Sax, D. S., Feldman, R. G., and Timberlake, W. H.: Sebaceous Gland Secretion in Parkinson's Disease During L-Dopa Treatment. J. Invest. Derm., *60*:134-136, 1973.
Decreased.

Plewig, G., and Kligman, A. M.: The Effect of Selenium Sulfide on Epidermal Turnover of Normal and Dandruff Scalps. J. Soc. Cos. Chem., *20*:767-775, 1969.
Objective count of epidermal cells being shed by stratum corneum (corneocytes) reveals that selenium acts by suppressing excessive epidermopoiesis associated with dandruff.

Harris, J. J.: A National Double-Blind Clinical Trial of a New Corticosteroid Lotion: A 12-Investigator Cooperative Analysis. Curr. Ther. Res., *14*:638-646, 1972.
Analyzed crusting, scaling, vesiculation, exudation, fissuring, maceration, pruritus, burning, pain and secondary bacterial infection to show that Valisone lotion is superior to placebo half the time.

Goette, D. K.: Dermatrophy from Long-Term Occlusive Topical Corticosteroid Therapy. Southern Med. J., *66*:542-546, 1973.

A hazard of long-term high-potency steroid therapy for seborrheic dermatitis of intertriginous areas.

Benaim-Pinto, C.: Topical Glycerin in Seborrheic Dermatitis. Lancet, *2*:1037-1038, 1972.
Use locally every fourth day.

Chesterman, K. W.: An Evaluation of O-T-C Dandruff and Seborrhea Products. J. Amer. Pharm. Assoc., *11*:578-581, 1972.
Stresses value of surfactants, antiseptics and keratolytics to remove the scales and their microflora.

Jacobs, J. C., and Miller, M. E.: Fatal Familial Leiner's Disease: A Deficiency of the Opsonic Activity of Serum Complement. Pediatrics, *49*:225-232, 1972.
Fresh plasma transfusions twice a month dramatically helpful in this exfoliative form of seborrheic dermatitis.

Readett, M.: Seborrhoeic Dermatitis. Practitioner, *196*:627-633, 1966.
Rx: topical antibiotic-steroid creams, rest, exercise and balanced diet.

Church, R.: Methyldopa Causing a Seborrheic Dermatitis-like Eruption. Brit. J. Derm., *89:Suppl. 9*:10-10, 1973.
Eleven of 13 patients cleared within two weeks of elimination of this anti-hypertensive.

50

Tattoo

A tattoo is not only a work of art but an experiment of man. It serves not only as an indelible identification mark but as a lifelong skin test. Not only a source of pride, it can be a source of transmissible disease. We can learn much from the study of tattoos.

Tattooing is a very ancient art, as its Polynesian name implies. Although it has always been a decorative act, it has had varying degrees of religious, in-group and psychiatric significance. Its attraction for man has never disappeared; only the trends vary. At times the tattoo has enjoyed the favor of the hierarchy, the nobility and the naval coterie. It has equally been the mark of the laity, the slave and the army reject. In this regard, just a century ago the English army tattooed "B.C." on its undesirables to indicate their bad character. At times the mania for tattoos runs high, 65 per cent of our navy men being tattooed in World War II, with over 500 a day standing in line to get into the Honolulu tattoo parlors. Now there is only a trickle of customers still asking for permanent hearts and flowers, eagles and panthers, or ships and anchors. For some the urge to be tattooed seems akin to the wish to adorn oneself, the desire to improve one's image. For others it is the search for peer approval or the status of personal souvenirs of the world's ports. It is sometimes the sign of immaturity, a rebellious nature, or a chance encounter after an evening "on the town." And in a few it is evidence of exhibitionism or a serious personality disorder.

The art of the tattoo is the introduction of colored metallic salts into the upper dermis by means of a high-speed vibrating needle. The professional skillfully patterns the powders into a pleasing design. His palette includes the white of titanium, the blue of cobalt, the red of mercury and the brown of iron. He may also introduce the yellow of cadmium, the green of chromium or the violet of manganese. Black is often simply

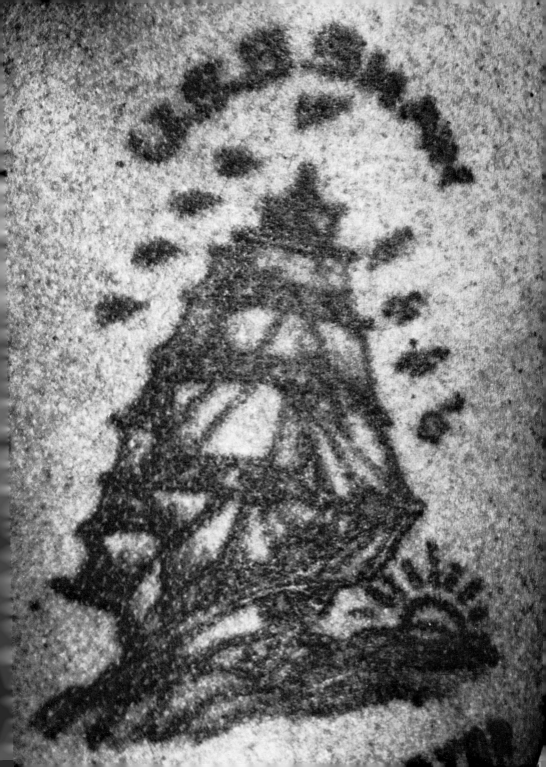

carbon itself. Any color thus can be reproduced by these inert, nonmetabolizable particles. Phagocytized by the macrophage they remain localized to the precise site of introduction within the skin. Thus, our patient's tattoo shows but little blurring of the rigging of sails that were set over a quarter of a century ago.

At times the tattooist's needle may carry more than the pigment, the patron receiving a lagniappe in the form of an infectious disease. This may range from a trivial pyoderma within a few days to a frightening leprosy, not evident until decades later. Tetanus and tuberculosis also are known to have been transmitted by the tattoo needle. In the viral group, infectious hepatitis is a special hazard as well as vaccinia and zoster. Even the chancre of syphilis can appear on the site of a fresh tattoo, though presumably not in one that is red with spirochetocidal mercury!

The tattoo is an experiment of man as well, for those who would study it. One of the most interesting observations is the swelling induced by sunlight in yellow tattoo sites such as in the Swedish flag. This is a phototoxic urticarial response induced by the irradiated cadmium sulfide. This same cadmium sulfide is often admixed with mercury sulfide, so that red areas may show a similar photosensitivity. Tattoos may also signal latent disease. In some the first evidence of psoriasis, lichen planus or sarcoidosis may come as a pathognomonic lesion within the traumatized site of the tattoo. In a few, the tattoo may trigger a local keloid, morphea or discoid lupus erythematosus. This latter may reflect the photosensitizing nature of certain of the tattoo pigments. Tumors can be another result of this experiment of man. Much more will have to be known before one can decide whether this is due to oncogenic metallic salts or to oncogenic viruses transmitted in this experimental way. Nevertheless, we know that Bowen's disease, squamous cell epitheliomas, keratoacanthomas, sarcomas and even malignant melanomas may rarely and strangely arise in tattooed sites.

Not only is the tattoo an experiment of man which gives us new clues to the nature of disease, but it is at once a permanent challenge and skin test for the immune sensitivity state. Of all the elements used, mercury seems to be the one with the highest capacity to induce sensitivity of both the immediate urticarial and delayed contact types. Once the hypersensitivity arises, the red areas selectively urticate on striking, or spontaneously develop an inflammatory eczematous delayed type reaction. Injury to the tattoo with release of the mercury into the blood stream can induce generalized eczematous reactions, a particularly vivid experience for those who have tried to remove such a sensitized area by dermabrasion. Cobalt is another element which can produce a similar hypersensitivity, at times manifesting itself also as a uveitis, with improvement in the latter when the cutaneous cobalt depot is excised. Chromium undoubtedly acts in the same antigenic way, remaining quiescent for years until the immune change occurs and the body finds the chromium to be an alien substance which it must deport.

But the most intriguing area of the tattoo as a skin test is in the field of sarcoidosis. We know that tattoos may develop local sarcoidal granulomas as seen histologically, and we know that the metallic salts of zirconium as well as of beryllium can induce late delayed hypersensitivity reactions in the form of sarcoid granulomas. It is evident that sarcoidal reactions in tattoos, if not due to leprosy, may well reflect such a specific acquired hypersensitivity to one of the elements within. Additional skin tests undertaken with an appropriate series of metallic antigens and examined histologically at six weeks, as with the Kveim test, must surely reveal the precise cause of such tattoo granulomas.

What can we do for the patient with the tattoo that bars him from genteel employment or from the affection of a Betty who might see his undying tattooed love for Jane? If the tattoo can be excised, this may be the best approach. Shaving the tattoo and grafting is an alternate plastic surgical approach for the life-size tattoo. Superficial dermabrasion has been commonly employed by dermatologists. This leads to postoperative extrusion of pigment and virtual obliteration of the details if not the design itself. This can be repeated months later with additional therapeutic gain. An alternate approach recommended by some workers is re-tattooing the tattoo with a caustic such as tannic acid. This also results in a sloughing out of much of the undesired pigment.

However, the simplest method of all is one time-honored home remedy, recently elevated to professional respectability. This consists of the inunction of wet table salt into the tattoo site until gross hemorrhage is evident. At this point the epidermis is gone and the salt is impregnated into the dermis. No further treatment is needed. Over the next week or two a crust forms which contains much of the tattoo pigment. This separates to leave a pink nonscarred skin with a much faded tattoo. An additional one or two salabrasions may be done at six-week intervals with complete clearing. In this, as in all abrasive or shaving techniques, results are much better with the professional tattoo than with the amateur or self-tattoo, in which the pigment is placed very deep.

With this tattoo we end our clinical odyssey around the world of dermatology, and reluctantly bid you adieu.

Roenigk, H. H.: Tattooing—History, Technics, Complications, Removal. Cleveland Clin. Quart., *38*:179-186, 1971.
Transmission and induction of disease by an art form 6000 years old.

Beerman, H., and Lane, R. A. G.: "Tattoo." A Survey of Some of the Literature Concerning the Medical Complications of Tattooing. Amer. J. Med. Sci.,*227*:444-465, 1954.
Monographic review of how body sequesters foreign nonmetabolizable metallic pigments in macrophages for life.

Gittleson, N. L., Wallen, G. D. P., and Dawson-Butterworth, K.: The Tattooed Psychiatric Patient. Brit. J. Psych.,*115*:1249-1253, 1969.
Rare in females; associated in males with personality disorder, especially if tattooed on more than one occasion.

Hamburger, E., and Lacovara, D. J.: A Study of Tattoos in Inmates at a Federal Correctional Institution. Its Physical and Psychological Implications. Milit. Med.,*128*:1205-1211, 1963.
Of 500 consecutive admissions, 65 per cent had tattoos; rare in blacks.

Thomson, H. G., and Wright, A. M.: Surgical Tattooing of the Port-Wine Stain. Operative Technique, Results and Critique. Plast. Reconstr. Surg., *48*:113-120, 1971.
Fifty per cent failure rate due largely to pigment leaching by vascular bed.

Baluyot, S. T., and Shumrick, D. A.: Pre-Irradiation Tattooing. Arch. Otolaryngol., *96*:151-153, 1972.
Marker technique: 19-gauge needle dipped in India ink.

Christensen, H. E., and Schmidt, H.: The Ultrastructure of Tattoo Marks. Acta Path. Microbiol. Scand., *80A*:573-576, 1972.
Colored macrophages remain in perivascular band in upper part of dermis.

Mowat, N. A. G., Albert-Recht, F., Brunt, P. W., and Walker, W.: Outbreak of Serum Hepatitis Associated with Tattooing. Lancet, *1*:33-34, 1973.
More than pigment may be introduced when needle moistened with saliva: 16 cases traced to single artist.

Watkins, D. B.: Viral Disease in Tattoos: Verruca Vulgaris. Arch. Derm., *84*:306-309, 1961.
Tattoo warts: more than was bargained for.

Cipollaro, V. A.: Keratoacanthoma Developing in a Tattoo. Cutis, *11*:809-810, 1973.
First case; cites also Bowen's disease, squamous cell carcinoma, reticulohistiosarcoma and malignant melanoma.

Kirsch, N.: Malignant Melanoma Developing in a Tattoo. Int. J. Derm., *11*:16-20, 1972.
In a blue tattoo, 27 years later.

Fields, J. P., Little, W. D., and Watson, P. E.: Discoid Lupus Erythematosus in Red Tattoo. Arch. Derm., *98*:667-669, 1968.
Triggered by photosensitivity state.

Fleischmajer, R., Lara, J. V., and Krol, S.: Localized Scleroderma. Arch. Derm., *94*:531-535, 1966.
Morphea extending out from tattoo faithfully reproduced contour!

Bjornberg, A.: Reactions to Light in Yellow Tattoos from Cadmium Sulfide. Arch. Derm., *88*:267-271, 1963.
Eighteen of 24 developed local urticaria on sunlight exposure. Phototoxic response reproduced by intradermal but not photo-patch tests.

Juhlin, L., and Ohman, S.: Allergic Reactions to Mercury in Red Tattoos and in Mucosa Adjacent to Amalgam Fillings. Acta Dermatovener., *48*:103-105, 1968.
The dentist, the tattoo artist and delayed contact type sensitivity to mercury.

Biro, L., and Klein, W. P.: Unusual Complications of Mercurial (Cinnabar) Tattoo. Generalized Eczematous Eruption Following Laceration of a Tattoo. Arch. Derm., *96*:165-167, 1967.
Excision followed by marked improvement.

Rorsman, H., Dahlquist, I., Jacobsson, S., Brehmer-Andersson, E., Ehinger, B., Linell, F., and Rorsman, G.: Tattoo Granuloma and Uveitis. Lancet, *2*:27-28, 1969.
Allergic sensitivity to cobalt in blue tattoo associated with uveitis which improved when tattoo excised.

Dickinson, J. A.: Sarcoidal Reactions in Tattoos. Arch. Derm., *100*:315-319, 1969.
Nodule in tattoo can herald systemic sarcoidosis.

Shelley, W. B., and Hurley, H. J., Jr.: The Immune Granuloma: Late Delayed Hypersensitivity to Zirconium and Beryllium. *In* Samter, M. (Ed.): Immunological Diseases, 2nd ed., Little, Brown and Co., Boston, 1971, pp. 722-734.
Zirconium and beryllium can induce local immune sarcoid response; should anticipate occurrence in tattoos with these and other metals.

Bailey, B. N.: Treatment of Tattoos. Plast. Reconstr. Surg., *40*:361-371, 1967.
Extensive tattoos in 150 patients treated by simple excision or shaving with or without grafting.

Goldman, L., Rockwell, J. R., Meyer, R., Otten, R., Wilson, R. G., and Kitzmiller, K. W.: Laser Treatment of Tattoos. J.A.M.A., *201*:841-844, 1967.
Selective thermal destruction of tattoo, still experimental.

Scutt, R. W. B.: The Chemical Removal of Tattoos. Brit. J. Plast. Surg., *25*:189-194, 1972.
Removal by re-tattooing with caustic: tannic acid and glycerine.

Grice, K. A.: The Removal of Tattoos with a Keratome. Brit. J. Derm., *76*:318-321, 1964.
Castroviejo unit allows precise removals at 0.7 to 1.2 mm. in depth.

Clabaugh, W.: Removal of Tattoos by Superficial Dermabrasion. Arch. Derm., *98*:515-521, 1968.
Underline — superficial!

Crittenden, F. M., Jr.: Salabrasion — Removal of Tattoos by Superficial Abrasion with Table Salt. Cutis, *7*:295-300, 1971.
Do it yourself kit consists of tap water, table salt, gauze sponge and a moving finger.

Index